HERBS IN THE
TREATMENT OF CHILDREN

Leading a Child to Health

HERBS IN THE TREATMENT OF CHILDREN

Leading a Child to Health

Julian Scott, PhD, and Teresa Barlow, BSc

Private Practitioners
Bath
England

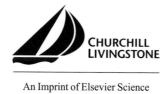

CHURCHILL
LIVINGSTONE

An Imprint of Elsevier Science

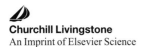
Churchill Livingstone
An Imprint of Elsevier Science

11830 Westline Industrial Drive
St. Louis, Missouri 63146

HERBS IN THE TREATMENT OF CHILDREN   ISBN 0-443-07163-2

Distributed in the United Kingdom by Churchill Livingstone, Robert Stevenson House, 1-3 Baxter's Place, Leith Walk, Edinburgh EH1 3AF, Scotland, and by associated companies, branches, and representatives throughout the world.

Churchill Livingstone and the sailboat design are registered trademarks.

Library of Congress Cataloging in Publication Data

Scott, Julian.
    Herbs in the treatment of children : leading a child to health / Julian Scott and Teresa Barlow.
        p. cm.
    Includes bibliographic references and index.
ISBN: 0-443-07163-2
    1. Herbs—Therapeutic use. 2. Children—Diseases—Alternative treatment. I. Barlow,
    Teresa. II. Title.

    RJ53.H47 S36 2003
    615′.321.083—dc 21

                                                            2002031578

Acquisitions Editor: Inta Ozols
Developmental Editor: Karen Gilmour
Publishing Services Manager: Peggy Fagen
Designer: Teresa Breckwoldt

KI/MVY

Printed in the United States of America

Last digit is the print number: 9   8   7   6   5   4   3   2   1

WARNING

A time of disease is distressing for the child and parents. A mild disease can become serious or life threatening. Always seek professional help if you have any uncertainties.

Preface

During the time we have been practicing there has been a great increase in chronic and recurrent illnesses affecting children. Asthma is almost an epidemic, and allergies and autoimmune diseases are becoming increasingly common. Many possible explanations exist: the rise in pollution, the degradation of the food supply, the side effects of the very medicines taken to cure another illness, and so forth. Whatever the reasons, parents now face greater difficulties in keeping their children healthy and in nursing them back to health once they become sick. It is against this background that we write this book. This book discusses how to treat the common diseases in babies and children with simple herbal remedies. We share the experience we have gained in the clinic, namely that herbal medicine is extremely powerful. When used wisely, it is safe, gentle, and yet very effective. The remedies we describe have been used for thousands of years with extraordinary success.

We show that treatment of simple illnesses with natural simple medicines dramatically reduces the need for antibiotics and strong orthodox drugs. What is more, the children will consequently be stronger, healthier, and happier, for we have observed that herbal medicines actually strengthen the body while curing the disease—in stark contrast to orthodox medicinal drugs.

Herbal medicine is based on somewhat different principles than is orthodox medicine. It supports the child rather than attacking the illness. It helps the child *through* an illness. It encourages the body to eliminate any toxins. It strengthens the immune system to evict bacteria and viruses and thereby lead the child to a better state of health. With this approach we have seen healthy children stay healthy and the chronically sick led back to health again.

■ CHOICE OF HERBS

A quick glance through this book will reveal that we use a very limited range of herbs. The ones that we discuss are those that we are familiar with and that we know to work. Some of these may be herbs that you, the reader, are not familiar with or cannot obtain. Fortunately, many different variations are possible, and we advise staying with the herbs that you know, rather than following too closely in our footsteps. It is much better to know a few herbs well than to have a superficial knowledge of many. It is for this reason that we have given an explanation of most of the suggested prescriptions and provided a brief materia medica. We hope this will be sufficient for the reader to work out satisfactory substitutes that are easily available.

■ SAFETY

Throughout this book we have tried to point out where the dangers lie. We think we have covered the most common ones, but inevitably there are rare conditions that may be dangerous that have not been specifically delineated in this book. We therefore advise parents to treat simple problems at home but never to hesitate in seeking advice from a competent practitioner.

THE BEST MEDICINE

We do not wish to downplay the extremely important role modern medicine has had in the world. Many millions of lives have been saved by the timely administration of drugs. We certainly do not want to give the message that Western drugs are bad and herbal medicine is good. We believe that one should take the *best* medicine for the illness. In acute conditions it may be orthodox drugs, such as the bronchodilators, which are so successful in stopping an asthma attack. However, there are many situations in which herbs provide quicker and longer-lasting relief. It is these conditions we discuss.

PRACTITIONER AND PARENT

We write for both the practitioner and the parent. Practitioners can use this book as a reference to help parents that come to their clinic and to aid in treating those conditions that cannot easily be treated at home. Parents will find this book helpful in enabling them to treat the simple diseases at home and to know when it is no longer simple and they need to go to the doctor.

THEORETICAL FOUNDATIONS: A UNIVERSAL MEDICINE

The theories on which this book are based are those of Chinese medicine, which are based on observation over many thousands of years. We have been using these theories for more than 25 years, and the longer we work with them, the more we are convinced of their usefulness in clinical practice. Our initial training was in Chinese medicine, but during the years we have been using it, we have come into contact with practitioners of other systems—Western herbalism, Ayurvedic medicine, Tibetan medicine, African medicine, and others. We have been struck by how much these systems have in common. All use a humoral system based

on the elements (three in the case of Ayurveda, four for Western herbalism, five for Chinese and Tibetan), and above all they all make a fundamental distinction between Strong patients and Weak patients. It is in Western herbalism that the tradition is weakest, but even here, Hot, Cold, Strong, and Weak have been at the foundations since the times of classical Greece, as the brief history that follows illustrates. They are at the core of the Physiomedical school of Western herbalism. Thus we can say that the principles that underpin this book are truly universal.

Origins of the Theories in This Book

The basic theories that underpin this book are those of Chinese medicine, but they are all to be found in various Western traditions:

- The ideas of Hot and Cold (which pervade all traditional medicines) were part of mainstream medicine as it used to be practiced in Europe and America up until about 100 years ago.
- The concepts of Strong and Weak patients needing different herbs run throughout classical medicine and were cornerstones of the Physiomedical system and other systems.
- The concept of an echo pattern is to be found in the writings of Hahnemann, the founder of homoeopathy. He gave them the name of *miasm*. (We have avoided the use of this name because later homeopaths such as Clark and Kent in the United States changed its meaning somewhat to include hereditary illnesses, particularly tuberculosis, syphilis, and gonorrhea.)

UPDATING THE TRADITION

We have found it necessary to introduce some changes to the traditional patterns when treating individual patients in the West because lifestyle is very different here from that of traditional China. The patterns seen in children who grow up under harsher physical circumstances and with iron discipline are somewhat different from those of a child brought up on a diet of cola and chips and relatively mild discipline.

The other great change we have made is to use Western herbs rather than Chinese herbs. We have done this for a variety of reasons. Partly it is their commercial availability compared with Chinese herbs, but mostly it is that they grow all around. It is possible to find the plant in the wild, watch it grow, and harvest it. Quite apart from the sheer joy of doing this, one comes to a much deeper understanding of the nature and uses of the herb than can possibly be obtained from a book.

We had a great impetus to this approach from the publication of the *Zhongyao Da Cidian* (*Greater Encyclopaedia of Chinese Herbs*, 1978),* which lists many of the Western herbs and their functions. Having worked with these herbs for many years, we can confidently say that this approach to using Western herbs has been very effective for the children of all ethnic backgrounds who have come through our clinics.

■ THE BASIS OF CHINESE MEDICINE: BODY, ENERGY, AND MIND

It is one of the basic tenets of Chinese medicine that human beings have a body, energy, and a mind (or spirit). This in itself is hardly revolutionary, and there are few who would disagree with this. What is different about Chinese medicine is the belief that all three are interconnected and interdependent. This means that an imbalance in the mind will in turn affect the energy and soon after will affect the body. These ideas are there in embryo in Western psychiatry, in the concept of psychosomatic disease, but only in embryo. In Chinese medicine there is no such thing as an illness that affects only one level of a person's being. If a person is ill, all three levels must be involved to

a certain extent. For example, if a person catches a cold, he or she may feel somewhat tired as the energy is affected and may temporarily have a slightly negative attitude in life as it affects his or her spirit.

The great strength of Chinese medicine is that after millennia of observation, they have come to find exactly how the imbalances on one level affect another level. In this way a clear connection can be established between the state of energy and behavior patterns. In a book of this size we do not have space to cover these connections in detail.

How Energy Affects Behavior

Throughout the text we refer to a child's behavior and how it gives an indication of the child's state of energy. It may come as a surprise that such a subjective indication could be used as the basis for preparing a prescription. Yet a moment's reflection will show how one's state of energy is reflected in mood and behavior. Imagine what it is like to be filled with energy and refreshed after going away for a good holiday. The problems that one faced before going away somehow seem less important. Even personality clashes, which still exist, are often easier to tolerate after a break. As time passes and the daily grind eats into reserves of energy, problems that should be small appear bigger and bigger. The activities that provided enjoyment when one was full of energy no longer seem so enjoyable and no longer seem to provide the same refreshment. According to one's temperament one's behavior may become more jumpy and irritable. One's general state of energy affects the way one views the world.

The same forces are at work in children, but fortunately the behavior patterns of children are relatively simple. Children with a lot of energy feel like doing things. They feel more outgoing and more able to take the knocks that life has. When their energy is decreased, they feel more vulnerable and more withdrawn. These ideas are fundamental to our approach because we have found that observation of a child's behavior and temperament may quickly lead to the correct prescription.

---

*Jiangsu New Herbal Research Institute: *Zhongyao Da Cidian* (*Greater Encyclopaedia of Chinese Herbs*), Shanghai, Hong Kong, 1978, Shanghai Technical Press.

■ OUR SOURCES
AND RESOURCES

This book grew from our experiences of treating and observing children in clinic over the last 25 years. During that time we have consulted many books and many practitioners. We have also had the opportunity to treat many children and see the suffering that they and their parents experience. If this book can relieve some of that suffering, it will have served its purpose.

BRIEF HISTORY OF HERBAL MEDICINE IN THE WEST

In this brief look at the history of herbal medicine we show that the fundamental ideas of Chinese medicine are part of the tradition of Western herbalism too. The ideas were developed gradually in classical times and reached their highest state of refinement in the second century ACE, when Galen, the physician to the Roman emperor, made a synthesis of the best from all the medical schools of the time.

By this time, all the ideas that are prevalent in modern medicine had been developed. There was drug therapy, surgery, anesthesiology, aromatherapy, psychotherapy, massage, dietary therapy, and exercise therapy. There was even a lively discussion of the merits of brown versus white bread. Studying the history of medicine, one is struck by the richness of the ideas that were debated and how much has been forgotten or ignored.

Classical Greece

The period that interests us starts in the fifth century BCE with the first books on medicine, for it is from this time that we can follow the development of the fundamental ideas of medicine. Before this, a sophisticated medicine was practiced in Egypt, but only tantalizing fragments have come down to us. The first extant writing of importance is the Hippocratic corpus. This is clearly written by more than one hand and suggests that at this time there was already lively discussion on the ideas of medicine. One part, the aphorisms, is a collection of traditional sayings; another part, on the "sacred disease," seeks to prove that epilepsy is not a visitation from the gods but is a purely physical illness.

The theoretical foundations of medicine in Hippocrates, as with most traditional medicines, are the humors—four in Greek thinking: Hot, Cold, Wet, and Dry. It was believed that illness arose when an imbalance of these occurred and that the role of medicine was to restore balance. Also implicit in most of the writings, and occasion-

ally explicit, was that the body was permeated by a life force ($\pi\nu\epsilon\upsilon\mu\alpha$).*

Sometime between 500 BCE and 300 BCE there was an integration of medicine and religion. In Hippocrates' time, medicine was clearly a liberal art and was no more (and no less) connected to religion than sculpture or pottery. By 300 BCE we see the development of Asklepions, healing temples dedicated to Asklepios. There were Asklepions in many places, the two greatest being at Epidaurus and at Kos. Here one went for a truly holistic cure.

The part of the cure in which Asklepios was invoked involved taking a sleeping draught, which was likely to induce dreams, and spending the night in the temple. Asklepios was expected to come in a dream and show the dreamer the solution to his or her problem. As with all dreams, the solution may have come in a coded message, and not surprisingly there grew a helpful team of dream interpreters who were resident in the temple. In this there is a similarity to one aspect of modern psychotherapy. We know that there were herbalists, masseurs, aromatherapists, and exercise consultants as well.

At the beginning of the third century BCE we see Kos again at the forefront of medicine, in the development of the empirical school of medicine, whose founder was Philias (fl 280 BCE). The basic principle of his school was the accumulation of medical knowledge through the "tripod" of observation, history, and analogy: observation of the patient and how he or she responded to treatment, history of the patient and his or her condition, and analogy of the patient's condition with that of other patients. This is the first time that we see a systematized database of patients.

Hellenistic and Roman Medicine

The Empirical school marks perhaps the high point of classical Greek medicine. There were still develop-

---

*In China the "Yellow Emperor's Classic of Internal Medicine" was being compiled at almost the same time as the Hippocratic corpus. In the Hippocratic corpus the life force is described as flowing along a "great vessel" ($\varphi\lambda\epsilon\beta\sigma\sigma$), which is very similar to the "great yang" vessel of Chinese medicine. One wonders whether the ancient Greek doctors had contact with Chinese medicine.

ments to come, but with the growth of the Roman empire, it was inevitable that Rome started to influence medicine. The next major development was characteristically Roman, the foundation of the Methodist school. This school was completely materialist in its approach. It even rejected the idea of a life force, which was known in Roman medicine as the *vis medicatrix naturae*. The theoretical foundation of this school was that the body is nourished by blood, which flows through "pores"—what we would now call *capillaries*. It was thought that there were three basic states of illness: relaxation of the pores, constriction of the pores, and mixed states. Moreover, they were uninterested in the causes of disease. Another development associated with this school is the idea of impurities in the blood as causes of disease. This idea is still with us in various guises—in the field of herbalism we have alteratives, which are for altering the impure condition of the blood, and in the naturopathic field we have the idea of impurities reaching the blood via the leaky gut syndrome.

Thus we see that by the end of the third century BCE we have nearly all the fundamental ideas that are current in medicine today. Anatomy was well developed, as was surgery. (Proof of this is in a surgeon's tool kit from Roman times, which was recently discovered in a sunken boat. The kit contains instruments that could be used today.) We have the humoral theory (which is still very much alive in modern medicine in the form of antiinflammatory drugs—medicines to reduce flame); we have the ideas of tension and relaxation, of tonics, and of lifestyle being both a cause and a cure of chronic disease. We have the interaction of mind and body as represented by the Asklepions, and we have materialism of the Methodist school, which so permeates orthodox medical thinking today. Interestingly, there were also very heated conflicts among the various schools.

These conflicts went on for some hundreds of years, until the foundation of the Eclectic school in the first century ACE. They sought to take the best of all systems and to try to reconcile differences between them. The reconciliation process continued for about a hundred years and found its fullest expression in the writings of Galen, who lived approximately from 130 to 210 ACE and became chief physician to the emperor Marcus Aurelius. Galen wrote an enormous number of books about all aspects of medicine, of which only a small proportion have survived. Among the books extant are descriptions of cures using herbs.

Tradition Maintained by the Arabs during the Dark Ages in Europe

After Galen there were many writers on medicine, but it seems that they were all derivative. No one had anything new to say after Galen. After his time, medicine went into a slow decline throughout most of Europe. During the Dark Ages, much of the medical knowledge of the Romans and Greeks disappeared from Europe, and it was left to the Arabs to carry the torch. It is to them that we owe the great debt of preserving the classical works, even they did not make great advances. In 925 AD we see Rhazes (Abu Bakr Muhammad Ibn Zakariya' Ar-Razi) writing in Baghdad a medical treatise that is essentially a compilation based on Galen and Hippocrates. Even the great Avicenna (Abu 'Ali Al-Husayn Ibn 'Abd Allah Ibn Sina) (980 to 1037) does not show a great advance, except in the description of the action of herbs.

The great virtue of the Arabs was that they did actually practice medicine. It was an art that had almost become extinct in Europe. It had to wait until the Renaissance for medicine to be revived as well. The works of Avicenna were translated into Latin, as was a huge *Materia Medica* written by Mesua, the younger of Damascus. This was translated under the title of *de simplicibus* and ran to 26 editions in the fifteenth century. Even in the time of King James I it was a standard medical textbook.

Revival in Europe

Also at the end of the fifteenth and beginning of the sixteenth centuries we see the foundation of the medical school at Montpellier (1593) and the turbulent life of Paracelsus, the name taken by Theophrastus Bombastus von Hohenheim (1490 to 1541 AD). Among his achievements, he is credited by some with being the founding father of allopathic medicine. He certainly experimented with a wide range of different medicines, even though his only enduring legacy is the use of crude antimony as a curative element. It was not until the nineteenth century that allopathic medicine really took root.

Before the nineteenth century, medicine in the West was herbal medicine. Unlike Chinese medicine, which used both animal and minerals, and Ayurvedic medicine, which used toxic minerals prepared in a way to render them nontoxic, Western medicine was almost entirely plant based. It changed little beyond gradually relearning what had been forgotten from the ancients. The milestones in British herbal medicine are books like Gerard's *Herball* (written at the end of the sixteenth century and revised in 1636). His book contains some lively interpolations based on his experience, but basically it is a compilation, in English, of the classical works. The same can be said of Culpeper's *A Physical Directory* (1649), although this has the interesting addition of the astrologic influences of plants. Both of these works are based on a humoral theory and give specific indications of the "temperature" of the herb, that is, whether it is Hot or Cold.

The Development of Herbal Medicine in North America

On the other side of the Atlantic ocean, there were more interesting developments. The Pilgrim Fathers had encountered the North American Indians, who had helped them enormously. Not only did they teach the Fathers how to survive, but they also taught them medicine. For the first time since ancient Greek times we see herbs used in a more sophisticated way. For the first time we see the ideas of toning and dispersing herbs and of stimulating and relaxing herbs. These are ideas that had not been seen for a long time and even to this day are not in widespread use in Europe. Not only were these ideas introduced, but also there were some wonderful new herbs added to the *Materia Medica*, such as golden seal *Hydrastis canadensis* and poke root *Phytolacca americana*.

As time passed, different schools of herbalism emerged. Foremost among these were the Thompsonians, the Physiomedicalists, and the Eclectics. The Thompsonians were the followers of Thompson, a fiery man who believed in heroic doses of herbs, especially of lobelia. For various reasons (some say because of his success, others simply because he had a difficult personality) he aroused the wrath of the American Medical Association (an allopathic group), which sought every means to discredit his work. The legacy of this is still with us, for in many countries lobelia, a very safe herb, is regarded as more harmful than the chemical paracetamol, which is known to be more toxic.

The Physiomedicalists were the closest followers of the early medical schools, being keenly aware of the difference between tonics, stimulants, and sedatives.* However, they were restricted in the range of remedies they used by the fear of

---

*The following quotation is from Cook WH: *Physio-medical dispensatory*, Sandy, Or, 1998, Eclectic Medical Publications (reprint of 1869 edition):

TONICS
Under the term Tonic are included all agents which impart a fuller vigor and a stronger acting power to the system. Cathartics, emetics, baths, and similar depurating measures, secure to the frame a sense of relief and increased strength, merely by ridding it of depressing accumulations. But these are not tonic in the true sense of the term; as under this are brought only such means as give, by their own action, slowly and permanently, greater firmness to the tissues.

Derangements of the stomach are the most prominent origins of general weakness; hence it is customary to look upon tonics as agents that improve the condition of the stomach; and as digestion is the one grand function of this organ, a tonic has come to be held as synonymous with a promoter of digestion. While these facts are true in part, they are not universal; for other tissues than the stomach frequently need the true tonic influence, and some of the purest tonics act upon remote structures without promoting digestion at all. Thus, after the acute stage of scarlatina, the system is not unfrequently contaminated with the peculiar virus of that malady; against the depressing influences of which the composition powder is a superior tonic—at once consolidating the tissues, sustaining the blood vessels, and eliminating the **virus** through tile natural channel of the skin. Cinchona and its alkaloid, (quinia,) are peculiarly tonic to the nervous centers, yet have only a limited action on the stomach, and quinia can scarcely be said to promote digestion at all. Juglans, in addition to being hepatic and cholagogue, exerts a very favorable tonic action throughout the bowels; but it has no influence in improving the function of the stomach, except through the relief it secures to the biliary organs. . . . Yet it is nevertheless the fact, that the great mass of tonics do act more or less upon the stomach. As the nourishment of the entire frame is dependent upon this organ, any general feebleness that arises from insufficient digestion is effectually reached by improving the digestion. . . . By making such a classification, and such discrimination, the practitioner will be enabled to employ his tonics with great accuracy, and with corresponding good effect.

ever using poisons. They could never grasp the fact that something could have healing properties in small doses while being a poison in large doses. They had a simple black and white approach: Something either was a poison or was not.*

The Eclectics, taking their name from the ancient Greek school, went down a different route and were prepared to experiment with all the new chemicals that were available. It seems that they took a position halfway between the Physiomedicalists and the allopaths. They used chemicals, but on the whole they did more good than harm. Their great contribution was the development of essential oils, which can be of great use in the treatment of acute coughs and in the treatment of those with digestions too weak to digest herbs.

Decline of Traditional Theories

The analysis of herbs and diseases into Hot and Cold was never questioned until well after the invention of the thermometer by Fahrenheit in 1708. Without a thermometer to measure the temperature inside the body, there is no way of knowing whether a person really is hotter or colder in objective terms. So if a person were lying sick in bed, white faced, shivering, with their skin cold to the touch, it seemed obvious that they were cold. Only by using a thermometer could you prove that their inner temperature was in fact raised. As the thermometer became increasingly used, it came to be relied on more and more and subjective symptoms of Hot and Cold less and less.

At the same time there was a shift in emphasis away from humoral theories of illness in favor of the new sciences of physics, chemistry, and microbiology. With the development of these new sciences came new objective tests for specific conditions, and as time has passed, more and more reliance has come to be placed on these tests and less on subjective sensations. The microscopic components of the body are seen as more important and real than the

hopes and fears of the patient, although to the patient the situation may be reversed. This emphasis on the physical level is very reminiscent of the stance taken by the Methodists of Roman times.

While traditional scientific theories were being discarded in favor of modern ones based on materially observable phenomena, there was a move in the opposite direction, with the discovery and development of homeopathy. Homeopathic remedies are potentiated to bring out the "energy" of the medicine, and many contain none of the original medicine from which they were prepared.

Herbal Medicine Today

The herbal tradition is still very much alive in Europe and in the United States, despite its low profile and low funding. The gentleness and efficacy of herbal remedies make them attractive to those whose constitutions are upset by the harsher pharmaceutical medicines. In Britain and the United States we are especially fortunate in having the tradition of using herbs from both continents* and having place for different schools of herbalism.

Throughout Europe and the United States, herbal medicine is experiencing a resurgence. In Britain herbal medicine can be studied to degree level at universities, as well as numerous flourishing private schools. In the United States it can be studied at many naturopathic colleges. Despite increasingly restrictive legislation, the demand and availability of plant medicines continue to grow.

■ ACKNOWLEDGMENTS

The authors would like to thank Monica Barlow for her invaluable help in reading the manuscript, Inta Ozols for suggesting the book in the first place, and all the staff of Elsevier Science who helped in the production of this book. We would also like to thank the many teachers we have had over the years from whom we have learned so much.

---

*Time has proved them wrong on this point, with a number of deaths in the last decades from an overdose of carrot juice. Carrots are one of the most beneficial foods, especially for young children, but when taken to extremes they become poisonous.

*Countries such as France and Italy, with a wider range of climate than Britain, have access to a wider range of indigenous herbs, but they do not benefit from the glorious North American herbs like golden seal *Hydrastis canadensis* or queen's delight *Stillingia sylvatica*.

Contents

Basic Concepts

1

Energy and Health

During the last 200 years, the application of newtonian science to everyday life has led to extraordinary advances. No area has been left untouched. The air we breathe; the food we drink; the way we digest, breathe, live, and much more have been analyzed. The mechanisms by which the internal organs work have been investigated in great detail. The resulting prosperity and longevity are in themselves proof of the truth of this approach. But do these discoveries describe the whole truth? Many Western scientists would have us believe so, but for those of us who have worked in the health profession with both sick and healthy, old and young, this picture is unsatisfactory. We believe that there is more to life. Newtonian science provides a good description of inanimate systems, but there is something missing when it is used to describe human beings. Humans are more than mere machines. They have likes and dislikes, hopes and fears. What is more, all people are different and react in different ways in sickness and in health.

When it comes to illness, these differences are important. Children in particular face very different problems than those of adults; therefore their illnesses are somewhat different and need different treatment. We give medicines based on how the individual is affected as well as on the organism that caused the disease. In this book we show how to prepare an individually tailored prescription to help them recover.

The foundation for this is developing an understanding of "energy" and how disturbances in energy open the way for illness. We show the factors in life that give rise to disturbances, and by so doing we are able to make the all-important connection between what is going on in a child's life and the illnesses that the child experiences as a result. We then go on to consider the basic types of children (Strong or Weak, Hot or Cold) and show how they need different basic treatments.

■ ENERGY

One of the basic concepts we use in this book is that of vitalizing energy, a concept overlooked in Western science. Everyone knows the feeling of having lots of energy—or of having very little, when we want to stay in bed all day. We live by virtue of this energy. It is this that dictates what we feel like doing every day. For children energy is even more important, and in healthy children it seems to overflow. In Oriental medicine this energy is called *qi*, *ki*, or *chi*; in Indian medicine it is called *prana*; in Ancient Greek medicine, $\pi\nu\varepsilon\upsilon\mu\alpha$ *(pneuma)*; in nineteenth century medicine, the *vis medicatrix naturae*. It used to always be an important part of medicine, for it was considered the basic life force that governs our state of health and how we respond to illness.

--- A Word of Caution ---

The majority of illness, especially common childhood illnesses, can be healed in the home, but this is not *always* the case. If you as a parent or practitioner do not know what is taking place or if you find yourself frightened or in a panic, do not hesitate to get help. In babies and young children, an illness can quickly get out of hand.

One of the great problems of the scientific approach is the reliance on instruments, which cannot measure energy. Unfortunately, there is an unstated assumption that if something cannot be measured with an instrument, then it does not exist. Consequently, something as basic as the patient's energy has been eliminated from science and, by extension, from modern medicine. Babies and children have small physical bodies but huge amounts of energy, so natural medicines that work mainly on the energy work best for them.

Energy Types in Healthy Children

We all know what it is like to have lots of energy, and similarly, we have all experienced periods of less energy. When it comes to practice, one can, as a first step, try to determine whether a child has a lot or little energy. When one asks this question time and time again, one comes to the conclusion that there really are two types of children. Some children have lots of energy; some have less. This does not mean that the child with lots of energy is healthy and that the one with less energy is not. Both may be healthy—they are simply different types of healthy children. Each type has a different way of reacting to life and its situations.

This division is also significant in relation to illness and the medicines children need. A Strong child, with a good appetite and good energy, will typically have a good, reactive immune system. The paler, weaker child will often have a slower immune response. It therefore makes sense to give the weaker child something to boost the immune system. A Strong child will not need medicines to strengthen the immune system but rather something directed toward fighting the disease.

HOW TO RECOGNIZE A HEALTHY CHILD'S ENERGY TYPE

We now discuss how to observe and recognize different energies in children. To simplify things for the purpose of this book, we have grouped children into the following three basic energetic types,

and throughout this book we refer to these types of children.

- Strong, full-energy type
- Delicate, low-energy type
- Delicate type with nervous, high energy

It is important to understand that these are energy types during times of health as much as during illness. A delicate, low-energy child may never be ill; a Strong, full-energy child may often be ill. We describe the children in this way because when a child does becomes ill, each type of child tends to react to illness in a characteristic way. The stronger children tend to have vigorous reactions and fight the disease. The weaker children tend to be more submissive.

Description

STRONG, FULL-ENERGY TYPE

Typically, Strong, full-energy children are strong in everything. They have sturdy bodies and strong likes and dislikes. They come into the world seeming to know what they want to get out of life, and with a determination to get it! They are not ones to give in easily and are not easily overwhelmed; rather it is their parents who get overwhelmed!

Appearance
- Sturdy
- Red complexion
- Well built, strong bones
- Good appetite for everything
- Lots of energy
- Strong voice
- Not easily hurt by falls, scrapes, and bruises

DELICATE, LOW-ENERGY TYPE

Children classified as delicate, low energy are not so strong. When they come into the world, they do not have the same ebullient enthusiasm, and their energy is not so strong. They tend to spend their time doing less energetic things like reading, coloring, or just sitting. They also tend to be quieter children. You may also notice that they easily feel overwhelmed and may need more comfort than other children.

Appearance
- Paler complexion
- Small appetite
- Thinner bones
- Affected badly by falls, scrapes, and bruises
- Notable preference for reading and drawing rather than running around and engaging in rough-and-tumble play

DELICATE TYPE WITH NERVOUS, HIGH ENERGY

Children who are considered delicate type with nervous, high energy are something of a paradox. On one hand, they are slight and delicately built; on the other hand, they often run around with the energy of a much physically stronger child. Their appearance and their energy levels do not match up. When they are still, they appear much like the delicate type, with a pale face and thinner bones. When they sit down to meals, their appetites are small, sometimes tiny. When they are away from the table, though, their energy seems boundless. They are on the go all the time. It is this discrepancy between the amount of food they consume and their energy that differentiates these children. The amount of energy they have could not possibly come from the small amount of food that they eat.

These children often exhibit a characteristic behavior: They like to be the center of attention. Most people like to be the center of attention some of the time, but these children like it all the time. They literally thrive on it. In extreme cases these children can become habitually irritating in a bid to be noticed.

Appearance
- Pale complexion
- Small appetite, often very picky eater
- Thin, stick legs
- Sensitive; easily cries at the smallest thing
- Attention needy; likes to be the center of attention
- On the move; runs around a lot, often out of control

- Often high-pitched scream, hysterical laughter
- Highly imaginative and creative, when given a chance

At the end of this section, we further discuss how this pattern arises.

■ HOT AND COLD

A factor of similar importance to the strength of children is whether they have Hot or Cold energy and, when it comes to illness, whether their illness is Hot or Cold in nature. Children with Hot energy look hot: They often perspire, they often have a red face, they cannot bear to have lots of clothes on, and they often throw off their clothes. At night, these children are often restless and may throw off their covers. The behavior of these children is often rather active. They tend to run around a lot and have difficulty in sitting still. They have a high metabolic rate (Box 1-1).

In contrast, children with Cold energy look pale, even white. They rarely perspire, even in hot weather, and they do not mind having lots of clothes on. At night they may wake up if they get the slightest bit cold. Their behavior tends to be rather less active, and they may prefer sitting still. They have a low metabolic rate (Box 1-2).

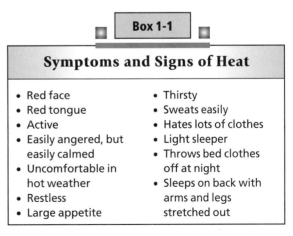

Box 1-1

Symptoms and Signs of Heat

- Red face
- Red tongue
- Active
- Easily angered, but easily calmed
- Uncomfortable in hot weather
- Restless
- Large appetite

- Thirsty
- Sweats easily
- Hates lots of clothes
- Light sleeper
- Throws bed clothes off at night
- Sleeps on back with arms and legs stretched out

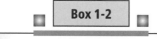

Box 1-2

Symptoms and Signs of Cold

- Pale face
- Pale tongue
- Rather passive
- Hatred for cold weather
- Often curled up in a ball
- Food has to be just right or will not eat it
- Often gets a tummy ache, especially after drinking cold water
- Does not drink much
- Does not sweat easily
- Wears thick clothes
- Deep sleep, but sometimes woken by colic
- Sleeps curled up or on tummy

Mixtures of Types

We have presented pure "stereotypes." In reality children are much more varied, but when all of the signs are considered together, you will usually find that there are clear signs of one of the types we have given.

Normal Variations

As the seasons change and the demands on the child come and go, the child's energy and balance between Hot and Cold fluctuate. For example, toward the end of winter semester, children become more tired. In spring and early summer, children become somewhat hotter; in autumn, they are somewhat cooler. Comparisons of Strong and Weak types and Hot and Cold types are provided in Tables 1-1 and 1-2, respectively.

DELICATE TYPE WITH NERVOUS, HIGH ENERGY: A FURTHER DISCUSSION

Before we leave this introduction to children's energy types, we shall spend a little time explaining how this pattern arises. It is a somewhat curious pattern, for these children manage to exhibit so much energy without the need for real food. They do it by living on nervous energy, or adrenaline. All children can do this to a certain extent; running around like crazy when very excited for a day or so while eating nothing, but the nervous energy type is in a state of more or less permanent stimulation. They keep

themselves in this state by all sorts of means, including watching television, using computers, and playing electronic games, all of which stimulate the brain and produce rushes of adrenaline.

These children tend to avoid physical games and hate quiet, reflective games, preferring to rush around but in a rather jumpy manner. The consequence is that children with this pattern tend to spend more time in their heads—that is, thinking—and not enough time "in their body"—to the extent that they are almost unaware of their bodily needs. They even avoid eating too much food because it would bring them back into their body too heavily.

Another way that some of these children get their energy rushes is by being the center of attention. Anyone who has had to speak in public is familiar with the energy rush that this can cause. On a smaller scale, the same is true for these children. Being the center of attention, with everyone watching them, gives a boost of energy and a feeling of well-being. In extreme cases this type of child will go to great lengths to get attention: crying at the slightest thing, disobeying every instruction, refusing to go to bed, and insisting on "treats" before doing anything.

We do not want to give the impression that this type of child is more difficult than others. These children, like all others, are adorable most of the time but still capable of exasperating us. With these children, if things go to extremes, they eat little and use up too much nervous energy in excitement, making them vulnerable to illness.

How Do Things Get This Way? The pattern often starts when, for some reason, the parents have no power or ability to say no or impose some measure of discipline. This may be because the parents are exhausted or ill or in a difficult emotional state. It may be because they are reacting against the way that they themselves were brought up. It may be because they have strong principles about the freedom that children need and believe that it is wrong ever to say no to a child. Sometimes it is because they love their child so much that they cannot bear to hear him or her cry and simply cannot say the word *no*. Whatever the reason, it is easy for the parent to let the child watch television or play on the

Table 1-1 Checklist for Strong or Weak

TYPE	STRONG		DELICATE		DELICATE WITH HIGH ENERGY	
Muscles	Sturdy	☐	Flaccid	☐	A bit weak	☐
Bones	Strong	☐	Thin	☐	Thin	☐
Boisterous, energetic games	Likes	☐	Dislikes	☐	Dislikes	☐
Voice	Loud	☐	Softer	☐	Piercing	☐
Rough games	Likes	☐	Dislikes	☐	Dislikes	☐
Appetite	Good	☐	Picky	☐	Minute	☐
Goes to bed	On time	☐	Early	☐	Late	☐
Needs to be center of attention	Maybe	☐	No	☐	Yes	☐
Hyperactive	Maybe	☐	No	☐	Yes	☐

Table 1-2 Checklist for Hot or Cold

TYPE	COLD		HOT	
Face color	Pale	☐	Red	☐
Lips and tongue	Pale	☐	Red	☐
Behavior	Quiet	☐	Restless	☐
Favored weather	Warm	☐	Cool	☐
Appetite	Small	☐	Large	☐
Stomachache	From cold water	☐	From eating too much	☐
Thirst	Rarely drinks cold water	☐	Likes cold water	☐
Sweats	Rarely	☐	Easily	☐
Clothes	Likes wearing a lot	☐	Hates wearing a lot	☐
Bed clothes	Likes to have lots	☐	Throws off	☐
Sleeps	On front	☐	On back	☐
Sleeps	Curled up	☐	Splayed out	☐
Sleeps	Heavily (except for colic)	☐	Light	☐

computer. It is easy for the child to refuse to eat or sit down to a meal. Every parent has experienced this at one time or another. No parent likes to battle with their child constantly and therefore occasionally gives in. If this happens once in a while or for a short period in life, then things will right themselves; if the situation is more or less continuous, habits start to form and the child never eats a decent meal, television becomes the normal after-school activity instead of playing outside, bedtime gets pushed later and later, and so on. When these children come to play, their brains are overstimulated and they tend to run around in a hyperactive, nervous fashion.

On a positive side, these children are often highly imaginative, given the chance. Take them away from the television and stimulation of the computer and they can draw and create extraordinary things. If the somewhat negative side to this type is controlled, these children have been found to be some of the most sensitive and loving children with great talent.

Routine and Boundaries in a Child's Life. In the nervous energy type of child it is common for the routine and discipline of life to become very vague. No one can deny that it is a good thing that the discipline of the Victorian age in bringing up children is over (at least, we hope it is!). Rigid and unforgiving rules at home and harsh schools were for the most part detrimental to child and family. Thank goodness we have returned to a more caring and loving form of parenting where children can express themselves in imagination, laughter, and even naughtiness!

A child must have some guidelines by which to live; for example, ensuring that children do not play near cars or play with electricity because doing so is wrong and dangerous. By imposing rules and boundaries, one makes children feel secure and safe. The other aspect of life that makes children feel secure is routine. As adults most of us have routines that we are trying to get away from. Most children do not have enough routine, though, and need to be gently guided into one. Following a routine gives children a feeling of being in the right place at the right time, a feeling of comfort. Regular meals and a regular bedtime contribute to a secure and confident child. No one is suggesting this routine be imposed with iron discipline or corporal punishment; gentle firmness is often more loving to children than letting them have their own way in everything.

We would like to stress that we are not writing a parenting book and are not concerned with whether one way of bringing a child up is better than another. There is no way that is "right." Different children respond better to different styles. Some need a very tight discipline, whereas others need great freedom and support. What we are concerned with is the way that upbringing affects health. If a child is perfectly healthy, then continue what you are doing. However, if one of these patterns emerges, it may be time to look at boundaries and decide whether they are too strict or too lax.

Energetic Approach. There is another way of explaining how this situation arises, from an energetic viewpoint. The relation between the mother* and the child is very strong. As a newborn, the two are virtually inseparable because the mother pro-

*In this book we tend to be rather old fashioned and refer to the mother as being the primary caregiver and energetic supporter of the child, as was the case in days gone by. We are well aware that there are different scenarios these days, and the main caregiver may be the father, partner, or grandmother or may be two or three people within the family unit. Please do not take offense at the term *mother*, by which we mean the main caregiver for the child.

vides milk and warmth for her baby. In those early days of a new life, a mother gives unreservedly of her time, her body, and her energy. This is even more pronounced when the baby or child becomes ill, when the mother willingly provides all she has to help her child through the illness. It is common to see an ill child in the clinic looking exhausted, but what is just as common is that the mother looks equally tired even though she remains healthy. This is because she tends to give even more at these times, thinking only of her child, not of herself. This is a natural mechanism by which the mother actually provides her own energy for the child to help her child get well. You might call it support, or simple love, but it translates into an energy that is essential for healing. This is completely natural because a baby has little in the way of reserves of energy and has difficulty getting through an illness without help from outside.

Usually, as children grow, dependence on their mothers' energy reduces. The children learn to live for themselves, feed themselves, and support themselves energetically. However, these nervous, energetic children continue to need their mothers' support and never learn to make enough of their own energy. They are constantly demanding in some way and are therefore able to take a little "energy" from those around them. If their mothers become unable to provide energy in some form, these children find someone else to provide it. This is interesting because what you may notice in these families is that the parents or caregivers of these children become very tired even though they are healthy. Providing constant energy and stimulation is draining.

▪ ENERGY OF HERBS

Herbs are living substances that grow, live, breathe, and die. It takes energy for them to do this, and consequently each herb has a particular energetic force. Moreover, human interaction with plants is a complex process. There are effects at different levels: emotions, energy, and the physical body. At the most refined level, plants, particularly flowers, have a powerful effect on our emotions, so much so that there is an entire industry devoted to their production. Woe betide the husband who does not give his wife flowers. There are florists in every town to supply the need. In the field of medicine, this has been put to great use by the pioneering work of the Welsh physician Dr. E. Bach. His flower remedies are based purely on the wonderful effect that flowers have on our feelings.*

At a slightly more material level, plants have an effect on our grosser moods. Some have long been used to cheer humans up when they get a bit down, hence the old saying "borage for courage." (At the time this saying was coined, the word *courage,* deriving from the Latin word for "heart," *cor,* meant having a light and cheerful heart.) Similar effects are noticed by sensitive people from aromatic herbs like rosemary and thyme, as well as rose petals.

At a more material level still, we can say that certain herbs are warming and others are cooling. Some are tonifying; some are dispersing. We can go even further and define the effects of herbs on specific organs. This is summarized in the *action* of a herb as given in the *Materia Medica.* So, for example, you will see in the *Materia Medica* that fennel *Foeniculum vulgaris* "aids digestion, relaxes spasms, soothes colic, mild expectorant, increases milk supply in nursing mothers." These actions are a starting point for understanding the energy of a plant and are about as far as one can go in a book of this kind. For the purposes of writing an effective prescription, this is enough for most patients.

A simple summary goes nowhere near describing the full qualities of a plant. For example, there are plants such as centaury *Centaurium erythraea* and

gentian *Gentiana amarella,** which have a very similar action at the physical level but which have a very different effect on the emotional level. It shows in their appearance: Looking at these two beautiful plants, one has a completely different feeling. Likewise, these plants are of benefit in very different emotional conditions, a fact that was put to great use by Dr. Bach in his flower remedies. Centaury is good for "those who are over-anxious to serve others," whereas gentian is good for "those who are easily discouraged."[†]

In this book, our use of herbs is based predominantly on the energetic properties of the herb. In our experience this is most useful in clinical practice because it describes how a plant actually affects the human body. In particular, it enables one to tailor a prescription to an individual who has a specific pattern of illness. These energetic properties are also a distillate of practitioners' experience over the centuries.

Active Principles

In the nineteenth century, when chemistry was in its infancy, there was great excitement when pure organic chemicals could be isolated from plants. Carrying out human experiments, researchers found that in many cases these isolated chemicals had effects similar to the plant itself—so much so that the belief arose that the effect of a plant could be summed up by the action of its "active principles" as these extracts were called.

This point of view is still with us. There are companies and research teams whose whole interest is to identify and extract active principles from plants. It is for this reason that many a *Materia Medica* will contain a brief summary of the main organic compounds to be found in a plant.

---

*Dr. Bach believed that all illness was preceded by an emotional imbalance and therefore the way to cure the illness was to restore the emotional balance. To this end he developed his system of flower remedies, which are prescribed on the basis of emotional disharmony. They are extraordinarily successful in treating a wide range of illness. Children respond well to them, and their timely use can often avert an illness by treating it before the emotional imbalance has taken a firm hold.

---

*The gentian normally used in medicine is *Gentiana lutea,* rather than *G. amarella* (or *Gentianella amarella*). However, their medicinal properties are very similar. *G. lutea* is preferred for medicine mainly because it is so much larger that it makes collection much easier.
[†]From Bach E: The twelve healers, Saffron Walden, England, 1941, CW Daniel (and reprints).

This is an interesting approach, but it is one that has yielded disappointing results. There are very few cases of an analysis of a plant's compounds pointing the way to new cures for illnesses. For the most part, all the scientific analysis has done is confirm results already known from experience. What is more, by separating one compound from a great many that make up a plant, it often happens that a nontoxic plant is rendered toxic. A case in point is aspirin, which can be obtained from the Spirea family (from which aspirin takes its name), particularly meadowsweet *Filipendula ulmaria*. Aspirin is known to cause stomach problems, but the whole plant actually cures stomach problems.

Here is a clash of cultures between orthodox science and experience. Our approach is to take the middle way. We believe that for clinical practice, the energy of the herb is of greater importance. After having worked with herbs for many years, we find it obvious that herbs are far more than a mass of chemicals. The entirety of the herb works in the body in a particular way, peculiar to that herb. On the other hand, measurements of the active principles of the herbs does provide us with new insights. Without these, we would not know about the similarities in the actions of foxglove *Digitalis purpurea* and squills *Urginea maritima*. It has been shown that the cardiac glycosides of these two herbs are almost identical. It is therefore pointless to give both herbs. One should choose one or the other. By contrast, the active principles of hyssop *Hyssopus officinalis* and coltsfoot *Tussilago farfara* are quite different, so one can give both in a prescription.

▪ BASIC CATEGORIES OF HERBS

The action of herbs may be categorized very simply to match the main categories of child that we have described. The children who are Strong, Weak, Hot, or Cold are matched by herbs that are tonic, dispersing, Hot, and Cold, respectively.

Tonic and Dispersing Herbs

Just as we can divide children into basic categories of Strong children (those who never seem to feel tired) and more delicate ones (those who tire easily and are more likely to burst into tears), we can also divide herbs into those that are appropriate to each category. The idea is simple, and a very old one. Tonic herbs are those that provide an extra bit of strength. They give the child that extra bit of energy. This enables the child to come back and face difficult situations in life, as well as to come back and fight a disease. One will use different medicines, so-called dispersing medicines, for stronger children. These medicines may tire the child out a bit, but they will have the effect of relieving an excess of intolerable buildup of pressure. Giving a dispersing medicine to a Strong child has few ill effects. The child has plenty of energy, so it does not matter if some energy is lost. It may calm the child down a bit, enabling him or her to sleep. The worst medicine to give such a child is a tonic because that would increase an already high pressure.

To give an illustration of these two types, first imagine a baby boy who is teething. He is very hot in the head. It is not just that the teeth are bothersome—he is irritated by everything. He cannot sleep and easily flies into a great rage. This child does not need a tonic because it might make things worse. A tonic might increase the pressure in the head and increase his temperature and rage. What this child needs is some way of "letting off steam" or some way of reducing the pressure in his head. This will enable him to relax enough to sleep. Once asleep, healing can take place. The dispersing herbs will do this.*

As another example, imagine a boy who is pale and floppy. He has a very poor appetite and is often constipated. A typical dispersing treatment would be a large dose of senna *Cassia angustifolia* to treat the constipation. Such a treatment could produce only bad results, for the child who is thin and eats poorly has no reserves. To give a purgative would be to drain him of

---

*Interestingly, the modern medicine paracetamol (sold under the brand names of Calpol and Tylenol) is a dispersing medicine and is appropriate for these children.

what little reserves are available. What he needs is herbs that strengthen and tone the muscles of the intestines.

Hot and Cold

The idea that the food we eat and the medicines we take can be Hot or Cold in energy is a very old one, but it has almost disappeared from our thinking. The idea was common in all the ancient writings. It was there in Gerard's *Herball* of 1636, and even there to some extent in Culpeper's writing in 1649. It only began to disappear in the eighteenth century with the invention of the thermometer. Although it is an old idea, we feel we need to present it again.

The idea is very simple. Something with a Hot energy is something that makes you feel hot! Something with a Cold energy is something that cools you down. As an obvious example, ginger *Zingiber officinalis* is Hot, whereas cucumber *Cucumis sativa* is Cold. It is not only herbs that are Hot and Cold, but foods too. Hot foods are those like lamb stew, which you would instinctively eat on a cold day, and the Cold foods are those like lettuce and cucumber, which you would instinctively eat on a hot day. (See Boxes 1-3 to 1-6 for examples.)

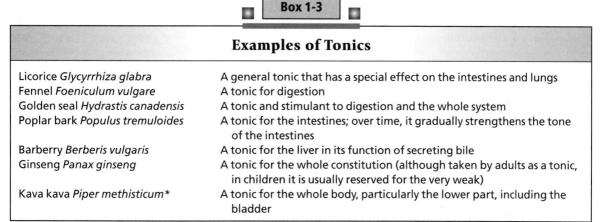

Box 1-3

Examples of Tonics

Licorice *Glycyrrhiza glabra*	A general tonic that has a special effect on the intestines and lungs
Fennel *Foeniculum vulgare*	A tonic for digestion
Golden seal *Hydrastis canadensis*	A tonic and stimulant to digestion and the whole system
Poplar bark *Populus tremuloides*	A tonic for the intestines; over time, it gradually strengthens the tone of the intestines
Barberry *Berberis vulgaris*	A tonic for the liver in its function of secreting bile
Ginseng *Panax ginseng*	A tonic for the whole constitution (although taken by adults as a tonic, in children it is usually reserved for the very weak)
Kava kava *Piper methisticum**	A tonic for the whole body, particularly the lower part, including the bladder

*Note that kava kava is banned in some countries.

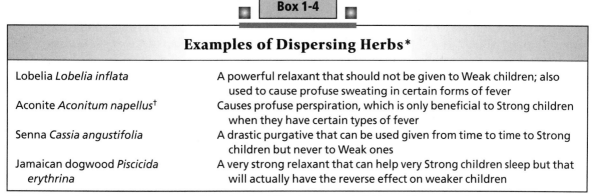

Box 1-4

Examples of Dispersing Herbs*

Lobelia *Lobelia inflata*	A powerful relaxant that should not be given to Weak children; also used to cause profuse sweating in certain forms of fever
Aconite *Aconitum napellus*[†]	Causes profuse perspiration, which is only beneficial to Strong children when they have certain types of fever
Senna *Cassia angustifolia*	A drastic purgative that can be used given from time to time to Strong children but never to Weak ones
Jamaican dogwood *Piscicida erythrina*	A very strong relaxant that can help very Strong children sleep but that will actually have the reverse effect on weaker children

*Dispersing herbs can be given to Strong children but should be given to Weak children with great caution.
[†] Give with caution. In medium doses, aconite is a poison.

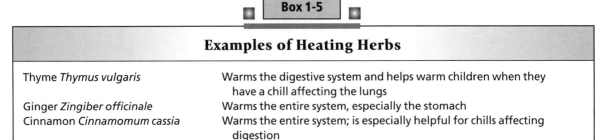

Box 1-5

Examples of Heating Herbs

Thyme *Thymus vulgaris*	Warms the digestive system and helps warm children when they have a chill affecting the lungs
Ginger *Zingiber officinale*	Warms the entire system, especially the stomach
Cinnamon *Cinnamomum cassia*	Warms the entire system; is especially helpful for chills affecting digestion
Chili pepper *Capsicum minimum*	Warms the entire system

Box 1-6

Examples of Cooling Herbs

Marshmallow *Althea officinalis*	Cools inflammations, especially in the lungs and digestive tract
Gentian *Gentiana glabra*	Reduces excess heat in the system, especially when the heat comes from liver problems, such as hepatitis
Barberry *Berberis vulgaris*	Reduces inflammation in the digestive system (as well as being tonic)
Violet *Viola odorata*	Reduces inflammation in the chest

The "temperature" of the herb is important because it describes the way that a child will react to that herb. For example, herbs with Cool energy, such as violet *Viola odorata* and echinacea *Echinacea angustifolia*, which are often given for bacterial infections with heat symptoms, would be fine on their own for a Strong red-faced child with a fever, but they may be inappropriate for a pale and Weak child, even if the child has a bacterial infection. These herbs would benefit the child only if they were combined with tonic and warming herbs. We will return to this in more detail when we cover each individual disease.

Dose

At this point we should mention that dose is all-important. The tonic and dispersing effects are not really so evident at small doses. For example, it takes large doses of lobelia to cause violent sweating, whereas smaller doses seem almost to be tonic for the lungs. It takes large doses of poplar bark to give adverse effects in Strong patients.

The same is true for Hot and Cold. For example, in large doses, gentian *Gentiana glabra* is very Cold, but in small doses, this effect does not really come into play.

2

Energetic Patterns of Illness

▣ THE WAY CHILDREN BECOME ILL: PROBLEMS FACING THE NEWBORN AND CHILD

Central to our understanding of illness is that there is a factor in the person's life that is causing the illness. This cause could loosely be termed *stress*. To begin with, stress acts as a stimulant to the system, but if it persists, it leads to an imbalance in energy. If it continues, it may lead to illness. Following this approach, the way to understand illness is to determine what the main stresses are in a person's life and the corresponding system that is likely to be stressed.

For adults there are two major stresses in life that may lead to disease: tension from emotional strain and exhaustion from overwork and lack of sleep. Therefore the two categories of medicine commonly used to combat these two conditions are relaxants (for tension) and tonics (for exhaustion). This is recognized in orthodox medicine as well, as evidenced by the vast prescribing of tranquilizers such as diazepam (Valium) for the treatment of tension. The street sales of ginseng and gota kola for the treatment of exhaustion are enormously high.

Before we discuss children's illness, we need to know which system is most likely to be under stress, and this requires an understanding of the life of a baby and child and how different their lives are from adults'. This knowledge provides the clue to the different patterns of illness seen in children. The main points of stress for children are digestion of food and protection against cold. Of these, digestion of food is the most important. The child needs to grow, and growing requires the absorption of nutrients. It is not only nutrients that are absorbed from food but also energy. The child needs energy for protection against cold, to learn, and to interact with the world. So, once again, the functioning of the digestive system is of paramount importance for the health of a child.

The main points of stress for children are as follows:
- Digestion of food
- Protection against the cold

What we have found in clinical practice is that a good digestion in children is the key to good health. Children in whom digestion is not working well may be prone to all sorts of disease. Likewise, in many diseases, as diverse as diarrhea, insomnia, chronic cough, and even convulsions, regulating digestion may be enough to cure the condition.

— Special Problems Facing Babies and Toddlers —

It may be suggested that the first 2 or 3 years of life, although important, amount to only a very short time in a person's life and that it is therefore somewhat out of proportion to focus on these very early years. However, we believe that these very early years are indeed of the greatest importance, for it has been our observation in clinic that ill health that appears in these early years is likely to remain with the child, perhaps even into adulthood.

There are various reasons why this is so. The baby's immune system is immature and easily set off balance. A simple illness can often cause a great deal of distress to a newborn, whereas a 6-year-old may overcome the same illness in a day. What is more, once the system is upset, it can be hard for the baby to set it right again.

☐ THREE INTERRELATED PROBLEMS

We are now going to look at the three main problems facing a newborn and a toddler:

- Digesting food
- Keeping warm
- Breathing

Before birth, babies do not have these problems, but after birth they do. They have spent 9 months in the warmth and security of the womb, and suddenly they have to eat, breathe, and keep warm. Of these, eating poses perhaps the greatest problem (and the greatest difference from adults) because babies need to consume vast quantities of food (relative to body weight) to grow. A moment's reflection will reveal how much food the baby needs to consume: A baby's birth weight doubles in the first 6 months of life and triples in the first year. The amount of food relative to body weight needed to double weight in 6 months is truly staggering.

Into this equation, we also have to add the problem of keeping warm. Once again, there is a difference between babies and adults in that babies have a much greater ratio of surface area to body weight, so relatively speaking they lose more heat. This interacts with digestion, for it means that babies have to consume yet more food to keep warm.

The third factor, breathing, comes into the equation too. Because breathing is such a new activity, it is easy for the child to acquire lung infections, and these, in turn, take energy to fight off. This means that the baby needs extra food to provide the extra energy, but it also means that there is less energy to digest the food.

From this brief discussion, we can see that these three factors are paramount in a baby's life. In principle, adults also have these problems, but in developed countries there are very few adults whose life is so harsh that they are truly exposed to the elements. Most adults face different problems in their life, usually related to social interaction and earning a living! (A further discussion of how children's problems evolve into adult problems is given in Chapter 6.)

This interaction is not merely theoretical. It is something we meet in the clinic: When a baby acquires an infection, it is normal for the digestive system to be upset too. In the mildest form it means that the baby's appetite will be reduced; in more severe forms it means that the baby may suffer from diarrhea. One also sees that if a child has a poor appetite, he or she becomes weak. The immune system does not develop or work properly, and the child becomes prone to lung infections. Likewise, it means that when a baby has a digestive disturbance, the baby often concurrently develops a cough or a runny nose. When a child presents with a cough, we always consider the state of the digestive system. If digestion is not working well, any improvement in the cough will be short term. The cough will almost certainly return as soon as the child stops taking the herbs.

Digestion and the Lungs Are Intimately Connected

In Western medical science, it is usually assumed that the lungs and digestion function independently. If you have a cough and seek medical attention, it is unlikely that the doctor will ask about what you eat! However, having observed many patients and having studied Chinese medicine, we find it obvious that the state of the digestive system and what we eat have a profound effect on the way the lungs function.

This is a fundamental tenet of Chinese medicine. At present, there is no commonly accepted scientific explanation for it. A possible reason may be that both the lungs and the intestines have a mucous membrane. When excess acids build up in the intestines (perhaps from eating excessively rich food), the digestive tract becomes mildly irritated and slightly inflamed.* In reaction to inflammation, the body produces a thicker layer of mucus

---

*This effect has been confirmed by scientists working on leaky gut syndrome, described later in this chapter.

for protection. As the levels of mucus increase locally, they also increase throughout the body and in the lungs. What starts out as an irritation in the digestive system can end up as excess mucus in the lungs. This gives rise to symptoms such as a rattly cough, some sinus congestion, a runny nose, and generalized catarrh.

The following three systems are interrelated in babies:
  • Digestion
  • Skin
  • Lungs
If one is disturbed, it is easy for the other two to become disturbed.

Digestion and Fluid Metabolism

Another consequence of a digestive disturbance is that the fluid metabolism goes wrong. If the digestive tract is impaired, inflamed, full of mucus, or damaged, the amount of fluid absorbed is altered, upsetting a fine equilibrium. This in turn affects the levels of mucus and inflammation in the body, for if the body is somewhat dehydrated, not through drinking too little but because the gut is absorbing badly, then inflammation will worsen. Similarly, mucus production will increase, which impairs water absorption. In contrast, if too much fluid is consumed and the kidneys do not function well, the child can easily become waterlogged and the kidneys overworked. It is common to see children thin and almost dehydrated simply because they do not absorb water properly. Likewise, children may retain water because more fluid is being absorbed than can be excreted by the kidneys.

SIGNS OF IMPAIRED FLUID METABOLISM

Children with impaired fluid metabolism may have squashy legs (i.e., slightly enlarged and soft to the touch), a puffy face, and a swollen abdomen. They may urinate little in the day but a lot at night, to the point of wetting their beds. Once again, When a child is waterlogged, do not just look to the kidney system and treat these problems with astringents or diuretics, but look to the digestive system. Is it working well? The digestive system may need to be treated, not the urogenital system.

--- **Signs of an Impaired Fluid Metabolism** ---
  • Squashy legs
  • Puffy face
  • Swollen abdomen
  • Little urination in the day but a lot at night, to the point of wetting the bed

---

In the next few sections, we discuss common ways that digestion can go wrong. It tends to go wrong in very simple ways, leading to commonly seen patterns or types of digestive disturbance.

▪ PATTERNS OF DIGESTIVE PROBLEMS

Although all children are different, their digestive systems seem to go wrong in very simple ways. In adults it is common to see one part of the digestive system, such as the gallbladder, go out of balance more or less in isolation. In children it is more common for the entire digestive system to be affected. As we have seen, when the digestive system is affected, the whole child is affected. Although the child may have a particular symptom such as continuous vomiting, constipation, or even chronic cough, we first of all look for one of the patterns discussed later in this chapter.

--- **About Patterns in General** ---
Patterns of illness are descriptions of a collection of symptoms and signs that often accompany one another. They are a way of classifying illness that helps in prescribing herbs. They are a sort of halfway between purely symptomatic prescribing and completely holistic prescribing. If you prescribe symptomatically (as is usually done in orthodox medicine), then the same medicine is used for the same symptom whenever it appears. Some herbalists use this approach too; for example, there are some who will always give gentian *Gentiana lutea*

Continued

——— **About Patterns in General—cont'd** ———

for nausea, irrespective of the cause. At the other extreme, there are those who say that each prescription should be individually tailored to each patient.

Patterns are a half-way between these two extremes and give one a starting point for deciding on which general category of herbs will or will not be suitable. Truly speaking, patterns are an energetic imbalance, and as such, they are hard to describe. Here we do our best by giving a list of symptoms and signs that commonly occur together.

What makes the use of patterns so special is that by identifying the main pattern, you have put your finger on the main energetic imbalance affecting the child. Sometimes you can give a herb simply for the pattern, without paying special attention to the main symptom. There is a saying that describes this: "One pattern has many symptoms, and one symptom may have many patterns."

The most common patterns affecting the whole digestion are the following:

- Stagnant food
- Weak digestion with low energy
- Weak digestion with nervous energy

SUMMARY
Stagnant Food. The child is Strong, has a good appetite, and therefore eats more than can be digested. The accumulated food then starts to ferment.

Weak Digestion with Low Energy. The child does not have much energy, so the digestive system does not work well. In addition, digestion is not working well, so the child does not have much energy.

Weak Digestion with Nervous Energy. The child does not get much energy from its food because he or she does not eat very much. Rather, the child lives off nervous energy.

▪ SYMPTOMS AND SIGNS

Stagnant Food

This is a pattern that affects Strong children more. These children come into the world with energy and enthusiasm. Their enthusiasm extends to food, and they normally have good appetites—so much so that some of these children will eat anything that is put in front of them. Sometimes they will go on eating long after they have had enough to eat. And it is this—overeating—that is one of the common causes of this pattern. What happens is that children continue to eat until their stomachs are bursting. The stomach contains more food than it can easily digest, and it is eliminated either undigested or partly digested and partly fermented. Children exhibiting this pattern share some common characteristics (see also Color Plate 2-1):

- They have red cheeks.
- They are irritable, touchy, and bad tempered.

The appearance of these children is simply due to a poorly functioning digestive system. They look like some adults feel after they have had a Christmas or Thanksgiving dinner!

After further questioning and examination, you will find the following:

- Swollen abdomen (often like a drum)
- Irregular stool pattern (diarrhea or constipation alternating with diarrhea; in mild cases the stools will smell of apples, as a result of fermentation, and in severe cases the stools will be really stinking)

In addition to the preceding findings, the following may also be present:

- Catarrhal symptoms
- Poor sleep

EXPLANATION OF THESE SYMPTOMS
- *Red cheeks:* Red cheeks can occur in both adults and children and often result from eating too much.

- *Irritability, touchiness, bad temper:* The stagnant food in the abdomen makes the child feel uncomfortable or even in pain, resulting in irritability.
- *Swollen abdomen:* If the food does not pass through the digestive system quickly enough, the warmth and moisture of the stomach allow the food to ferment. When there is fermentation gas accumulates, which results in distention. This fermentation also causes the stools to smell. If there is mild fermentation, the stools smell like cider; if fermentation is severe, the stools smell putrid. Constipation occurs because the food moves slowly and becomes stuck; it then ferments in the abdomen and is eliminated as loose stools.
- *Catarrhal symptoms:* These symptoms arise as a result of the systemic inflammatory process that causes mucus production, as explained previously.
- *Poor sleeping:* These children often have difficultly sleeping because of discomfort, nasal congestion, slight coughs, and so forth; in addition, heat in the system agitates the brain.

CAUSES

There are three main causes for this pattern: overfeeding, irregular feeding, and unsuitable food.

Overfeeding. These children have an enthusiasm for food, or perhaps are a little greedy, and take more food than can easily be digested. The food that is not digested begins to ferment and decompose.

Irregular Feeding. The digestive system works best when it is given food on a regular basis. If there are set times for meals, then the digestive organs start to accommodate to these. If the diet is very irregular, with large variations in the amount and time, then digestion never has time to settle down into a good rhythm and it starts to function poorly.

Unsuitable Food. When we talk about unsuitable food, we are not speaking moralistically. We are simply talking about food that does not suit an individual child. There are no absolute rules. What suits one child may not suit another. One child may have a gargantuan appetite and eat a wide range of "adult" foods and be perfectly well, whereas another child may have to be very careful about diet. In Chapter 3, we give a fuller discussion of what constitutes a suitable diet. Here we merely point out that high-fiber foods are often difficult for toddlers and children to digest, as are gluten and cow's milk products.

───── **Main Causes of Disruption of Digestion** ─────
- Overfeeding
- Irregular feeding
- Unsuitable food

Weak Digestion with Low Energy

This pattern is much more likely to affect the weaker children, although occasionally it may occur in Strong children who have been ill or who are eating food that they are allergic to. What happens is that something (e.g., an illness) causes their energy to drop. This means that they do not have much energy to devote to digestion. The lack of energy for digestion results in these children not being able to eat much food, and consequently, they do not obtain much energy from food. Thus a vicious circle is established, and they get stuck in the condition of low energy (see Color Plate 3-5).

When you first see these children, you will notice the following characteristics:

- Pale face; maybe slight yellow tinge
- Rather droopy
- Often shy
- Do not appear very forceful

When you ask questions and start to feel the child, you will find the following:

- Poor appetite, very picky and choosy over food (Box 2-1)
- Often constipated; occasionally loose stools
- Sensitive (cries easily)

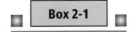

What Does *Poor Appetite* Mean?

When the child is younger than 3 years old, a poor appetite means simply that he or she does not eat much food. Some children eat so little, you wonder how it is that they manage to grow at all. However, when these children reach about 9 or 10 years of age, they are often more active and will need to eat a lot more. Here the key sign is not so much the quantity of food that they eat but the range of foods that they eat. At 10 years old, a child with a poor appetite might eat a lot but be restricted to a diet of burgers and chips, with occasional frozen peas.

- Thin arms and legs or rather squashy arms and legs—without good tone
- Easily tired
- May want to sleep in the day

EXPLANATION OF THESE SYMPTOMS

All of these symptoms are simply the result of not having much energy. There are few that need explanation.

- The behavioral pattern of being shy and easily crying is because these children do not have enough energy to cope with the ups and downs of life.
- Constipation can occur because the energy in the intestines is low, so peristalsis is weak and slow.
- Thin arms and legs are common because these children are somewhat undernourished—simply because they do not eat much food.
- Squashy arms and legs are common because of mild water retention. When the digestive system is not working well, the fluid balance may be affected.

CAUSES

- Long labor
- Exhaustion of the mother
- Long illness

- Excessive immunization
- Unstructured nursing and feeding

The first three factors are ones that tire the mother and child and weaken their energy. Excessive immunization causes the same types of problems as long illnesses, leaving the child feeling weak. This problem is discussed further in Chapter 5. The reason why unstructured nursing and feeding weaken digestion is given in Chapter 3.

> Take time to find a regular schedule and suitable food for your child.

Weak Digestion with Nervous Energy

When you first see children with weak digestion and nervous energy, you will notice the following characteristics:

- Pale face
- Often shy
- Do not appear very forceful

When you ask questions and start to feel the child, you will find the following:

- Poor appetite, very picky and choosy over food
- Often constipated; occasionally loose stools
- Sensitive (cries easily)
- Thin arms and legs or rather squashy arms and legs—without good tone

When these children get to know you a bit, you will discover the following:

- Never tired
- Always on the go
- Never want to go to bed at night
- Like to be the center of attention

EXPLANATION OF THESE SYMPTOMS

The explanation of most of the symptoms is the same as listed previously. The difference, the behavior pattern, arises because these children live off nervous energy. Another way of looking at it is that this behavior pattern allows these children to attract energy toward themselves. By being the center of attention and irritating people, they find that they can pick up vital energy from those around them.

CAUSES

The causes are the same as for weak digestion:

- Long labor
- Exhaustion of the mother after childbirth
- Long illness
- Excessive immunization
- Unstructured nursing and feeding

In addition to the preceding, another cause may be the following:

- Lack of routine

The reasons for the first four factors are the same as for the previous pattern. The reason why lack of routine encourages this pattern is discussed in Chapter 1.

■ THE PARENTS' ENERGY DURING ILLNESS

During our discussions on energy, we have spent most of the time concentrating on the energy of the child. This is not really a "holistic" picture, for a child's energy cannot be considered in isolation from his or her parents, especially when the child is very young. This is more true during illness, because when a child is ill, extra energy is needed. What this means for parents is that when their children are ill, they are likely to feel exhausted from providing the extra energy needed to cope with the illness.

This can pose problems for working mothers and fathers, who may be unable to take time off work to provide the time and space for a sick child. Being stretched to the limits, they may not have much energy to spare.

■ LEAKY GUT SYNDROME

In recent years, discoveries have been made about the malfunctioning of the intestines, and this has led to the idea of leaky gut syndrome. A possible explanation for food intolerance and allergy has been put forward under the heading of the leaky gut. It has been shown that in many people who have low-grade health problems, the villi in the intestines become slightly inflamed and that when they are in this condition food is not absorbed properly. Normally, the intestines absorb only food that has been broken down into molecules small enough for the liver to transform. When the intestines are inflamed, much larger molecules are absorbed into the bloodstream. Molecules that should remain in the intestines leak into the bloodstream. These cannot easily be further digested, and it becomes the task of the immune system to break them down. Thus what should have been food is seen by the immune system as foreign and becomes a poison. There is a lot of research to back up this proposition. In particular, the involvement of the immune system can be shown by the presence of antibodies to certain foods in the blood.

Leaky Gut and Patterns

In leaky gut syndrome, the digestive system becomes disturbed, as does the immune system. This means that from a disturbance in the gut, the whole body can be set off balance. The particular imbalance varies among children. Some children react by developing the stagnant food pattern, whereas others react by developing the weak digestion pattern. In yet others, the main symptom may be food allergy or respiratory allergy.

When it comes to treating with herbs, we normally do not focus on the fact that the gut is leaky; rather, we focus on the way the leaky gut has affected the child. The condition typically rights itself when the child is given the appropriate herbs, and the gut no longer leaks.

Leaky Gut and Antibiotics

Antibiotics have been shown to be an aggravating factor for leaky gut because the bacteria in the intestines are mostly beneficial. There are bacteria for breaking down bile and other large molecules such as hormones that are excreted into the bowels. When antibiotics are taken, the intestinal bacteria are seriously disturbed and the breakdown is no longer complete. The consequence of this is that bile and hormones that should have been broken down are reabsorbed through the leaky gut. The effect of antibiotics is to magnify the harmful effects of a leaky gut.

Candida

Candida albicans is a yeast that thrives in the gut and other moist places, especially the mouth and the vagina. Once it has taken hold, it can be difficult to eliminate. It affects many adults and a lot of children and is a factor in oral thrush. *Candida* can be caused by the leaky gut syndrome and can also exacerbate it. It exacerbates it by damaging the epithelial cells. Moreover, the toxins that it generates enter and affect other organs, including the brain, which can in turn predispose children to attention-deficit/hyperactivity disorder and autism. Additional information on candidal infection is given in Chapter 15.

Using Patterns to Maintain Health

These patterns return again and again throughout this book. They are patterns that underlie many different conditions and diseases. However, your child, or a child brought to you, may have one of these patterns and, as yet, have no definite illness. If this happens, you do not have to wait for illness to come along in order to treat. We think it is much better to start treatment while a child is well, to prevent disease from occurring. One of the great uses of these patterns is that they show the way to an appropriate diet, prescription, or treatment.

As far as details are concerned, these are given in different chapters. In particular, if your child has weak digestion or the stagnant food pattern, refer to Chapters 10, 11, and 14 . Even though the particular child's symptoms may be relatively mild, these chapters contain useful prescriptions and the effects of taking the herbs.

☐ MAIN POINTS FROM THIS CHAPTER

- A good digestion is crucial for a child's health.
- Digestion and the lungs are related.
- There are three commonly seen digestive patterns.
    Stagnant food
    Weak digestion
    Weak digestion and nervous energy

3

Diet

By the time parents come for a consultation, most are aware that diet is important for the health of their child. We are often asked to advise regarding a suitable diet and a suitable weaning pattern. In this chapter we briefly touch on these subjects, although we do not provide much in the way of definite answers! Our experience has been that there are a few don'ts but not so many do's. When it comes to getting a child to eat, the child often has a much stronger voice than you as a practitioner or parent. Most children will not eat what they do not want to eat, and they will be very vociferous about demanding the foods that they do want.

We also have found that most parents give their children food that is suitable (with a few exceptions mentioned in the following sections). Rather than giving their children unsuitable food, parents are much more likely to initiate a poor feeding schedule; therefore in this chapter we discuss this before anything else.

▪ OVERFEEDING

One common problem is simply eating too much food (or milk in the case of a nursing baby). Some children are enthusiastic about eating, and their mothers are delighted to see them eating so much. There is something satisfying in giving food, and conversely, it is almost impossible to resist the demands of a child crying for food, even if the child is known to be full.

The pattern of overfeeding is less common among breast-fed babies, for there is a limit to the quantity of milk a mother can produce. It is possible for breast-fed babies to overconsume milk, though, if their mothers produce very large quantities of very rich milk.

▪ IRREGULAR FEEDING

In the past, overfeeding was the most common cause of digestive complaints. Fast catching up is irregular feeding. This is simply because the whole pattern of life is becoming more irregular and less disciplined. Not long ago it was normal for the family to sit down to three meals a day. Nothing was eaten between meals, except perhaps a snack at well-defined times for the children. This pattern has now been replaced in many families by food taken directly from the freezer to the microwave, with each person eating when he or she feels like it. In some families, "grazing" is the norm; that is, everyone in the family continually snacks, but they do not really sit down to a proper meal. With this background it is not surprising that the same feeding patterns are extended to babies and toddlers. For some babies and toddlers, this is not a problem; however, there are many babies and toddlers whose digestive systems do not cope well. Their stomachs never completely empty, and they never feel properly hungry. This leads to one of two patterns: the stagnant food pattern or the weak pattern.

How Irregular Feeding Leads to the Stagnant Food Pattern

Children who develop the stagnant food pattern are, once again, the enthusiastic children. Although they do not feel really hungry, at the sight of food they react with enthusiasm and gladly take some more. This results in undigested food being added to already partly digested food in their stomachs, which can lead to fermentation.

This applies to breast-fed and bottle-fed babies as well. Regular feedings in very young children are actually better for digestion. Feedings may be given as frequently as every $1\frac{1}{2}$ or 2 hours in young babies, but it is important to wait at least 1 hour between feedings. When the baby is ill or needs special comfort, providing regular feedings may be difficult, but in general, if the child has a regular feeding pattern from the very start, then a much healthier digestion develops than if the child is fed irregularly and very frequently.

How Irregular Feeding Leads to the Weak Pattern

Children who develop the weak pattern are those who never really eat a proper meal. They are not hungry at mealtimes and often eat next to nothing. Half an hour later, however, they start to feel hungry and then fill up on a snack. They snack all the time and consequently never get a full meal and never give their stomachs time to rest. Unlike other organs in the body, the stomach needs time to rest, so if it has to work all the time, it becomes weak. Over time, this weakness can spread to the rest of the body.

▪ UNSTRUCTURED NURSING

Unstructed nursing is really an extension of irregular feeding, but we mention it as a separate cause because it often gives rise to the weak digestion pattern. The reason is that the initial milk produced during suckling is thinner milk, called *foremilk*. The foremilk, which is more watery, helps quench thirst. Only after the baby has been suckling for several minutes does the richer milk, called *hindmilk*, start to flow. This means that if a baby sucks for just a minute at a time and then stops, soon returning for another minute, he or she receives only foremilk and never benefits from the richer hindmilk. Leaving an hour to an hour and a half between feeds and then giving a full feed will mean that the baby gets the full range of milk.

What Is a Suitable Regular Feeding Pattern?

In babies and toddlers, the feeding pattern is necessarily different than that of adults. Babies' and toddlers' sleeping patterns do not correspond with those of adults, so they often eat at different times as well. This is even more true for nursing babies in the first months of life. What is a suitable feeding pattern? There are few absolute rules here, but there is one that we find is very helpful, especially if the baby is unwell: to make sure that between feedings, the stomach has enough time to empty completely. In practice this means that there should be *at least* 1 hour, preferably $1\frac{1}{2}$ hours, between feedings—a period when the child consumes no food or water. For some mothers this is a hard rule to adopt, but for some children, it is absolutely essential if they are ever to get well.

There should be *at least* 1 hour, preferably $1\frac{1}{2}$ hours, between feedings to allow the stomach time to empty.

▪ Case History

When we first moved to the United States, one of our first patients was a child who had "absences." These had been diagnosed by the doctor as mild epileptic attacks. Her normal pattern was to stop what she was doing and stare blankly. Sometimes she would tremble, and sometimes, when the seizures continued for a long time, she would stumble and fall over. She was brought to us when she was about 21 months old. She was still breast-fed on demand. In her case this meant that she would return to her mother to take a sip at the breast every 3 to 5 minutes. She would take a suck or two and then return to her play.

Her type of epilepsy is related to weakness, and we came to the conclusion that the weakness was in part the result of the child's feeding habits—the child was receiving only the thinner foremilk and never the more nourishing hindmilk. We therefore advised the mother of the need to wait at least 1 hour between feedings. This advice fell on deaf ears, for the mother had a deep belief in the correctness of her child's instincts, combined with a deep dislike of discipline and a craving for liberty. Although we explained the difficulty in curing her child without some change being made in the feeding pattern, the mother was unable to make the necessary changes.

Our fears about the difficulty in curing the child were well founded. She underwent many months of treatment with both acupuncture and herbs—treatment that would be expected to cure her completely, but she improved little. The turning point came eventually. There was a period when the mother fell ill with mild food poisoning, and during this illness, she felt unable to feed her daughter every time the child was hungry. For the first time the child had at least 1 hour between feedings.

The mother noticed that her child was already getting better, and she was so encouraged by the results that she continued this practice. From this time on, the child started to get better, and within a few weeks, the seizures stopped.

▪ DIET AND HEALTH IN PREGNANCY AND NURSING

We will not go into great detail but rather confine ourselves to a few of the most important foods and how they affect the baby through the mother. We wish merely to state the obvious—diet in pregnancy affects the baby! There are a few general principles to bear in mind:

- *Eat good-quality organic food.* The residues left in the food from nonorganic agriculture definitely affect the baby. In addition, nonorganic food is often deficient in trace minerals such as boron. Even important minerals such as calcium are often much reduced in nonorganic food. Locally grown fresh food may be a good second best if organic food is not obtainable.
- *Take supplements during pregnancy.* This advice applies especially to women who cannot obtain organic food. The vitamin and mineral content of food produced with fertilizers is now greatly reduced from what it was 25 years ago because the soil in which it is grown

has been depleted. Fortunately, this deficiency can be repaired by taking a good-quality broad-spectrum vitamin and mineral supplement. (*Caution*: Never exceed the recommended dose. It is possible to overdose on vitamins and minerals.)

- *Look after your energy as much as possible.* If you are very tired during pregnancy, it makes sense to rest as much as possible. It will help the new baby and make life easier for you after the baby is born by ensuring that you have energy for all of the extra work that will need to be done.
- *Seek alternative medicines for ailments of pregnancy.* Many therapies can help alleviate the common ailments of pregnancy (e.g., nausea, sickness, anemia, high blood pressure). Herbs, acupuncture, and homoeopathy are of enormous benefit. These are noninvasive therapies that have been used for centuries and are actually beneficial for the newborn.
- *Remember that the baby lives your life.* After about 4.5 months, everything you do is registered by the baby. The emotions you feel are directly felt by the baby too.
- *Avoid oranges during pregnancy.* Overconsumption of oranges is associated with babies becoming restless to the point of being hyperactive. There are not usually many long-term problems (after the first 3 years) for the child, but it is certainly a problem for the family to have a sleepless child.

Breast-Feeding

Numerous studies have shown the benefits of breast milk over all other forms of milk.* Not all mothers want to breast-feed their babies, but those who do often find that they have little support to overcome the difficulties. In our experience there are very few, if any, mothers who cannot produce enough milk if they are given help and encouragement and, if needed, help from herbs.

---

*There are certain exceptions, for example, when the mother is obliged to take medicines that may pass through into the milk.

This is a book about children, so we will not go into a full discussion of the best ways of overcoming common breast-feeding problems. Here we would encourage mothers who wish to breast-feed not to give up easily. Read about likely problems beforehand. Get assistance from a herbalist, a homeopath, an acupuncturist, or a breast-feeding adviser. All of these therapists can help in the treatment of common problems, such as sore or cracked nipples, inflamed breasts (milk fever), and insufficient milk. Excellent information can be found in McIntyre's book *The Complete Woman's Herbal* (1994) and many other herbal books related to treatment of women's problems.

There is one remedy that we cannot resist mentioning—dill seed *Anethum graveolens*, which is a wonder herb for promoting milk production. Make tea from one heaping teaspoon of seeds in as much water as you would like to drink. Drink all of the tea. Take this three times a day or more if you like.

Mother's Diet When Nursing

Just as the mother's diet during pregnancy is important, so is her diet when nursing. Obviously, the mother has to take in enough food to keep both herself and her baby alive. What is not so generally realized is that the energy of the food goes immediately into the milk. It continues to surprise us that the stimulating or sedating effect of some foods goes into the milk well before there has been time for the food to be digested (Table 3-1).

The comments we gave in our discussion of pregnancy apply to nursing as well: Consider taking supplements, eat organic foods, rest as much as possible, use natural therapies for ailments when possible, and avoid eating oranges.

FORMULA MILK

Formula milk is not as good as human milk. Formulas that are currently available are much closer to human milk than before, but they are still nowhere as good. Part of the problem is that

Table 3-1   Possible Adverse Effects of Foods When Nursing

FOOD	POSSIBLE ADVERSE EFFECT
Cow's milk	The mucus-producing effect of cow's milk can be passed directly onto the nursing baby.
Wheat	The gluten in wheat gets passed on through the milk and can also give rise to a lot of mucus in some children. The mucus that is produced tends to be greenish, as opposed to the mucus from milk, which tends to be colorless.
Peanuts	The mucus-forming effect is passed on through the milk.
Coffee, tea	The stimulating effect can be passed on to the baby, although this varies from mother to mother. One mother we knew could not even take one cup of pale tea, much less coffee, without the child being sleepless for 3 nights. With other mothers and children, this effect can be much less pronounced, even nonexistent.
Oranges	Oranges are thought to contain a chemical that affects the nervous system. They can cause hyperactivity.
Shellfish (oysters, prawns, mussels)	Shellfish can cause sleeplessness and irritability amounting to hyperactivity in the baby.
Brassica	Some mothers find that Brassica gives their baby indigestion and colic.
Beans	Beans can cause flatulence and colic in the baby.

the organic compounds must come from something organic. In particular, the protein usually comes from an animal, and animal protein is simply not the same as human protein. It is a relatively recent discovery that the shape of a protein molecule is important in determining whether an enzyme can break it down. Protein from cows has a different shape than human protein and cannot be digested in the same way. Even protein from vegetables such as soy beans is different and cannot be digested as easily as human protein.

There are also other factors. Rarely is the mother aware of where the protein in the formula comes from. A little-advertised fact is that many formula milks used to contain protein from the brain and spinal cord of cows. This type of formula was not withdrawn until the mid-1990s, well after the BSE (bovine spongiform encephalopathy; mad cow disease) crisis had gathered momentum.

Quite apart from this, it is believed that the child's immune system can benefit from taking human milk, for antibodies in the mother's blood enter breast milk. This means that the child is receiving the benefit of the mother's fully developed immune system and receiving antibodies for many of the current viruses and bacteria that the mother is exposed to. These antibodies are not found in formula milk.

COW'S MILK AND CALCIUM

We are inundated with information telling us that we need cow's milk for healthy bones to develop. It is for this reason all schools serve it and even as adults we are encouraged to drink cow's milk to prevent osteoporosis, to keep strong teeth, and so forth.

This is a position with which we strongly disagree. Cow's milk is not essential. In fact, many people are actually intolerant to it, even allergic. Cow's milk is ideal food for calves, but it is not good for humans. Of course a growing child needs calcium and vitamins, but these are available in a variety of foods, which are listed at the end of this book in Appendix 1. In a well-balanced diet, be it vegetarian or not, all vitamins, minerals, and calcium can be obtained without the need for cow's milk. What is more, recent research has shown that the calcium in milk cannot be easily absorbed and that some people who are calcium deficient become even more calcium deficient when they drink cow's milk.*

We believe that most children would benefit from reducing or eliminating cow's milk from their diets. Furthermore, we believe that giving up cow's milk would result in a large majority of diseases in young children being reduced or even disappearing! This is a subject we will return to in Chapter 15.

The main problem is that cow's milk contains proteins that are very hard for many children to digest. These proteins are made even more indigestible through pasteurization. They put a strain on the developing digestive system, overloading it and causing it to become slightly inflamed. This in turn creates mucus and weakens the gut.

What is more, most cow's milk today is the milk of an unhealthy cow—one that has been fed monoculture grass with the addition of chemical feeds, hormones, and antibiotics. Many of the cows are kept in appallingly overcrowded conditions, which also affects the milk. So many of the hormones and antibiotics pass from the cow into the milk that normal milk is unsuitable for making cheese. This quality of milk cannot be good for a young child.

Effect of Pasteurization. Pasteurizing milk has become so common that it is now difficult to obtain raw, untreated milk. There are obvious benefits to pasteurization: The process kills tuberculosis bacteria, and the milk lasts longer before going sour. The side effects have never been seriously considered, though, except by a few. It is worth mentioning one or two here.

---

*Sellmeyer DE, Stone KL, Sebastian A et al: A high ratio of dietary animal to vegetable protein increases the rate of bone loss and the risk of fracture in postmenopausal women. Study of Osteoporotic Fractures Research Group, *Am J Clin Nutr* 2001;73:118. Other interesting facts about the dairy industry may be found on the website www.notmilk.com.

First, pasteurized milk is harder to digest. This is partly because the process of pasteurization alters the structure of the proteins. It is also partly because there are beneficial bacteria in milk from a healthy cow, which assist in digestion. These beneficial bacteria are killed along with the harmful ones.

Second, there can be both short- and long-term effects on health. If animal experiments are anything to go by (and they are used as evidence for banning certain herbs), the effects are surprisingly profound. Experiments were done on cats and on rats, feeding them pasteurized and sterilized milk. It was found that in the short term, susceptibility to disease was decreased and that, in the long term, after two generations, birth abnormalities increased.* These results are so shocking that it is astonishing that they are ignored.

Alternatives to Cow's Milk

- *Goat's milk:* Goat's milk is a good alternative for those who like it. It is much more digestible than cow's milk because the proteins contained in goat's milk are more akin to human milk proteins. We have seen many chronic problems resolved by merely changing from cow's milk to goat's milk. Moreover, at present, goats are not so intensively farmed, so the quality of the milk is better. The main problem is that some people hate the taste and smell. Some doctors strongly advise against goat's milk on the grounds that it contains much more sodium than cow's milk, claiming that this causes a threat. In children younger than 1 year, excess sodium can overload the immature kidneys and cause renal dysfunction. We are not in a position to comment on this, apart from saying that we have seen no negative side effects from goat's milk in any of the children we have treated.

---

*Katase A: Der Einfluss der Ernährung auf die Konstitution des Organismus, *Path Inst Med Acad Osaka*, 1931; Pottenger FM: The effect of heat-processing of food on the dento-facial structures of experimental animals, *Am J Orthodon Oral Surg* 32:467-485, 1946; and Price WA: Nutrition and physical degeneration, New York, 1939, PB Hoeber. Quoted in Husemann F, Wolff O (ed): *Anthroposophical approach to medicine*, vol 3, Spring Valley, NY, 1989, Anthroposophic Press, p 94.

- *Sheep's milk:* Another good alternative is sheep's milk. The main disadvantage is that it is very fatty. In some children this can cause mild diarrhea.
- *Soy milk:* This is an excellent alternative to cow's milk. Most organic soy milk products contain added vitamins and calcium. Some children find this hard to digest. A common problem babies have with soy is flatulence and colic. You will find these children have difficulty digesting all bean products, including soy. Also watch out for rather smelly stools. This is normal; smelly stools occur from the higher proportion of protein. It may be distressing to the parents or those who have to change the diapers, but it usually is not indicative of a health problem.
- *Rice milk, oat milk:* These are also available with added calcium and vitamins and are usually very well tolerated. The main disadvantage is that it is very low in fat. Some milks made from cereals have added fats, making them good substitutes.

Weaning to Solid Foods

We have much experience in watching the effects of different approaches to weaning. The following advice is thus based on observation rather than just theory.

There are no firm rules, but the following principles usually apply:

- Weaning should start between 5 and 12 months. Generally speaking, a baby should start to show some interest in taking something other than milk at about 6 months, but for some it is as late as 9 or 10 months. If by the age of 12 months there is still no interest, the child probably has a weak digestive pattern. This is something we would consider treating. Some children start to show an interest in solid food at 4 months, but usually this interest should be curbed or at least restrained. Starting solid foods at this age can easily lead to the stagnant food pattern.
- Weaning should finish sometime between 9 months and 5 years. This may seem like a long period, but it is based on our observations. If a

child weans completely before the age of 9 months, some digestive complaints are likely to develop. It seems that the digestive system is not developed enough before 9 months to cope with a diet of solid food only. The child may also get more minor infections because the immune system is far from developed at this age, and if the child stops breast-feeding, a supply of immunity is cut off.

- As for the upper end, a range of opinions is available. Some believe that breast-feeding longer than 1 year encourages the strengthening of family ties at the expense of individual development. Others believe that a child should have the opportunity to continue breast-feeding until the age of 5 years. Although this is not what we normally advise, there are no strong medical grounds for advising against it. Children who are weaned at this later age do not seem to develop significantly more medical problems. Many mothers might want "their bodies back" long before this, but that is a matter of the mother's preference and does not seem to affect the child's health adversely.

First Foods

First solid foods should be very simple, for example, well-cooked cereal. Finely ground white rice, or white rice cooked until it is mushy, is well tolerated by most children. Wheat in various forms can also be given, although many children find it harder to digest. This is partly because there is more gluten in wheat and partly because modern strains of wheat are harder to digest. If wheat is given, the bran should be removed because it is also difficult for babies to digest. Spelt is an easier-to-digest alternative to wheat.

For those who are committed to giving only whole foods, whole-grain millet is the easiest to digest. It is not as easy to digest as white rice, but it is the easiest to digest of the whole grains and substantially easier to digest than whole wheat. Some people criticize the use of millet because it is very low in protein, but in our practice, we have not

noted any protein deficiencies resulting from a child being weaned on millet.

▪ HOT AND COLD FOODS

In Chapter 1 we mentioned that children are either Hot or Cold in energy; the same can be true of herbs and food. One knows this instinctively: Most people prefer to eat a warming stew on a cold day and to eat a cooling salad on a hot day. The study of the energy and medical effects of foods is very interesting but beyond the scope of this book. Here we confine ourselves to the very basics. Table 3-2 lists the energy and function of a few of the most important foods.

▪ A SUMMARY OF OUR DIET SUGGESTIONS

- *Watch out for high-fiber foods.* In the field of alternative medicine, we meet many parents who have read about the benefits of whole food for adults, and they naturally extend this to their children. In our experience there are some children who can cope with this rough food, but the children who come to the clinic—those who are somewhat unwell—often have difficulty digesting fiber. There are many possible reasons for this, one of them being that the digestive tract is much shorter in children, meaning the food goes through much more quickly and there is not enough time for the fiber to be digested.
- *Eat organic food if possible.* Food that has been grown using modern methods contains pesticides and other poisons and is deficient in minerals and other substances essential for health. If organic food is unobtainable, fresh local produce is a good second best. (See following under Essential Fatty Acids.)
- *Encourage breast-feeding.* Numerous studies have proven the benefits of breast milk over all other forms of milk.
- *Watch out for cow's milk.* Many children have difficulty digesting cow's milk, even pure, unprocessed, organic cow's milk. Many are even allergic to it. What is worse is that much of the milk sold today is very low quality, with

Table 3-2   The Energy of Some Common Foods*

FOOD	ENERGY	COMMENT
Rice	Neutral	This is one of the best first foods to start weaning.
Oats	Slightly warm	Oats are very suitable in cold weather.
Bread	Neutral	Bread tends to create fluid imbalances and mucus in many children. It is difficult for many children to digest.
Bananas	Cold	The Cold energy of bananas is often the reason for colic, especially in children who are already cold. On the other hand, they can be the secret of successful stools in babies and children who are constipated because of being too Hot internally.
Yogurt	Cold	Yogurt can also cause colic in Cold children. On the whole, we advise against yogurt unless it is both live and comes from organically fed cows. If you can get this sort of yogurt, it has a special use in restoring the intestinal flora during and after a course of antibiotics.
Milk	Cool	Organic, or better still biodynamic, milk is suitable for those who can digest it without problems. Other milk should not be used. Even good-quality milk can cause excess mucus production in many children.
Cheese	Variable; most cheeses tend to be Cool, but the more pungent cheeses, and those which crawl off the plate, tend to be Warm	Cheese should be given only after about 2 years of age. If given late at night, it can cause nightmares, especially if given as grilled cheese sandwiches or Welsh rarebit. Once again, take great care over the quality of the cheese. Highly processed and sterilized cheese is better not eaten.
Haricot beans	Neutral	All beans and bean products tend to cause abdominal wind and flatulence and therefore colic in babies and toddlers. This effect can be minimized if the beans are cooked with cloves.
Fruit	Cool to Cold	All fruit is Cool to Cold, with the possible exception of peaches. Raw apples are particularly Cold and can cause indigestion. They are better when cooked with cloves.

antibiotics and pesticides in it. Signs of milk problems are overproduction of mucus, chronic cough, and asthma. We return to this later.

- *Watch out for peanuts and peanuts butter.* Peanuts and peanut butter tend to produce phlegm. In addition, we have seen many children who are allergic to them break out in a rash or even progress to anaphylactic shock.
- *Watch out for gluten in foods for the first year of life.* Gluten is hard for many babies and children to digest. A lot of children even have a mild allergy to it. Even for those who are not allergic, it may put too great a load on the digestive system.

Gluten is found in wheat and other cereals, particularly rye and, to a lesser extent, oats.
- *Bananas and yogurt can cause colic.* These foods are commonly given as first foods. Many children tolerate them well, but they may cause colic in others.
- *Do not worry about protein from meat.* This is advice that runs contrary to orthodox dietary theory, which emphasizes proteins. (The very word *protein* means "first.") In our experience children often find proteins in the form of meat and eggs rather hard to digest. It is easy for them to develop the stagnant food pattern. This is not to say that protein is not necessary! Of course

Table 3-2   The Energetic Properties of Some Common Foods*—cont'd

FOOD	ENERGY	COMMENT
Fruit juice	Cool to Cold	Their cool effect is deliciously refreshing on a hot day, but if taken to excess, fruit juice can be a major cause of diarrhea.
Carbonated drinks	Usually Cold	The majority of carbonated drinks contain sugar, colorings, and sweeteners and should therefore be kept to a minimum.
Hamburgers	Warm	Hamburgers made from organic ingredients are an acceptable food for many children. The ingredients for hamburgers sold in fast-food chains is rarely of this quality and should be avoided.
Ices and ice creams	Cold (obviously)	Keep ices and ice creams to a minimum and try to give those made with good-quality ingredients. Although ices and ice creams are Cold, there are some herbalists who give their herbs in ice sorbet or ice cream as a way of getting the herbs down the children with a minimum of fuss. The prescription is usually altered to include some extra ginger *Zingiber officinalis* to overcome the cooling effect of the ice.
Sugar	Neutral	Although it is neutral in small doses, in large doses it gives a "rush." The children first become hyperactive, then about half an hour later become distressed and weepy. A small amount of sugar has always been thought to be beneficial for children, although we have treated some children who cannot take more than a teaspoon a week without becoming overwhelmed by runny nose and cough.
Chocolate	Warm	Chocolate can cause hyperactivity, although for some rather pale-faced children, it can help them get a bit of a grip on the world. This may be due to the caffeine that it contains.

*We were first alerted to the effects of food in children by Chinese sources, but the information given in this table is based on our own experience in clinic. For those who wish to learn more about the effects of food, we recommend Pitchford.

protein is essential for growth, but nearly all that a baby or child needs can be obtained from a diet of mainly grains with a little milk.

- *Keep refined sugar and junk* food to a minimum.* This has to be said, although once again, most parents who seek alternative treatment have already taken this step. We advise keeping junk food to a minimum rather than cutting it out altogether because most families find this impossible. Having said this, some children (particularly those who are hyperactive or who are chronically exhausted) must eliminate *all* sugar and junk food from their diets.

- *Keep fruit juice to a minimum.* Organic fruit juice is vastly to be preferred to artificial carbonated drinks, but fruit juice should be kept to one or two glasses a day, unless there is a good reason to the contrary. If children are really thirsty, they will typically drink water. The problem with drinking too much fruit juice is that it contains a lot of sugar (fruit sugar, to be sure, but still sugar), and it is easy for this to become the main source of carbohydrate for the child. Fruit juice should especially be avoided if the child is prone to diarrhea or if the child has a poor appetite.

- *Limit consumption of oranges and orange juice.* Many children become hyperactive if they drink too much orange juice. For some, even one teaspoon is too much!

*There is no exact definition of *junk food.* Foods that qualify for this description include highly processed food, food containing artificial colorings and flavorings, food with poor-quality ingredients, foods containing cheap cooking oils, and mass-produced meat. This sort of combination is often found in pre-prepared frozen meals.

Essential Fatty Acids: Omega-3 and Omega-6 Fatty Acids

Essential fatty acids (EFAs), as the name implies, are essential for a healthy body. There are two main families—omega-3 and omega-6—and research is now beginning to show that if the EFAs of the omega-6 family are taken in high amounts, they can have disastrous inflammatory effect on the body.

For these EFAs to be of optimal benefit to health, they must be taken in the correct proportions: a ratio of approximately 1 part omega-3 to 4 parts omega-6 (a ratio of 0.25). What we find today is that we are consuming relatively more omega-6 in our diets. In many diets the ratio is as low as 0.09. One of the reasons for this is modern farming methods. The ratio of 1:4 is found in nature in the whole plants from which many oils are extracted and in organic, naturally farmed food. As an example, in organic eggs the ratio of omega-3 to omega-6 is found to be near 1:4. In factory farmed eggs, it is near 1:100. Similar statistics are found when comparing organic and intensively reared beef. Moreover, omega-6 is found in oils extracted from soy bean, sunflower, and safflower, the main oils used in the preparation of fast foods.

It is especially important for people who have allergies and skin problems to increase their dietary intake of omega-3 and reduce their intake of omega-6. This simple change can have startling effects in the treatment of these problems. Other conditions associated with deficient omega-3 are echo pattern, allergies, hayfever, premenstrual tension, and many of the autoimmune diseases.

Omega-3 is found in flaxseed, borage seed, evening primrose, canola, pumpkin, and walnut oils. Omega-6 is found in sunflower, safflower, corn, sesame, and wheat germ oils.

Difficulties Mothers Face When Trying to Change Their Child's Diet

If the cause of the child's problem is overeating, the obvious advice is to reduce the quantity of food given. This is not to say that it is not always easy to put this into practice. If the child is in the habit of eating a lot, it requires willpower and determination to reduce the quantity of food. This is especially true when the child is being breast-fed. If the baby is screaming and is normally comforted by being given the breast, it is very difficult to break the habit. The urgency of a screaming baby may override logical reactions.

If you are intending to make a change in your baby's feeding pattern, do not expect it to be trouble free. Make small changes at first, and choose a time when you know you can implement the changes. What we have heard from many mothers is that any complaints about a new diet or feeding pattern can last 5 to 7 days, but after that the going is easy. Prepare for 5 to 7 days of struggle.

■ MAIN POINTS FROM THIS CHAPTER

- Overfeeding and irregular feeding are common causes of digestive disturbance.
- Breast milk is the best milk for babies.
- Some children do not do well on demand feeding and need to be taught a rhythm.
- Wean onto very simple foods.
- Children younger than 3 years find bran and fiber hard to digest.
- Many children find cow's milk hard to digest.
- If there is a lot of mucus, suspect cow's milk, peanuts, or sugar intolerance.

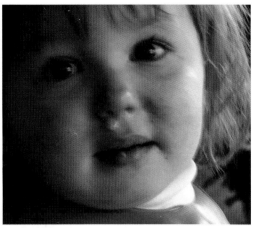

Color Plate 1-1 This child has a fever, with the complication of the stagnant food pattern, as can be seen from the red cheeks and the green, gluelike nasal discharge. The mucus discharge gave her a slight cough.

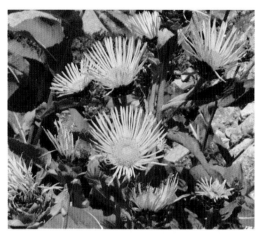

Color Plate 1-2 Elecampane *Inula helenium* helps clear thick, gluelike mucus and moves the digestive system. It is of benefit in treating coughs and the stagnant food pattern.

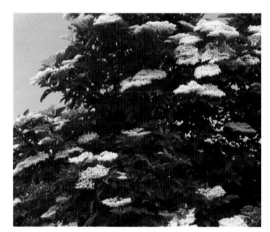

Color Plate 1-3 Elderflower *Sambucus nigra* is specific for fevers in children and also clears mucus from the upper respiratory tract. However, it does nothing for the stagnant food pattern and needs to be combined with elecampane (see Color Plate 1-2).

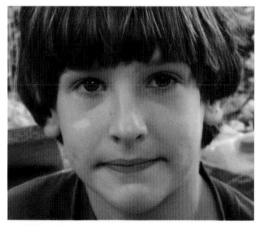

Color Plate 1-4 This boy has many of the signs of an echo pattern. In particular, he has swollen glands and the characteristic patch of slightly depigmented skin on his right cheek. The dark shadows under his eyes are a sign of exhaustion and possibly of food allergy.

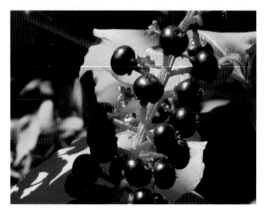

Color Plate 1-5 The berries of poke root *Phytolacca decandra*. The root has wonderful effects in softening the thick phlegm of an echo pattern and is therefore suitable for the boy shown in Color Plate 1-4.

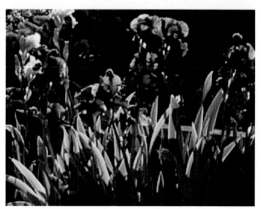

Color Plate 1-6 Blue flag *Iris versicolor* is often combined with poke root for treatment of an echo pattern.

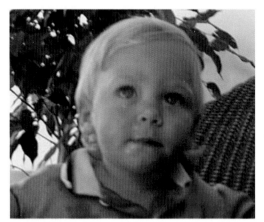

Color Plate 2-1 This boy is just lovely to be with when he is well.

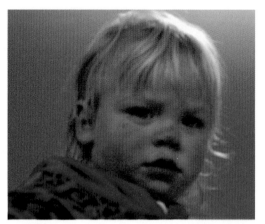

Color Plate 2-2 This is the same boy as shown in Color Plate 2-1. He now has the stagnant food pattern from overeating, and it has turned a lovely boy into a rather difficult one. Notice the characteristic red cheeks. His problem was food allergies, but the mother overcame these merely by controlling the amount of food he ate, so the stagnant food pattern never returned.

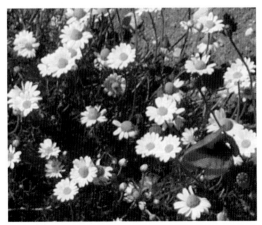

Color Plate 2-3 German chamomile *Chamomilla matricaria*. This herb does not taste so great, but it is very good for mild cases of the stagnant food pattern, such as the boy shown in Color Plate 2-2.

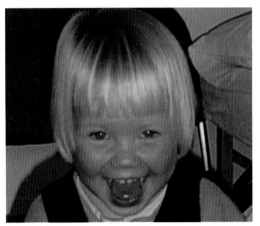

Color Plate 2-4 This child has the signs of Heat in the system: red cheeks and red tongue. Her behavior was somewhat impetuous also. She had the Heat pattern of chronic cough and was well on the way to becoming asthmatic.

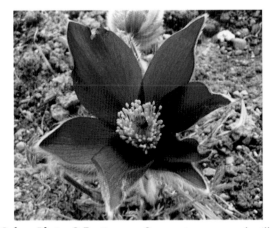

Color Plate 2-5 Pasque flower *Anemone pulsatilla*. This herb helps bring heat to the surface and would therefore be useful to bring heat out of the lungs of the child shown in Color Plate 2-4.

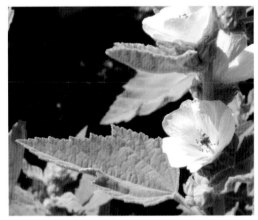

Color Plate 2-6 Marshmallow *Althea officinalis* is specific for Heat conditions in the lungs, such as bronchitis, both acute and chronic.

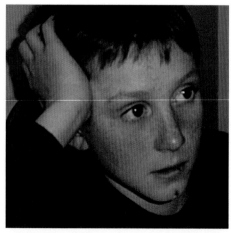

Color Plate 3-1 This boy has a large forehead and a small jaw, indicating that his energy is in his brain. When he was young he slept only 4 hours a night. He was very pale at this time. At about the age of 9, he went through a rather bad fever, with chills, and after that he slept much better and developed a warmer personality.

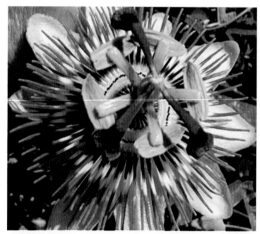

Color Plate 3-2 Passion flower *Passiflora incarnata* is a nerve tonic and is very useful for treating insomnia in children who are very imaginative and who easily become overstimulated (such as the boy shown in Color Plate 3-1).

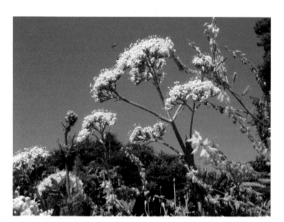

Color Plate 3-3 Valerian *Valeriana officinalis* helps relax children who are very tense. It is one of the herbs used for insomnia.

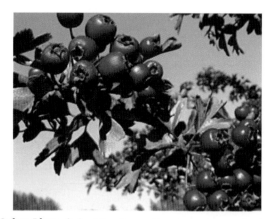

Color Plate 3-4 Hawthorn *Crataegus oxyacantha* improves circulation and is a mild relaxant. It is used for children who have insomnia of the Weak type.

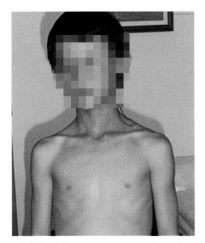

Color Plate 3-5 This boy has the weak digestion pattern. His appetite has always been poor, and now he is small for his age.

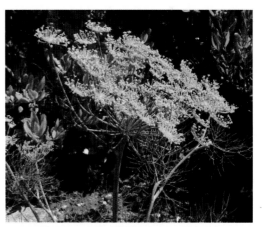

Color Plate 3-6 Fennel *Foeniculum vulgaris* is specific for weak digestion and, combined with other herbs, would be suitable for the boy shown in Color Plate 3-5. Because he is 10, progress will be much slower than if he had started taking herbs at a younger age.

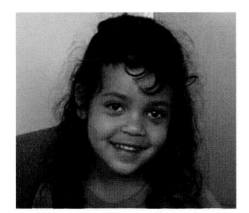

Color Plate 4-1 When the skin is more darkly pigmented, one needs to look closer to see the underlying colors—white in this case, showing a tendency to lung complaints and asthma.

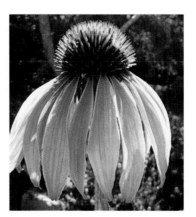

Color Plate 4-2 Echinacea *Echinacea angustifolia* "rallies" the immune system. If taken in the first day or two of a cold or fever, it may stop the illness dead in its tracks. Normally, it should not be taken for a long period, for it does not have a long-term effect of boosting the immune system.

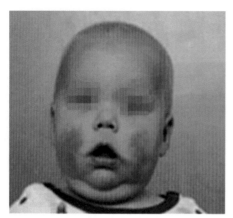

Color Plate 4-3 This boy has a severe skin rash. It was improved by herbs and homeopathy, but not cured. The cure came some 3 months after this picture was taken, when he contracted whooping cough. His mother nursed him well, and he came out of it much healthier and with no skin rash.

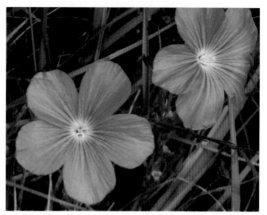

Color Plate 4-4 Flax *Linum usitatissimum*. Flax seed oil, made from this plant, is an excellent source of omega-3 fatty acids and is of great benefit in treating many skin conditions and conditions of allergy.

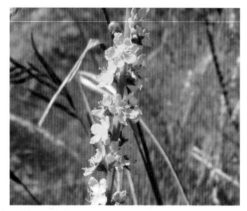

Color Plate 4-5 Agrimony *Agrimonia eupatoria* is one of the best herbs for the treatment of diarrhea, both acute and chronic, because it is drying and also tones the digestive system.

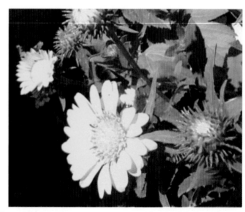

Color Plate 4-6 Gum weed *Grindelia camporum* (together with thyme *Thymus vulgaris*) is one of the herbs used for whooping cough. With this at hand, there is little to fear from the disease, even in babies as young as the one shown in Color Plate 4-3. The only children at risk are the very weak.

4

Fevers and Infectious Diseases

In this chapter we discuss the role of fevers and infectious diseases. We show that they are an indispensable part of childhood and that, in certain circumstances, they can make a child stronger. At the very least they present the possibility of strengthening the immune system.

■ A DIFFERENT VIEW ON DISEASE

Infectious diseases such as fevers, coughs, and colds are common in early childhood and generally diminish with age. The commonly given explanation is that the immune system gradually "learns" to recognize different viruses and bacteria and develops protection against them. Although this is true, it is clearly only part of the picture. It does not explain why some children acquire diseases such as whooping cough and suffer very badly while others have only a mild form of the disease. In this section we look at this question and offer some answers. The view that we present is that there are really two types of infectious disease. One type is caused by attack by an infecting agent, such as a virulent strain that attacks even the healthiest body. The other type is the result of the body being already out of balance before the infecting agent came along. The resulting illnesses appear similar but need to be treated differently.

In orthodox medicine there is an unwritten assumption that most diseases are caused by viruses or bacteria. Bacteria and viruses are associated with many infectious diseases, from pneumonia and tuberculosis to whooping cough and the common cold. Recently, bacteria have even been associated with the development of stomach ulcers. The involvement of bacteria in disease was shown by Pasteur, and it soon became held as a general truth that it was the bacteria that actually caused the disease. It was assumed that if only we could avoid contact with these bacteria or viruses, we would not get ill. This view has now taken hold so completely that every supermarket is lined with rows of antibacterial soaps, washing powders, and so on. This theory is also the basis behind immunization. The unspoken assumption is that if we can boost our immune system to fight a virus or bacteria, we will never get ill.

We believe that this approach is too simplistic. There are many other forces at work that determine whether the infecting agent can take hold or not. This is not a new idea. Even in Pasteur's time, opposing opinions were voiced. Pasteur's great rival, Beauchamp, always maintained "c'est le terrain" (that it was the "ground" that was all important); in fact, in a celebrated public demonstration, he drank a glass of water known to contain cholera germs but did not contract cholera.

Since then there have been many other demonstrations that disease requires more than just an infecting agent. For example, *Streptococcus* bacteria can be found in the throats of many healthy people, and *Pneumonococcus* bacteria is found in the lungs of many healthy people. The bacteria are living there quite happily for month after month, but not causing disease.

More recently, research has been conducted by doctors in the Anthroposophical movement that more or less confirms Beauchamp's position, rather than Pasteur's. Their results imply that diseased tissue can cause otherwise beneficial bacteria to mutate into harmful ones.*

The conclusion one is forced to is that infectious diseases require both an infecting agent *and* a suitable ground for the infection to flourish. If the body is healthy, the ground is not suitable and there is no infection. Similarly, if there is no infecting agent, then there is no disease. This explains why some people contract certain infectious diseases when exposed to an infecting agent while others do not.

Likewise, this goes some way to explaining the progress of an epidemic through a school. It is obvious that the children most likely to become ill during an epidemic are those with a significant imbalance, such as those who are very weak or very tired. Children of a robust constitution often suffer little or not at all.

When it comes to clinical practice, the underlying, unstated assumptions have an enormous impact on the way disease is treated. If the infecting agent is considered the primary cause of disease, as in orthodox medicine, then the treatment of disease is focused on killing the infecting agent, for example, with the use of antibiotics. In our approach the state of the body is considered more important, so treatment is focused on strengthening and rebalancing the body. Only in desperate situations are antibiotics and antivirals needed. This approach also shows the way to prevent disease by strengthening and balancing the body in a way unimagined by orthodox medicine.

The Disease Process

So far we have described the circumstances for a disease to take hold. There must be an imbalance present, and there also must be some virus or bacterium to take advantage of that imbalance. How the disease progresses from here depends on a number of factors, and there are a number of possible outcomes. What we find is that there are circumstances when disease can lead to a worse state of health and

---

*Quoted in Husemann F, Wolff O (ed): *Anthroposophical approach to medicine*, vol 3, Spring Valley, NY, 1989, Anthroposophic Press, p 10.

some circumstances when it leads to a better state. Which way it goes depends very much on the strength of the child before the disease process begins, whether the full immune response is evoked, and whether the child is allowed to recuperate. Let us look at the following situations.

- Strong child, full immune response, allowed to recuperate
- Strong child, full immune response, no time to recuperate
- Weaker child, partial immune response
- Weaker child, stronger disease factor

1. STRONG CHILD, FULL IMMUNE RESPONSE, ALLOWED TO RECUPERATE

If the child is strong and is basically healthy, there is likely to be a full immune response. This may mean that the child is quite ill, for a full immune response often involves a very high fever. However, while the child has this fever, the underlying imbalance that allowed the infection to take hold is being corrected; to put it in naturopathic terms, the body is being cleansed.

The child will be tired after the fever, so at this stage it is important that the child be allowed to rest and recuperate. This was well understood in the past, when it was common to send a child away to the country to recover after a severe illness. The rule that we now give our patients is to keep their child home from school for at least as many days as the child had the fever. If the fever lasted 3 days, then the child should be kept out of school for at least 3 days after the fever has resolved.

The eventual outcome is that the child is much stronger. The basic imbalance has been corrected, and the child has had an opportunity to recover his or her energy and health.

Example. During the spring, a girl gets influenza and has a high fever. The fever lasts 3 days, peaking at 104° F (40° C). She is treated with herbs such as yarrow *Achillea millefolium* and sweats profusely. After the illness subsides, she is exhausted but is allowed to stay at home. The yarrow is continued until she is again feeling marvelous.

2. STRONG CHILD, FULL IMMUNE RESPONSE, NO TIME TO RECUPERATE

In a strong child who has a full immune response but is not allowed time to recuperate, the first part of the disease process (i.e., the disease proper) is the same as that of the previous child. The key difference is that the child does not have the opportunity to recover. This is very common today, as evidenced by children being sent back to school as soon as they can get out of bed!

The eventual outcome of this is not as favorable. The balance of the body is better in some ways, but the child is left weak, and when back at school, the energy recovers slowly. This means that the child will be prone to illness, for if the next epidemic appears before strength has returned, he or she may easily succumb.

Example. A boy gets a cough in autumn during a time when the coughs are going around the school. Although relatively strong, he is not given time to recover but rather sent back to play on the school football team. To be on the safe side, the doctor prescribes antibiotics. After this, the child is not quite right for a long time and has a cough that comes and goes.

3. WEAKER CHILD, PARTIAL IMMUNE RESPONSE

In a weaker child who experiences only a partial immune response, the child starts off somewhat weaker and therefore the immune response is not as strong. When a fever develops, it is not as violent and the child does not have a great deal of energy to put into fighting the illness. The immune response is only partial.

Another possible way in which the immune response is "partial" is when the normal progress of the disease is halted by antibiotics. In such cases the entire process never goes to completion, and the body never has an opportunity to recover its balance. Put in naturopathic terms, the body never has an opportunity to cleanse properly, for the process is halted halfway through.

The outcome is that the child who has had a partial disease process only gets partially better. There is an imbalance left behind. The "ground" has not been cleansed properly, and the way is open for another disease soon after. In contrast, if the disease is allowed to run its full course, the child supported and nursed throughout and allowed time to recuperate, a weak child can become stronger than before.

Example. A 6-month-old baby developed a cough during a period of unseasonably wet weather. The cough was watery and slightly productive, and the child had a slight fever. Even so, the baby was coping well. The mother became concerned and went to the local doctor, who then prescribed antibiotics. This cleared the problem up quickly, but it was only a month later that the child again developed a very similar cough because the original balance was never cleared.

4. WEAKER CHILD, STRONGER DISEASE FACTOR

A weak child with a strong disease factor represents the worst situation. Either the child does not have access to medicine, or the medicines are ineffective or inappropriate, allowing the disease to take a strong grip. The disease wracks the body and leaves it injured.

The outcome of this is that the child's health is injured. One or more organs are seriously affected, and it may take many years to recover fully.

Example. A 2-year-old boy has had a bad appetite all of his life. By this age he is very thin and has no reserves of energy. The child then has the misfortune to get whooping cough and has no access to alternative medicine. To be on the safe side, the doctor prescribes prophylactic antibiotics. Unfortunately, the antibiotics do nothing for the whooping cough, which goes on and on, week after week. The child loses more and more weight, for he vomits what little food he does eat. The continuous coughing gradually weakens the lungs and leaves the child with a poor constitution and weak lungs for the rest of his life. The disease processes are summarized in Table 4-1.

The Role of the Herbalist

Herbalists have a great many remedies at their disposal. There are herbs for restoring imbalances,

Table 4-1 Table of Possible Outcomes of the Disease Process

TYPE OF CHILD	IMMUNE RESPONSE	RECUPERATION	OUTCOME
Strong	Strong 104° F (40° C)	Plenty of time	Body is more healthy than before
Strong	Strong 104°F (40° C)	No time to recover	Balance of body is better, but child is left weak and therefore prone to more disease
Weak	Incomplete 100° F (38.5° C) or interrupted by antibiotics	No time to recover	Child is only partially well and has a partial illness for a long time after
Weak	Weak; disease rages	Enough time	Even though there is enough time to recuperate, the child's health has been seriously affected

and there are also herbal antibiotics and antivirals (see following discussion). The antibiotics and antivirals are the remedies to use if it looks as though the disease is getting out of hand. These are appropriate to use in children prone to asthma who are developing an all-too-familiar infection. For most children, herbs for restoring imbalances are appropriate. When the child is pale and shivering with cold, herbs that provide warmth with help relieve the symptoms far more quickly than any antibiotic or antiviral and will leave the child much healthier. When a child has a raging fever, herbs that promote cooling through sweating will provide the quickest cure.

This does not make the herbalist's life easy. The herbalist must make fine judgments regarding a child's state of health and whether a child can overcome an illness without antivirals or antibiotics. The herbalist has to lead the child to a state of health. On the other hand, the herbalist's reward is to witness children get much stronger and ultimately become healthy adults.

SUMMARY

We believe that the majority of minor infections are actually beneficial to a child and that to try and stop them is an error, unless there is a real danger of the infecting agent getting the upper hand. Moreover, we believe that it is beneficial for the disease to continue until the imbalance that allowed it to take hold has been corrected. That is, it should

continue until the "ground" is no longer suitable for disease to flourish.

For example, if a person catches a "cold" and has symptoms of a runny nose, watery cough, and puffy skin, this means that the excess dampness is being eliminated from the body. The imbalance that has allowed the water to accumulate is being corrected. Likewise, when a person has an infection characterized by feelings of cold and shivering, then during the fever the Hot-Cold balance is being corrected. When this is finally corrected, the fever will resolve—but not before.

Epidemics

What we have described so far relates to the normal coughs, colds, and fevers that are part of everyday life. This type of illness is often a beneficial illness and comes about when a body that is out of balance meets the appropriate infecting agent. The relatively mild irritant of the infecting agent provides the means whereby the child can get back to health. However, some truly virulent infecting agents exist and can cause dreadful diseases, such as the *Ebola* virus, against which the body has no protection. When the common cold was first introduced to the Eskimo population, there were widespread deaths because the population was being exposed to a completely new virus. In situations such as this, the orthodox model of being "attacked" by a disease really is appropriate. If the invading factor really is strong, do not hesitate to use antivirals or antibiotics.

▪ FACTORS IN LIFE THAT CAUSE DISEASE

We now discuss factors that influence the "ground," the imbalances that enable an infection to take hold.

Influence of the Weather

Traditionally, the influence of weather has always been considered one of the foremost causes of disease. The very word *influence* has given its name (via Italian) to the disease influenza. It is still true that sudden changes in weather and extremes of weather can give rise to the imbalances that cause disease. To obtain some understanding of this, we consider what happens when the weather turns suddenly cold and damp.

Normally, the adult human body loses between 500 ml and 1 L of water through the skin each day through mild perspiration. If the weather turns suddenly cold and damp, there will be less evaporation from the skin and less water will be lost. At first the same amount of water reaches the skin, so one of two things will happen: either the skin becomes damp, or the dampness accumulates under the skin, making it somewhat puffy. If the damp weather persists, the body should soon adapt, with the excess water being excreted through the kidneys. If this adaptation is too slow, the whole of the skin may stay too damp. This dampness may even affect the skin's related organ, the lungs, resulting in the lungs also becoming too moist. When this occurs, the way is open for viruses or bacteria that thrive in damp conditions. Typically, the accumulated dampness will give rise to symptoms of watery cough and a runny nose.

We have chosen the example of dampness because this is the problem that affects so many people in the British Isles, but a similar process takes place with other weather changes, giving rise to diseases that are characterized by dryness, heat, or cold.

▪ Case History

This story relates to an epidemic at a boy's boarding school. In this true story the influence of the weather was assisted by humans! The event occurred at the end of February, which is a dismal month in England. The weather had been exceptionally cold, and to make matters worse, the heating failed for a week. Fortunately, the boys were sturdy, and the classrooms were normally kept cold, with the express idea of toughening the boys. At the end of a week without central heating, the weather turned suddenly very mild. At the same time the heating was repaired. However, not content with just repairing it, the heating engineer insisted that the heating stay on at full strength for several days. So for these days, after the weather had been exceptionally cold, the boys were all sweltering. On the fourth day, most of the schoolchildren came down with tonsillitis with high fever. More than three fourths of the boys were ill at one time, as the heat imbalance corrected itself!

Boosting the Immune System

How does this discussion fit in with the idea of boosting the immune system? Surely, if a child repeatedly has minor infections, something must be wrong with the immune system, so it makes sense to boost it.

This may be appropriate for some children, but for others it makes little sense simply to boost the immune system if the child does not have the energy to maintain health. What makes more sense is to strengthen the child and correct any imbalance while simultaneously strengthening the immune system. What we usually find is that by simply strengthening the child or righting the imbalance, the immune system becomes stronger without the need for "immune boosters" such as echinacea *Echinacea angustifolia*.

How This Affects Treatment

This has great importance in the clinic, for it throws an entirely new light on the way to prevent and treat coughs, colds, and minor infections.

- The aim of prevention is not merely to strengthen the immune system but to keep the body in a state of balance so that illness cannot occur, or so that when it does, the illness is only mild because there is only a small imbalance to correct.
- The aim of treatment is not to kill the infecting agent but to minimize the unpleasant symptoms and to speed the process of righting the imbalance. A secondary aim is to prevent the imbalance from becoming more severe.

■ CHILDHOOD DISEASES

Following on from our discussion of infectious diseases, we turn to the childhood diseases. Once again, we present an alternative point of view: If properly handled, the childhood diseases of mumps, measles, and whooping cough can all be beneficial to the body. Far from being diseases that come purely from outside and that should be eradicated, these diseases represent necessary stages in the development of a child.

During these disease processes the body is being cleansed of any imbalances present at birth. Thus the childhood diseases are not primarily caused by outside infecting agents but rather are a process of restoring balance to the body, where the outside infecting agent simply provides the opportunity for cleansing.*

In this context it is interesting to note that each of these three illnesses is connected to a different system. Measles is connected to the brain and ner-

---

*It is interesting to note that new viruses are evolving to take the place of old ones. Most children in the United Kingdom have been immunized against whooping cough, so there are few who get it. However, many get a cough that is very similar to whooping cough but that is caused by an adenovirus. Although the child does not have exactly the same symptoms, the effect of the illness is very similar.

vous system, mumps to the glandular system, and whooping cough to the lungs and digestive system. Each illness clears out imbalances in a different system. The beneficial results are further discussed under each individual disease in Part 3.

Potential Dangers

This discussion of the childhood illnesses does not mean that we do not take them seriously. We take them very seriously. Like any infectious disease, the childhood diseases can go the "wrong way," and children can end up in a much worse state after the illness rather than in a better state. In circumstances of deprivation and poverty, such as are common in the developing world, many children die from the childhood illnesses.

What this means in practice is that there may be times when you want to prevent a child from getting a particular disease. If the child is very weak and there is a real danger of meningitis as a complication of getting measles, obviously you should do everything possible to prevent the child from having contact with measles. If the child is not really at risk (as the huge majority are not), then a properly nursed case of measles gives nothing but benefit to the long-term health of the child.

■ THINGS PEOPLE TAKE TO FIGHT DISEASE

Echinacea

Echinacea has recently been promoted as the wonder way to health. One sees advertisements with beautiful bodies side by side with this beautiful flower, and one is led to believe that the combination of bee pollen and echinacea will boost the immune system and increase health and longevity. We believe that these implied claims are misleading. The proper time to use echinacea is in the early stages of an infection, just before the infection has really taken hold. It has the effect of "rallying" the immune system, thereby temporarily activating it. If echinacea is taken continually, this effect wears off. Echinacea also has the special use, which was of great value in the past, of treating conditions in which much pus and discharge are produced, such as boils and purulent tonsillitis.

Research has been conducted on the subject, but the results are variable. Research sponsored by the echinacea suppliers produces the result that echinacea is indeed a panacea. More objective research seems to show that far from reducing susceptibility to colds, long-term use of echinacea might actually increase it.

Vitamins and Minerals

Some people take vitamin and mineral supplements regularly, and these people are likely to give their own children similar preparations. We used to believe that one does not need any medicine on a long-term basis, even vitamins and minerals, unless one has a chronic disease. We have had to change our position after observing some patients. In some cases a food supplement of this kind can make a big difference to the health of a child. There are two situations when supplements are called for: (1) when the child has a poor appetite and (2) when the available food is of poor quality.

Some children never really develop a good appetite, despite being treated by many alternative therapists. If these children are truly healthy and have plenty of energy, they do not need to take minerals and vitamins. More often than not, they easily get tired and are relatively prone to minor infections. This can be because they are simply not taking in enough minerals and vitamins to remain healthy and grow. In this case a supplement can be beneficial.

Similarly, poor-quality or "factory-farmed" food is depleted of minerals and vitamins. If this is all the family has access to, once again, the child has a general lack, even though the quantity of food consumed is adequate. This pattern is becoming more and more common because food is produced by the use of increasing amounts of fertilizer on increasingly depleted soil. An example of this is broccoli, which now contains less

than one fourth of the amount of calcium it used to. The exception to this is organic food, although even here one has to chose truly organic food. Much food sold as organic is organic in name only. It is grown by hydroponic methods with organic nutrients but without ever growing in soil. This food may be free of pesticides, but it often does not contain the full range of minerals and vitamins. In these circumstances a supplement may be beneficial.

Which Supplement?

Even choosing a supplement is not without its problems, for although the supplement labels imply that they are produced in a natural way, this is often far from the truth. The vitamins may be produced industrially and the minerals made from animal waste products. Once again, one should take care in selecting a supplement to be given daily. At the very least, supplements should come from organic vegetables. A promising new development is a supplement made from concentrated extracts of organic vegetables and fruits made into sweets or candies.

▪ USE OF ANTIBIOTICS

Antibiotics have many uses. They have saved millions of lives. In addition, they have reduced the incidence of a whole class of illnesses—those caused by exhaustion from long fevers. However, let us not blind ourselves to their shortcomings. They have very pronounced side effects. The antibiotics commonly used today have the near disastrous effect of killing all of the beneficial flora in the body, as well as the disease-causing ones. In certain circumstances it may be worth tolerating this. Certainly, if a man is dying and the antibiotics will save his life, minor side effects are insignificant. On the other hand, if a child has an illness that she can easily get over by herself, then why give antibiotics? The illness may resolve a few days earlier with antibiotic use, but the body is put out of balance for weeks or months. Other problems may arise, such as the illness coming back again in the same form a few weeks later or leaky gut syndrome (mentioned in Chapter 2); in addition, the likelihood of resistant strains of bacteria developing is increased.

Plant Antibiotics

The antibiotics used by orthodox medicine are broad spectrum. They kill a wide range of bacteria (although as time passes, resistant strains develop). Commonly, these antibiotics are made from very lowly plant forms, such as molds. It is not generally realized that there are other antibiotics that are developed from higher plant forms. Examples of these include the antibiotics found in horseradish *Cochlearia armoracia*, elecampane *Inula helenium*, and ribwort *Plantago lanceolata*. These antibiotics have a much more specific action. They are not like machine guns that destroy everything in their path. They are more akin to the magic bullet that was sought in the 1950s. For example, the *Cochlearia armoracia* antibiotic has a specific effect on bacterial cystitis. Extract of *Inula helenium* has a specific effect on the tuberculosis bacillus and *Plantago lanceolata* on *Pneumonococcus*. Because their action is so specific, they do not upset the balance of the body.

Plant Antivirals

As is clear by now, our approach to viral illness is to give children herbs that restore the balance of the body; Weak children are given tonics. In this way it encourages the child's immune system to do the work. However, there are times when the child simply does not have the strength to overcome a disease or when a disease has run down such a well-worn path that it is likely to go down the same path again unless something is done to combat the specific virus. It is here that plant antivirals have their great use. By this we mean plant substances that have been shown to have an antiviral effect in laboratory settings. Foremost among these is ti-tree oil *Melaleuca alternifolia*.

When to Use Allopathic Antibiotics

It is sometimes appropriate to use broad-spectrum antibiotics such as penicillin, which are derived from lower plant forms. The obvious situation is when a child has a life-threatening bacterial disease and is not responding to other medicines. Another situation is when time is of the essence. If a child is weak and has a dangerous disease (e.g., nephritis), it may be judged that there is no time to waste. It may be believed that the risks in trying a gentle treatment first are too great. In most other situations, broad-spectrum antibiotics are found to be inferior to plant remedies, even for conditions such as chronic urinary reflux for which prophylactic doses of antibiotics are commonly given. With such conditions, plant antibiotics such as that produced from horseradish are just as effective against the bacteria, without the damaging effects to the beneficial flora in the body.

Overcoming the Bad Effects of Broad-Spectrum Antibiotics

The worst of the side effects of broad-spectrum antibiotics can be mitigated to a certain extent by eating live yogurt. Live yogurt contains a variety of bacteria, and once the child has stopped taking antibiotics, these will thrive in the intestines. By taking 1 teaspoon of live yogurt three times a day during a course of antibiotics and for 3 days after, complications such as diarrhea and fungal infections can often be avoided. Another way, recently developed, is to take a powder consisting of dried concentrated intestinal flora.

■ GENERAL GUIDELINES ON WHEN TO SEEK HELP

Being a parent can be very hard at times, and when a child is ill is perhaps the most trying and exhausting of all. We have discussed some of the more subtle reasons for this in great detail in Chapter 2, but it does not take much imagination to see that when a child is ill, the parents are worried and often exhausted because of their sleepless nights. It is often at these times that you will be called on as a practitioner to help the child. What we frequently see in the clinic is that the parent really does want to help the child with the use of natural medicines, but at some point in the course of treatment, something happens. For example, the child may start screaming uncontrollably in the middle of the night with an earache. The parent has invested much time and money in coming to see you and feels bad about giving antibiotics, but she is tired, the child is miserable, and she starts to imagine her child going deaf. She wants to phone but knows you are not there. What should she do?

As practitioners and parents we will all have our own approach as to how to deal with this situation, but we would like to share with you what we do. When we take on a child patient, we also take on the parents. A big part of our practice is to educate parents about how to take care of these emergency situations. We explain emergency cures and helpful things to do for earaches, asthma flare-ups, coughs, and so on. This is very important in the treatment of children. Most herbal practitioners are not available 24 hours a day, and educating and empowering our patients to heal themselves and their children is one of the most valuable parts of treatment.

These powerful home remedies usually are enough, but we also advise parents that they should seek help from a doctor, hospital, or us if we are available in the following circumstances:

- The child simply is not responding, and the condition is getting worse. (See individual illnesses for specifics on danger signs.)
- The fever begins to rise very rapidly, making it difficult for the child to breathe, and the parent cannot help quickly and efficiently.

- The child suddenly becomes lethargic and floppy.
- The parent starts to panic uncontrollably. Any illness is difficult, but there are times when things seem to be getting completely out of hand. If it is your own child who appears to be seriously ill, it is likely for panic to set in. When this happens, the child make pick up on your panic. The very presence of panic makes the illness much harder to cure (a point that is discussed in Chapter 16).
- The parent simply does not know what is going on. This is a new illness, and the parent is completely lost as to what to do and is subject to fears. When this happens, he or she should seek help. Even a friend or relation may be able to see things more clearly and so lead to the correct course of action.

■ MAIN POINTS FROM THIS CHAPTER

- Bacteria and viruses are not the sole causes of disease. They are only part of a complex process.
- Equally important in disease is the ground or state of body, which enables the illness to take hold.
- Many infectious illnesses in children are a sign of the body's balance being restored and can be beneficial in the long run.
- The childhood illnesses of mumps, measles, and whooping cough are beneficial, if managed properly.
- Use herbs to lead a child through a disease.
- Keep antibiotics for really life-threatening disease.

5

Echo Patterns

In this chapter we present a way of looking at long-term problems of health. We introduce the idea of an echo pattern and show how it originates. We also show how immunizations can easily lead to echo patterns. Understanding echo patterns opens the way for completely curing many long-standing problems and also for clearing out any unwanted effects of immunizations.

■ WHAT IS AN ECHO PATTERN?

An echo pattern is a pattern that comes again and again, just like an echo. It may start with a major disease such as whooping cough, which exhausts the child. Then for months or even years, the child has a cough from time to time. Typically, the cough comes and goes, being worse in the winter and during times of stress and tiredness; then it seems to disappear altogether. When the next period of stress occurs or when the child tires again, the symptoms return. As the child gets older and stronger, the symptoms may get fainter and fainter, like an echo dying out.

In some ways it is not a real disease but more of a predisposition, for there may be long periods when the child does not have any apparent symptoms. Even when the symptoms do return, they may be mild and not enough to be called a real disease. It may seem as though the child is perfectly healthy between attacks. However, to the trained eye, it is obvious that the imbalance is always present. It is for this reason that we call it a pattern rather than a disease, although at times it can return with the full force of the original disease.

Echo patterns can affect any part of the body. Chronic coughs that come and go are the most common. Also common are ear infections, tonsillitis, and sinusitis. Less common are chronic diarrhea and urinary tract infections.

Echo patterns may manifest in the following ways:
- Chronic cough
- Asthma
- Eczema
- Tonsillitis
- Otitis media
- Glandular fever

■ HOW DO ECHO PATTERNS ARISE?

Echo patterns occur when an illness is not completely expelled. They occur after a child has had a serious illness and has not had enough time to recuperate. They also are seen after immunizations and courses of antibiotics. The reason for this is not entirely clear, but it may be because the child never has quite a strong enough fever to expel the pathogen that is introduced.

Why Echo Patterns Are Important

Echo patterns are important in a number of different ways.

- They are key to understanding chronic illnesses. In the clinic we often see children who have a cough every winter. Their parents have discovered that herbs help alleviate the symptom but do not cure the child. Understanding the nature of echo patterns opens the way to eradicating the illness.

- Echo patterns can become more serious. The illness becomes stronger rather than weaker each time the pattern appears. For example, what starts out as a cough may become worse each time it appears, until eventually the child has asthma.
- Echo patterns are often seen during the late stages of treating an illness. When a child has an acute or chronic cough, it is usually relatively easy to cure the worst of the symptoms, but the last stage of getting rid of the cough completely usually involves expelling the echo pattern.
- Even when the echo becomes fainter and fainter, to the point that the symptoms have disappeared, the pattern may nevertheless remain. It may remain unnoticed year after year and resurface only at another time of life when the adult becomes severely stressed. A common pattern is for the disease to return as glandular fever (mononucleosis) or chronic fatigue when the child reaches the late teenage years. In some cases the symptoms may reappear with the onset of old age—the adult may start to experience symptoms that he or she had not had since childhood.
- The character changes that accompany this pattern can also stay with a person for life and cause difficulties and problems that could otherwise be avoided.

We now provide a description of the pattern, with an explanation of the symptoms and signs.

Distinguishing Features

There are some characteristic signs that indicate an echo pattern in a child. These include the following:

- Slightly glazed look in the eyes
- Slightly depigmented patches on the cheek

On questioning, you will often find the following:

- Chronic illness
- A cough with thick mucus
- Enlarged tonsils
- Occasional drops of energy for no apparent reason
- Intermittent abdominal aches
- Allergies

On examination, you will find the following:

- Glandular congestion—enlarged lymph nodes
- Rough skin or slightly powdery skin (seen occasionally)
- Subtle behavior changes

Box 5-1 discusses each of these symptoms in detail.

■ CURING THE PATTERN

The details of treatment for long-standing patterns are given in the Part 3 of this book under the separate headings for each symptom. Obviously, the treatment of chronic otitis is different from the treatment of chronic cough. No matter where the site of the main symptom is, though, certain aspects of treatment for an echo pattern are the same:

- Treat any weakness with tonics.
- Clear out phlegm.
- Soften thick phlegm.

Treat Any Weakness with Tonics

When a child first comes for treatment, one should simply treat the obvious symptoms. In particular, if the child is weak, tonics must be given first. This cannot be overstressed. If the child does not have enough strength, there is no chance of clearing out an old illness. It takes energy to change and to extirpate an old illness. Likewise, if any pronounced symptoms are present, such as cough or vomiting, these must be treated. Getting over this first stage can take many months.

Box 5-1

Explanation of Symptoms

Glandular Congestion—
Swelling of the Lymph Nodes

When the body is exposed to infection, it is normal for the lymph nodes to become enlarged. It is thought that there is first an increase in the production of lymphocytes. Newly formed lymphocytes migrate to the lymph nodes, which therefore become enlarged. Once the active infection is over, one would expect the swelling to go down, but it is a curious feature of the echo pattern that the lymph nodes (or lymph glands in common parlance) remain enlarged. It thus seems as though the infection has never quite left the system.

Once you start to look for swollen lymph nodes, you often find that many are swollen throughout the body and that the lymph system in general is congested. When performing a thorough examination, one first notices that the submaxillary nodes are enlarged. Posteriorly, one often finds that the cervical nodes are also enlarged. Continuing, one discovers that it is not only the lymph nodes in the neck that are swollen but rather all the nodes that are palpable, including the inguinal nodes. It is probable that even the abdominal nodes are enlarged, for children with this pattern often complain of a diffused abdominal ache that comes and goes.

Thick Mucus

Associated with this pattern there is always some very thick, viscid mucus. This mucus production often gives rise to the symptom of a harsh cough that comes and goes. In general, the cough is nonproductive, except after a long period of coughing, when a very small amount of thick mucus is expectorated (i.e., when mucus "comes up"). In many children the mucus is so thick that it cannot be expectorated at all, and it may be so congealed that there do not seem to be any signs of it. The parents will say that their child has no mucus problems.

This has very great significance clinically, for it provides valuable in formation about the prognosis and treatment. The treatment of this condition requires herbs that were traditionally used for lymphatic congestion. Among these one finds poke root *Phytolacca decandra* and queen's delight *Stillingia sylvatica* in the American pharmacopeia and blue flag *Iris versicolor,* cleavers *Galium aparine,* and figwort *Scrophularia nodosa* in Europe.

As far as prognosis is concerned, the quality of the swelling indicates how difficult the problem is to cure. In general, smaller nodes indicate a better prognosis than larger one. On the other hand, if the nodes are very hard and small, somewhat like 5-mm ball bearings, they are much harder to cure, for the first step is to "soften" the mucus that is causing these hard swellings.

Allergies

An echo pattern is often to be found in children with allergies. The child may have an obvious allergy to food or an allergy to something airborne, characteristic of hayfever. In these allergic cases it has been shown that the immune system is already working overtime, and it is the allergen that tips the balance and leads the body to a crisis. This is discussed more fully in Chapter 15.

Continued

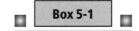

Explanation of Symptoms—cont'd

Behavior Changes

One of the symptoms commonly associated with echo pattern is a "glazed look in the eyes." This goes hand in hand with a change in the child's behavior. If you saw a child in a classroom with glazed eyes, you would naturally assume that he or she was daydreaming, and it is something similar that happens to children with this pattern. They are "not quite there." There is a certain distance between them and the world. This is not to say that there is anything wrong with them mentally or that they cannot interact socially. It is more that they are not properly in touch with their feelings, and consequently, there can be a lack of spontaneity about their behavior.

In some children the behavior changes are even more pronounced. If the thick phlegm is accompanied by Hot energy, these children are often very irritable and restless as well. They feel more or less permanently "out of sorts" or even permanently angry. In extreme cases they can become hyperactive or autistic.

Sudden Drops in Energy

Some children with an echo pattern experience sudden drops in their energy. There seems to be no obvious cause for these periods of tiredness, which can occur at any time of day. At first, one looks for an allergen, but the drops in energy do not seem to be associated with one. We have no satisfactory explanation for this symptom, which is nevertheless characteristic of the pattern.

Intermittent Abdominal Aches

Another symptom associated with glandular congestion is intermittent abdominal aches. Like the drops in energy, these may come at any time and for no obvious reason. We believe that the aches result from the lymphatic circulation in the abdomen, which becomes more or less tender from time to time.

Small Patch of Depigmentation on the Cheek

Equally characteristic is a small patch of reduced pigmentation on the cheek. It looks as though the child has been in the sun some time ago and a little area was sun burned and later peeled. Since then the child has been back in the sun, and some, but not all, of the pigmentation has returned. An example of this is given in Color Plate 1-4.

Rough Skin

One often finds that there are patches of rough skin somewhere on the body. It is a low-grade form of eczema. It may appear anywhere—on the face, the arms, or often the abdomen or legs. The feeling you have when you touch the skin in this area is that it is not quite smooth, as though there is sand just beneath the skin. The explanation of this is that the thick mucus associated with this pattern stops the free flow of nutrients to the skin.

Clear Out Phlegm

If the child has any signs of phlegm, such as a productive cough or loose stools with phlegm, this must be cleared before continuing to the next phase because the next phase of treatment involves softening hard phlegm and may increase the symptoms of productive cough.

Soften Thick Phlegm

The image we have given of mucus that has congealed or become hard also helps explain what happens during treatment. As the treatment progresses, it is common for the very hard mucus to soften and then become apparent. In a clinic it is common to see children who present with no cough and have only a mild skin complaint or possibly just swollen tonsils. As the treatment progresses, the mucus softens and a cough begins to develop.

This development of a cough can cause parents to complain if they do not understand what is happening. From their point of view, they had a child with swollen tonsils before the treatment started. Now that the treatment is halfway through, they have a child with swollen tonsils *and* a cough! At this stage they may often even have very bad behavior (as discussed next)!

■ BEHAVIOR CHANGES DURING THE HEALING PROCESS

When these children start to get well, they often go through a period during which they exhibit very difficult behavior. Typically, after 3 to 6 weeks, these children start to be obstinate and assertive in a way that they had not been before. This can be disconcerting for the parents and in some cases can lead to the parents deciding to discontinue treatment. However, the parents should be encouraged to continue treatment. After a few more weeks the difficult behavior settles down, and at the end of treatment, the child is much more open and happy. It seems that this period of difficulty is a necessary part of getting better. One can say that when a child behaves in this way, the

treatment is going in the right direction. All that is needed is to continue for a bit longer, and the child will certainly be well. It is only a question of time.

The reason for this apparently aggressive behavior is not difficult to understand. These children have been separated from their feelings for a long time, and this may have led to them doing things that they really did not want to do. When at last they get in touch with their feelings, they realize that the balance of their life is all wrong! To change it, they may find that they need to make quite a fuss!

■ DIFFICULTIES IN CURING LONG-STANDING ECHO PATTERNS

Long-standing Echo patterns are more difficult to cure, especially when the child has had the pattern over one or more of the great transitions in life (the 7- and 14-year transitions; see the following chapter). Each time a child goes through one of these transitions, any imbalance becomes more deeply ingrained. What starts as merely a physical imbalance can lead to an emotional imbalance and then become a habit. As time goes on, this starts to color the child's attitude to life itself. This makes the condition much harder to cure.*

■ FAMILY DYNAMICS IN ILLNESS

When one member of the family has a chronic illness (e.g., asthma), it changes the family dynamics. The child who is ill inevitably gets different

---

*As a guide, if the problem is recent, it needs only one therapy. If it has been present over one major transition, then it needs two therapies (e.g., herbs and acupuncture); if it has been present over two transitions, it needs three therapies (e.g., herbs, homeopathy, and acupuncture). This is not a hard-and-fast rule, but it gives some idea of how imbalances can become deeper. If an imbalance persists over a transition, it affects another level of the child's being; the child may therefore require a therapy that works more specifically on the newly affected level.

attention from other family members. The sick child is likely to be treated more leniently and given special privileges not accorded to his or her brothers and sisters. It is easy to see why. When the parents sit by the bedside in the hospital wondering if their child will live or die, they would give anything for the child to live and get well. When they return home with a child who is still fragile, they find it difficult to impose boundaries, even when the occasion demands it.

When it comes to curing the child, this will affect the family dynamics. The child who was sick is no longer so and no longer deserves special privileges. For the child this can be quite difficult. Even for the parents it can be surprisingly difficult to let go of the idea that the child is sick. There is something so defenseless about a sick child that for many parents the idea of their child being well is strangely disturbing. Of course they want their child to be well, but it can be difficult to change from a pattern of indulging the child to a pattern of imposing boundaries.

These problems are even more severe when treating the echo pattern, for, as we have seen, the child can become somewhat rebellious for a month or two during the period when toxins are being eliminated from the body. Obviously, the people they will rebel against are the main authority figures in their life—their parents!

It is this that is one of the chief problems in treating your own child. If there is a third party involved, he or she can often be of help in guiding the family through such a transition.

▪ Case History

Master H., at 9 years of age, came for treatment for a chronic cough. It had been with him since very early in life. Also from the earliest time, he had been a bit of a "mama's boy," never wanting to let mom out of his sight. He had always been very polite and had always helped his mother in many ways. In particular, he liked (or appeared to like) helping wash the dishes.

The treatment went well for the first few weeks, but then the mother started to complain of a new and unpleasant feature in her child's behavior. He was starting to be quite aggressive, and from time to time, he was quite rude to her. He was becoming more and more difficult about helping in the kitchen, and one day he flatly refused to wash any dishes. The mother was most distressed.

When the child came to the clinic, we started to talk about these things, and he came out straight away with the fact that he had always hated doing the dishes and had previously helped with them only to please his mother. He still wanted to please his mother, of course, but he would much rather do it in another way. With no prodding, he volunteered to help with getting the wood for the fire and cleaning the fires out after. He felt much more at home with this and was even prepared to do help some with the dishes if he could be allowed to look after the fire.

This is a typical example of how an echo pattern can lead to a child being somewhat separated from his feelings. Then as the treatment progresses and the child gradually comes back into contact with himself, there is a period of difficult behavior, followed by a much greater openness.

▪ MAIN POINTS FROM THIS CHAPTER

- Echo patterns are common and last a long time.
- A key sign is swollen lymph nodes.
- Thick mucus is often seen in association with echo patterns.
- Immunizations, a severe illness, and courses of antibiotics can all cause an echo pattern.
- The child may behave badly while the echo pattern is being released.

6

Stages of Growth and Their Relation to Illness

Most of this book discusses how to treat illnesses after they have already appeared. In this chapter we focus on the longer view and the prevention of illness before it occurs. We look at the first 21 years of life and show how there are times in life when certain illnesses are more likely to appear. We show how problems that start at one time may evolve into different problems later in life. We also discuss the optimum times for clearing out old imbalances.

This chapter is therefore for the parent, who naturally cares about the long-term future of their child. It is also for the family practitioner, who also has the opportunity to help patients over many years. With the understanding of the broad sweep of life, you will be able to help children through the major problems of their life in a way unimagined by orthodox medicine.

◼ GATES IN LIFE: THE 7- AND 14-YEAR TRANSITIONS

Central to our theme is the idea of a gate in life. A gate is a time of life when many changes are taking place, and with the changes, many opportunities. In the West we perceive these gates as major life events, but to call them this is to miss their true significance. They are more than just events. The events are the points of change in life. At these points health and happiness may take a turn for the better or may take a turn for the worse. Which way it goes depends on the circumstances. For women, one of these gates is childbirth. Childbirth is a major event in a woman's life, a time when her character undergoes a significant change. When

childbirth is difficult, the woman's health may be adversely affected, requiring many years to recover. On the positive side, other women, who were somewhat timid and weak before childbirth, may suddenly uncover unexpected reserves of personal strength.

For those younger than 21, there are two gates or transitions: a minor one at 7 years and a major one at 14 years. At these gates there can be a change in a child's health: It can improve, or it can worsen.

The 7-Year Transition

At the 7-year transition children become aware of their emotions for the first time. Before this age, they are not truly aware of emotions at all. A 3-year-old never stops to think about whether he or she is happy or sad; the child just *is* happy or sad. Similarly, at this age children are not aware of being tired. When they are tired they just sit down—on the stairs, in the road, anywhere! They do not analyze it; in fact, they really have just a dim awareness of these feelings.

At 7 years of age, this changes. For the first time children are aware of being angry or tired. They experience the feelings as being something different from themselves. Then, human nature being what it is, they seek to control what they perceive as different. When they become restless, they may seek to control it and make themselves sit down. When they are tired, they use their willpower to carry on. Society expects it. At 7 years old, children are expected to be able to sit still at their desks. When they are sad or angry, they may try to repress their tears or their rage.

In some senses, this is the end of childhood. Certainly in terms of disease processes, it is at this age that the adult disease patterns first appear. The ability to restrain anger opens the way for the tension that adults experience. The ability to use the willpower to endure even when tired opens the way for exhaustion from overwork. Both of these internal conditions can lead to illnesses characteristic in adults (e.g., tension headaches)—illness that really do not have a counterpart in young children.

The 14-Year Transition

At 14 years there is an even more momentous change. This period is roughly the time that puberty starts, marking the enormous surge of hormonal energy. On the physical level this age is somewhat variable because the age of onset of puberty is now much earlier than it was in the past. Some girls have their first period as young as age 9. On a mental-emotional level, the really profound changes, those related to the maturity of the person, still happen around age 14. It is at this age that individuality starts to be more and more important. Before 14 years it is rare for children to have ideas that they could truly call their own. Their ideas are usually a blend of their parents' ideas and their teachers'. Then at 14 they start to have their own opinions. Their true nature begins to appear. They start to have ideas that are different from those of their parents—a feature of teenagers that many parents find difficult to handle.

Now if a child has a significant imbalance or illness while passing through these transitions, that imbalance or illness becomes even more ingrained. What begins as a feeling of unwellness and irritability becomes a habit if it remains present for too long. If this habit persists throughout puberty, it becomes embedded into the child's life and perspective of the world.

The easiest way to understand this concept is to imagine a boy who has a Hot echo pattern. Typically, one will see the symptoms of a red face and light, or perhaps broken, sleep. The boy will have a tendency toward hyperactivity and will run around all the time. At the age of 4 or 5 years, he has only a Hot echo pattern, which at this age is easily treated. Now think what happens when this boy goes to school. Before he began attending school, he could give free rein to its urges to run around all the time, but now he has to sit still during class. A lot of his energy has to be directed at doing this, and he will find himself spending much of his energy on simply sitting still. Initially, this does not have any serious effects, but over the next few years, the constant effort of restraining himself develops into a habit and creates a lot of tension. What was an ebullient, if overactive, child up to the age of 7 has become a rather tense and angry child. Unless given huge amounts of exercise (which is rare now), he will be prone to outbursts of rage.

What has happened is that the imbalance of energy has now become an imbalance of energy *and* emotions. As if this were not bad enough, the changes that take place at age 14 are even more profound. At 14 years, individuality emerges. If this boy is angry, this emotion colors his entire outlook on life. He will enter into his teenage years already angry. The consequence of this is that his outlook on life becomes somewhat warped. Feeling angry all the time, he looks to the outside world for the origin of his anger. Instead of seeing a world that is composed of good mixed with bad, he sees a world that is mainly bad. Of course all teenagers have this outlook to a certain extent, but if an echo pattern is present, this feeling may completely dominate the teenager's life.

What has happened is that the imbalance that started out as merely an imbalance of energy and then developed into an imbalance of energy and emotions has now become an imbalance in the whole of the person's life. The problem is no longer one that is easily cured. One can see clearly that once the imbalance has been embedded so deeply, it is going to take much more than merely herbs to clear the echo pattern to restore the body's balance. The person has to find a new way of relating to the world, one that is not based on anger.

This thumbnail sketch is not meant to be taken completely literally but rather as an illustration of how the echo pattern can influence one's life view and what the implications of this are. In particular, we wish to point out that if the imbalances are treated when the child is still young, they are very easy to treat. If the imbalances are left untreated while the child progresses through the major transitions in life, they take a stronger and stronger hold and become much more difficult to cure.

What This Means Clinically

So far we have painted a depressing picture of a disease taking a stronger and stronger hold. It is hoped that with the help of an herbalist, this hold can be loosened, even to the point that it is expelled altogether. There are some points to notice here:

- If the child is younger than 7 years, clearing the echo pattern is usually relatively easy. Of course, it may require some time if the child has become very weak or very thin or if the child does not have significant reserves of energy. In a case such as this it may take more than a year to build up the child's energy to the point that the echo pattern can be expelled, but there are no real obstacles to the treatment.
- If the child is between 7 and 14 years old and the echo has been with the child through the 7-year transition, the pattern is relatively hard to dislodge. This should be approached by gradually building up the child's strength and gradually trying to loosen the grip the echo pattern has over these intervening years. Then when the child is 12 years old, treatment can start in earnest, taking advantage of the huge surge of energy that accompanies puberty.
- From 12 to 14 years is a time of great change. It is possible at this time to redress very deep imbalances. If a child has the proper treatment before (to build up strength) and the proper treatment and support during these years, there is the possibility of completely eliminating the imbalances that have been there since early childhood.
- Some children are able to eradicate an old illness by itself, without the aid of any therapist.

This happens with children who are basically healthy and have a good constitution. Common signs of the echo pattern leaving once and for all are inexplicable skin rashes that occasionally appear in healthy children during puberty.

▪ Case History

Roy, at 12 years old, was a pleasant boy to be with, always obliging and friendly. He also had a great interest in mechanical things and hoped to build a hovercraft. However, he was hampered by being very tired. He had the enthusiasm to do the work of building his hovercraft, but he had to rest so often that not much got done after he had completed his schoolwork. Upon seeing the child, one could easily see the tiredness, for he even had difficulty in sitting up straight in his chair.

As he approached age 12, he came for treatment. When I examined him, I did not find anything especially wrong, except that his lymph nodes were swollen. In addition, the saliva on his tongue was very sticky, showing that all the body fluids were thickened and that he had an echo pattern. He continued treatment for nearly a year and a half. During that time he initially got a little better, but then he had a series of minor fevers. It seemed as though he was always ill. In fact, he was ill at least once a month, sometime twice. His mother started to despair.

Fortunately, we were able to point out the small signs that showed he was really getting better. His appetite was improving; far from being tired after his fevers, he actually had more energy. Throughout, his spirit was good.

By the time he reached 13½ years, he was in full strength. He had no difficulty in sitting up straight in his chair—in fact, he preferred not to sit at all but to be doing something.

▪ IMBALANCES CAUSED BY LIFE EVENTS

Imbalances Present at Birth

It is our observation that some children are born with an imbalance. It is not entirely clear to us why this should be so, but this is the way it is. Some children are born with a lot of mucus in the system, some with excessive amounts of Heat, and others with Cold energy already present. Sometimes there is a hereditary component: One can see a reflection of the parent's imbalance in the child. Other times, the child is simply born with imbalances, for no apparent reason.

There are also causes in pregnancy that can affect the unborn child. Foremost among these is shock or emotional trauma. If the mother witnesses some sudden terrifying event, such as a car accident, this can also affect the child, resulting in the child being born with "jarred nerves." A typical symptom associated with this is insomnia with nightmares.

Birth Trauma

Birth trauma, such as long or difficult labor, is now known to be a significant cause of problems. Surprisingly, it does not usually give rise to the jarred nerves pattern that we have just mentioned. More commonly, it gives rise to Weak energy. It seems that the most common effect is to reduce the child's enthusiasm for life. It is as though the child was expecting to enjoy life when coming into the world but finds it to be a much nastier place than expected. The resulting lack of enthusiasm often manifests in a poor appetite, and following from that the Weak energy pattern.

Rapid Birth, Painful Birth

When birth happens very rapidly, either naturally or from excessive birth-inducing drugs, the baby may have too much pressure on the cranium during birth. This can affect the craniosacral rhythms, giving rise to symptoms such as crossed eyes, headaches, insomnia from the cranial disturbance, and urinary or anal dysfunction from the sacral disturbance.

Teething

Some pediatricians still believe that all problems attributed to teething are unavoidable or are merely in the mind of the mother! We do not hold this view. We believe that many problems arise from teething, some small, some serious. Most of these can be helped with herbs and a simple change in diet.

Growing Diseases

Energy is necessary for growth. The absorption and redistribution of the physical substance of the body and the emotional changes that must take place as child matures strain the body's systems. Consequently, when a child goes through a growth spurt or an emotional transition, the child is prone to illness. The changes that take place on the physical, emotional, and spiritual levels can all lead to imbalances.

For example, when a child reaches the age of 2 years, the child's determination to do things his or her own way commonly leads to tantrums and rages. When these come, the child gets very hot during struggles against the parents. A child in a rage can turn bright red in the face and be covered in perspiration. The heat produced in this way can produce an imbalance in the same way as hot weather, and this is one explanation for the fevers that are so common at this age.

Growing Too Fast

Every mother has watched her child go through growth spurts and has noticed how the child's health and appetite change. A common pattern is for children to eat an enormous amount of food in preparation for the growth spurt; then when the actual growing takes place, it is common for the child to lose interest in food. At this time, all of the body's energy is devoted to growing and restructing the body. Children are often vulnerable at this time, and it is easy for them to get coughs and colds and other minor infections. If they are already somewhat unhealthy (e.g., if they have asthma), it is common for their chronic problem to be aggravated. The asthmatic child is likely to have a series of attacks during a growth spurt.

Children need two things during this time. The first is rest, and the second is tonic herbs. Often, it is easier to give the herbs because the education system has leaned far in the direction of continuous assessment and makes little allowance for children who go through a growth spurt and need some "time out" when they have outgrown their strength.

Growing Pains

Growing pains are very real to the child who experiences them. They feel wracking pains in their limbs, most commonly the lower parts of the legs. It feels as if the bones are being stretched. These pains do in fact accompany periods of rapid growth, but in our opinion they are not actually caused by the stretching of bones. We believe that the pain is a sort of rheumatism, caused by an imbalance of damp and mucus in the system. It can be effectively treated with medicines similar to those one would use for older adults who had rheumatism in damp weather.

Puberty and Teenage

The energy of puberty and teenage is volcanic and craves to be free. The corresponding emotional state is one of frustration and feelings of constriction. It seems grossly unfair to the teenager that parents should require them to be home by midnight every night, even earlier some nights! When this is added to the very real constrictions imposed upon them by school schedules, homework, and examinations, it can give rise to feelings of hopelessness. In some children this manifests as violent antisocial behavior. In other children the suppression of these feelings opens the way for odd illnesses, the most common being glandular fever (mononucleosis). This illness is especially common among those who already have an echo pattern.

▪ IMBALANCES CAUSED BY LIFESTYLE

It seems odd at first to talk about the lifestyle of a child, but it has to be mentioned, for the life of a child is very different from what it used to be. In our opinion this is one of the reasons why certain types of children and certain patterns of illness are much more common today. The main changes can be summarized as follows:

- More brain, less body
- Less freedom and less responsibility

More Brain, Less Body

More and more gadgets that encourage the development of brain rather than of body are available today. Among these are GameBoys, computers, computer games, and mobile phones. By contrast there is a reduction in the amount of exercise that children participate in. They rarely walk anywhere; it is not safe for them to play on the streets; and some schools discourage competitive games, thereby eliminating exercise altogether. The reader can provide his or her own list.

There are some good aspects to this. There is no question that such activities help intellectual development, and it can broaden the mind from the blinkered parochial mentality that one still finds in some areas. On the downside, this emphasis on mental activity opens the way for problems that affect the brain, such as hyperactivity and attention-deficit disorder or, more seriously, meningitis and other serious brain diseases. These problems are not new in themselves. What is new is that the conditions are much more prevalent today.

Less Freedom and Less Responsibility

Children have much less freedom to roam than they used to. It is not safe for them even to cross the road outside their houses, and they cannot play in the park unsupervised for fear of attack. Very few children have the freedom to travel anywhere on their own. Most are carried around by the taxi service provided by their long-suffering parents. All this comes with less responsibility for their actions as well. The trend is away from giving children clear consequences if they do something wrong and giving clear rewards if they do something good.

Surprisingly to many, these two factors also contribute to the new patterns of illness. The lungs are especially nourished by freedom. To understand this, imagine taking great lungfuls of air when you have reached some particularly beautiful wide-open space. Imagine also what effect it would have on your breathing to be completely stuck and constrained in a small space. It is this constrained feeling that many young people have now, and it is one of the factors contributing to asthma in the rising generation.

▣ MAIN POINTS FROM THIS CHAPTER

- There are major transitions at 7 and 14 years.
- At the transitions, imbalances can be expelled or can take a firmer hold.
- These transitions are good times to treat.

7

Diagnosis

In this chapter we cover a small part of the information that can easily be obtained in the clinic either through observation or through asking some simple questions. There are many books on the art of orthodox diagnosis, and there is no point in us repeating those here. What concerns us here are the signs that indicate a child's state of energy, for we believe that this aspect of medicine has been progressively ignored over the years. We describe what can easily be taken in through the four senses of looking, feeling (palpation), hearing (listening), and smelling as used in clinical examination.*

◻ LOOKING

Looking at a child is the first step in diagnosis because one has the opportunity to see a child even before any questions have been asked. It is also an important step because merely looking at the child's behavior, facial color, and overall shape tells an enormous amount about the energy of a child. Often, one can know what the mother is going to say before she has spoken.

How to Look

Children are very sensitive to the mood and feelings of those around them. When they first meet you, they will be assessing you as much as you are assessing them. What they are looking for are signs that they can trust you. Looking is typically the first initial contact, and therefore the actual

way in which you look at the child has an effect on his or her perception of you. If you look with the cold eye of a scientist, the child will feel that coldness and shrink away. If you look with eyes of love and with a genuine desire to get to know the person opposite you, the child will quickly warm to you.

This is true even for the babies. For those who have not worked with babies, it may be easy to forget that inside that tiny body is a real person. Babies do not have the ability to relate to others in the way that adults do, so it is up to us as practitioners to develop a way of connecting with them.

If you are a parent, you know your baby is a real person and you do not need to find special ways of communicating—you are well tuned to your child most of the time. For a practitioner, who is a stranger, it obviously takes some time to make this contact.

Behavior

If you are a parent, you will have studied your child's behavior. What you may not have realized is how closely the child's behavior is connected to his or her state of health.

As a practitioner, the child's behavior is likely to be the first thing you notice. The child will probably be shy and timid at first, but if your clinic is child-friendly, with a lot of toys, the child will soon relax and become engrossed. If you are meeting a child for the first time, it is often helpful to spend a few minutes in the waiting room, observing the child and family. Over time, one can learn to

---

*The sense of taste is rarely used for diagnostic purposes in the West.

diagnose much of a child's condition merely by behavior and appearance. In this book we can just point the way, with a few headings.

Timid	Often relates to insufficient energy. This is because the child does not have enough energy to overcome new obstacles.
Aggressive	Usually goes with excess energy. In addition, heat is often present, which results in the child becoming restless.
Generous	Usually goes with a child who has plenty of energy. It is common in a child who has a warm nature. When out of balance, this child may easily become overheated and aggressive.
Restless	Can mean that the child has much heat in the system, in which case the child's face will be red. The other condition is the overstimulated pattern, which results in the child having a pale or slightly green face.
Passive	Nearly always means Weak energy. The child does not have enough energy to do what he or she wants to do and prefers to sit and watch.

Note that these behavior traits may be normal and just part of the child's character.

Colors on the Face

The colors on the face, both the overall color and the details of the distribution of color, give significant indications concerning the child's health and any imbalances.

FACIAL COLORS IN ASIANS AND AFRICANS

Although color differences are easiest to see in lightly pigmented skin, they can also be seen in even the darkest skin—with practice. It can be helpful to compare the child's color with the parents'. This will help give a reliable assessment of the true color.

Red. An **overall red** color means Hot energy, just as people turn red on a hot day and after eating a very hot curry. This is of great importance in hyperactivity/attention-deficit disorder, a condition in which the color of the face allows discrimination between the different patterns immediately.

Redness of both cheeks usually indicates a stagnant food pattern, but it is also seen with lung conditions such as chronic cough and asthma, in which case it indicates a subacute inflammation of the lungs.

Redness of just one cheek is seen in babies when they are teething and may also be an indication of the stagnant food pattern.

Pale. A **pale** face usually means weakness of energy, or sometimes Cold energy affecting the body. Sometimes the pale color results from something blocking the energy, rather than there not being enough. This is seen when a child has an infection and also is seen in an echo pattern.

White. White can mean two things:

- The **lungs** have been affected (the white color is very common in children with asthma), *or*
- There is great **Cold energy** in the body, as is commonly seen in colic. (In colic the face sometimes turns red *while* the child is screaming in pain but is white when the child is calm.)

Pale Patches on the Face (See Color Plate 1-4). Pale patches seen on the face are most commonly a sign of an echo pattern. The reason is that the lymphatic circulation is congested, and the skin does not get nourished properly.

These patches are also a sign of intestinal worms. When worms are present, the patches may seem to be covered with a fine powder.

Between the Eyes. If a child has suffered a sudden emotional shock that remains unresolved, he or she may have a **blue** color on the bridge of the nose, between the eyes. Shock may also be evident as anxiety and fear in the child's eyes.

This color should not be confused with the **green** color, which indicates a sluggish digestion, usually with mucus. When the color is questionable, whether it is greenish blue or bluish green, the significance of the color can be distinguished by looking *into* the child's eyes. The shocked child looks frightened, whereas the child with a sluggish digestion tends to have a slightly muddy look.

Blue-Gray above the Lips. A **blue-gray** discoloration above the lips often is a sign of pain in the stomach (i.e., indigestion). It is commonly seen in babies after they have been feeding and before they have been "burped"; it also may be seen in babies with Cold energy in the stomach.

DROOLING FROM THE MOUTH
Drooling is a sign that the fluid metabolism is disturbed. The digestive system is commonly affected as well. One possible cause is food intolerance, especially to "damp" energy foods (e.g., cow's milk, peanut butter, sugar). This symptom is also seen when a baby is teething.

Nasal Discharge

GENERAL
All nasal discharges are made worse by too many "damp" foods. "Damp" foods include cow's milk, cheese, peanut butter, bananas, and sometimes oranges.

GREEN
A green gluelike substance coming from the nose is usually attributable to sluggish digestion. This color also occasionally relates to chronic inflammation of the sinuses, without sluggish digestion.

YELLOW
A yellow gluelike substance usually indicates sinusitis and is a sign of infection.

CLEAR
Nasal discharge that is clear points to a disturbance of water metabolism. This happens when a child has a cold, but it is also seen in a child with a chronic condition.

THICK, BLUE-WHITE
Thick, blue-white discharge is sometimes seen a month or so after a polio immunization. It is also seen with echo patterns.

Mouth Breathing

If a child breathes through the mouth instead of the nose, it means that the nasal cavities are blocked by thick phlegm (usually attributable to an echo pattern). This is also seen when the adenoids are enlarged (a condition commonly seen in the echo pattern).

Discharge from the Ears

Discharge of dark brown wax from the ears often accompanies otitis media. When it occurs on its own, without inflammation in the ears, it is a sign of phlegm and stagnation in the system. Usually, there is an underlying stagnant food pattern in children younger than 3 years.

Sweating

ON HEAD ONLY
If a child sweats on the head only, it may be a sign of heat in the stomach. This is often seen after feeding or at night. If there is perspiration over the whole body after feeding, this is a sign of heart weakness and must be taken seriously.

AT NIGHT
Recurring sweating at night is commonly the result of a stagnant food pattern or Hot energy echo pattern.

Shape of the Face

The brain is housed in the upper part of the head, most of it above the eyes. If this part of the head is relatively large, it means that the child's energy is

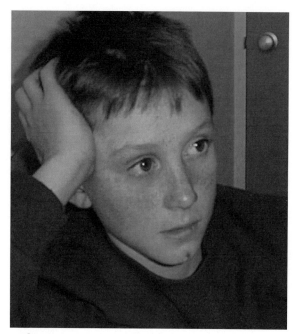

Figure 7-1   Child with energy mainly in the brain.

Shape of the Back

The back should be more or less vertical, especially in young children. Up to the age of 7 year, children's energy should be good and they should actually want to sit up straight. Even up until about 12 years of age, children should normally want to sit up straight; if they do not, something is certainly wrong with their energy. After puberty all of this changes, and it is normal (in our society at least) for teenagers to slouch.

Following are some fairly reliable signs of an energy imbalance and what these signs may indicate:

Sign	Problem
Child does not enjoy sitting up straight or truly has difficulty doing so	Overall weakness of energy
Upper thoracic is bent over	Lung weakness
Lower thoracic is bent in	Digestive weakness
Lumbar area is bent in	Weakness in the lower part of the body, usually of the urinary system

The reason for these changes in shape is simple: The energy in the affected part of the body is the same energy that nourishes the muscles in that area. If the energy is weak, the muscles do not function as well and a certain sagging takes place. In the following photographs (Figures 7-2 to 7-8), we give illustrations of these points.

mainly in his or her brain.* The mental energy of these children is likely to be very quick, but their physical body and energy are less developed. It is easy for them to develop the Weak digestion pattern. Such children are likely to be pale, but this is not an indication of a pathologic condition. A picture of such a child is given in Figure 7-1 and Color Plate 3-1.

Signs on the Back and Abdomen

The areas on the back correspond to the same organs mentioned earlier: The upper thoracic area relates to the lungs, the middle of the back (lower thoracic) relates to the digestive system, and the lumbar region relates to the urinary tract.

Growth of Down or Fine Hair

Sick children often have a growth of down or very fine hair in a particular area of the back. This hair

---

*It may come as a surprise to some readers that the shape of the head is influenced by the thoughts that go on inside it. This view was fashionable in the nineteenth century, when professional phrenologists arose. In the latter part of the twentieth century the maps that had been developed by the phrenologist were shown to have little correlation with reality. However, now that the twenty-first century has dawned, interest has turned again to this subject. The work of Doman and Delacato on children with brain damage has shown unequivocally that when a child's brain is exercised, it grows faster than average. In a completely different kind of study, it was shown that London taxi drivers have a part of their brain (the part thought to be connected to spatial awareness) significantly enlarged.

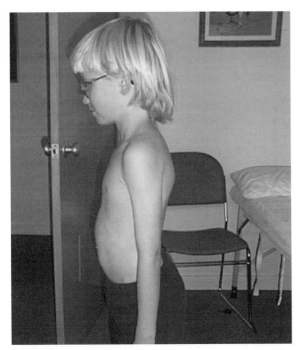

Figure 7-2 This child's main problem was sinusitis. It can be seen that the upper part of the child's back is bent over, indicating weakness of the respiratory system. The lumbar back is hollow, which is a sign overall weakness. This means that the problem will take a long time to cure because the child's constitution must first be built up before major changes can take place.

grows in response to a local coldness and is correlated to weakness of energy in that area. For example, if the hair grows in the upper thoracic area, it is usually a sign of lung weakness; this is commonly seen in patients with asthma.

Network of Tiny Blue Capillaries

A network of tiny blue capillaries does not indicate weakness so much as stagnation of energy. Once again, the appearance of these capillaries in the upper thoracic area suggests that the lung energy is not moving well, as seen in some children with asthma. In children with a stagnant food pattern, these capillaries may be seen on the abdomen.

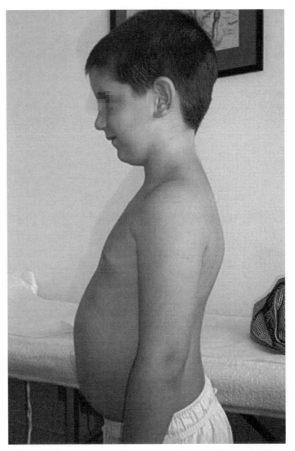

Figure 7-3 The overall energy of this child is good, but his digestion is out of balance. His large waist is an indication of water being retained. His main symptom was bedwetting, and he is a good example of bedwetting caused primarily by poor digestion.

■ FEELING (PALPATION)

Palpation is usually done after most of the questions have been asked and the child thoroughly examined. Palpation provides more reliable information about the energy of a child than do other methods. Here we are not referring to the rather heavy-handed palpation that is necessary to examine the internal organs. This technique is altogether lighter, especially for children younger than 3 years. The techniques we use are described in the following sections.

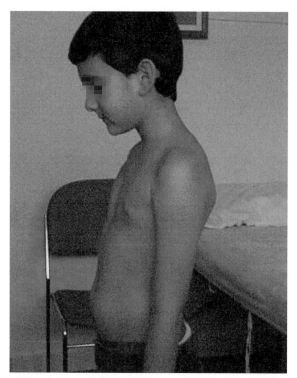

Figure 7-4   This child had bedwetting as a main symptom. His digestion was good, but as can be seen, his back was weak in the lumbar area.

Legs (for Babies)

Babies do not like having their "personal space" invaded, so if examination can begin with the legs, the babies will feel less threatened. When you grasp the legs, you will learn two things. First, the strength and tone of the legs are determined. In particular we find the following:

- Strong, sturdy, muscular legs are a sign of Strong energy.
- Thin, matchstick legs with thin bones are a sign of Weak energy.
- Squashy, flabby legs without much tone are a sign of excess fluid and often occur when there is a lot of phlegm in the system.

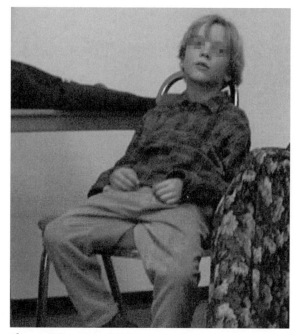

Figure 7-5   This child does not have the energy to sit up straight.

Second, note the reaction to your grasp:

- Violent, angry objection to grasping is a sign of a Strong child.
- Submissiveness or withdrawing without much fight is a sign of a Weak child.

After the legs have been palpated, the order of the remaining examination is not that important. The following should be included, however:

- Abdomen
- Back
- Lymph nodes in the neck

Abdomen

The abdomen is especially worth palpating in children younger than 3 years, for much can be learned about the state of the digestion. In particular, in

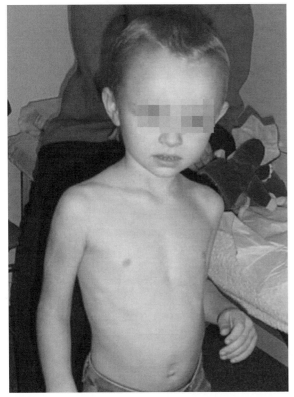

Figure 7-6 The head appears to be too big, but in fact, it is the body that is too small. The combination of weak digestive energy and poor-quality food have led to this child being undernourished and under-sized.

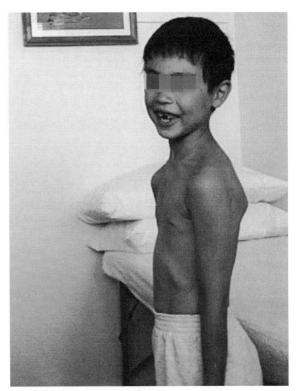

Figure 7-7 This child had a good enough appetite, but he lived on preserved food. He had never eaten any fresh food in his life. The combination of this and hyperactivity has led to him being very thin. The severely rounded shoulders are a sign of Weak energy, despite the hyperactivity.

younger children a swollen abdomen is seen with the stagnant food pattern, and with it usually constipation. In older children it is a sign of fluid accumulation related to poor digestion (see Figure 7-8 for an example).

Back

Palpating the back for the muscle tone is especially helpful in the examination of children older than 5 years, an age at which adult patterns start to develop. The technique is to run a hand briefly over the back, from top to bottom, trying to assess the energy and tone in each part. The significance is the same as for the observation of the back, and it should confirm what you already know—or if you do not want the child to take his or her clothes off, it can replace the observation of the back.

Lymph Nodes in the Neck

We *always* palpate the lymph nodes to determine whether an echo pattern is present, and, if so, how severe it is.

Large lymph nodes indicate an excess of mucus.
Hard lymph nodes indicate that the mucus is very hard and will be correspondingly difficult to clear out of the system.

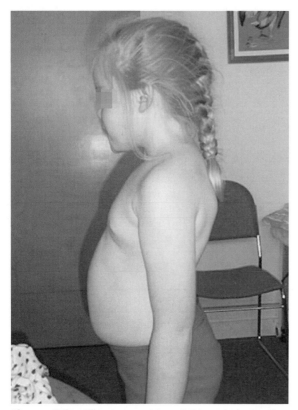

Figure 7-8   This is an older child with a swollen abdomen. At this age one thinks less of the stagnant food pattern and more of accumulation of fluids. In this child the main problem was bedwetting, which occurred when the fluids began to circulate at night.

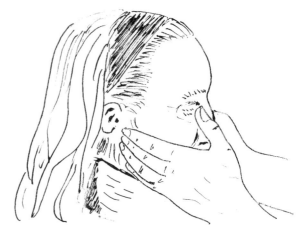

Figure 7-9   Palpating the cervical glands.

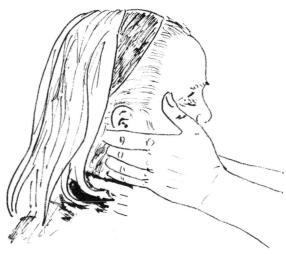

Figure 7-10   Palpating the occipital glands.

There are four sets in the neck that we commonly examine:

The **submaxillary,** midway between the angle and the tip of the mandible
The **occipital** lymph nodes
The **cervical** chains
The **tonsillar nodes,** at the angle of the mandible.

Figures 7-9 to 7-11 demonstrate how to palpate these glands.

How to Perform Palpation

Use the pads of your fingers to perform palpation. Move the skin over the underlying tissue in each area rather than moving your fingers over the skin. The child should be relaxed, with the neck flexed slightly forward, and if necessary slightly toward the side. You can usually examine both sides at once.

Potential Problems

The most important thing to remember is to *be gentle;* a child will not take kindly to you if you almost strangle him or her! If the child does not want you

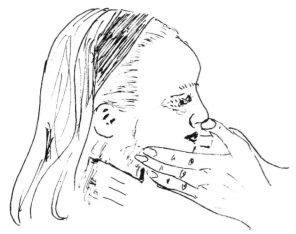

Figure 7-11 Palpating the mandibular and tonsillar glands.

touching the neck, there are possible reasons for this:

- The child is simply being difficult and did not want to be here in the first place.
- The child's neck hurts. You will find this in young babies who cannot tell you that their throat is sore. They try to wriggle away and are in obvious distress.

▪ HEARING (LISTENING)

Voice

First and foremost, one notes the strength of the child's voice. This means different things at different ages. After about 3 years of age, when children start to interact with adults more or less normally, a strong voice simply means a loud voice; that is, the child has the potential to shout loudly if not overcome by shyness.

In children younger than that age, and especially in babies, one has to listen for different signs. A baby is a small being, so the voice is also somewhat small. What can be noted is the *emotional strength* of the cry. There is something about the cry of a Strong baby that is very moving. When a Strong child cries, you immediately want to do something. It is a cry that you cannot ignore, for

you feel the suffering of the baby. It is this emotional reaction that you feel that gives a good indication of the true energy of the child.

This is in contrast to Weak babies, who evoke a reduced emotional reaction. If you must choose between attending to one child or another, the child with the weaker cry might find himself or herself in second place. (If you are trying to diagnose your own child, this aspect is somewhat unreliable. The emotional ties you have with your child will produce a strong reaction in you, whether objectively the child's energy is strong or weak.)

Sometimes children learn to attract attention by developing a piercing cry. Their cry seems to hit the resonant frequency of the ears, causing you to feel pain in the ear. This means that you have to stop what you are doing to stop the pain that you feel (rather than because you are emotionally moved). Although this seems like a "cry with strength," it is usually seen in the children with less energy. (We are referring to the normal cry that the child develops, not the piercing cry associated with intense pain in the head such as might be encountered in children with meningitis.)

Cough

When a child is brought in with a cough, it is helpful if you can get the child to cough in front of you. Cough can sometimes be provoked by tickling the child or enraging the child (the former is obviously preferable). The strength and sound of the cough reveal whether there is enough energy in the lungs and provide information regarding the quality of the mucus in the lungs. A harsh cough is a sign of very hard phlegm; a gurgling cough is a sign of watery mucus. Likewise, if the child does not have enough strength and needs to be toned, you will notice that the cough is nonproductive, even though the lungs are obviously congested.

▪ SMELLING

Smells are a less useful guide in diagnosis than they once were because people wash so frequently now. It is only those with a very keen sense of smell who can distinguish clearly the genuine body smell underneath the smell of soap. However, some smells are so strong that they cannot be washed off, and other smells may be reported by the mother.

Ears Smell Peculiar

Various smells may be emitted from the ear, and some mothers are unduly upset by them. The most common smell is that of pus, which indicates either an infection in the outer ear or pus escaping from the middle ear from a burst eardrum. Sometimes one may note a rotten smell coming from the ear. This is usually a sign of a stagnant food pattern.

Breath Smells Like Rotten Eggs

If the breath smells like rotten eggs, heat is affecting the stomach. Often, this originates in the stagnant food pattern.

Burps Smell of Sour Gas

When food is stagnating in the stomach, burps may smell of sour gas. Again, this often originates in the stagnant food pattern. Usually, it means that the child is being fed food that is too rich or that the child is not getting enough exercise.

Stools Smell Sour or of Apples

Stools that smell sour (or of apples) mark the beginnings of the stagnant food pattern. The sour smell is the beginning stage of fermentation.

Stools Smell Foul

Foul-smelling stools indicate either further progression of the stagnant food pattern or possible infectious diarrhea.

PART

2

Using Herbs

8

Administering Herbs

■ FORMS IN WHICH HERBS ARE ADMINISTERED

There are many ways of preparing herbs to combine effectiveness with ease of administration. Here we describe the ones that are mentioned in this book.

Tinctures

Throughout this book we normally specify tinctures. These are alcoholic extracts. We recommend these because of their convenience to use and their long shelf lives (most tinctures last for many years before losing their effectiveness). Commercially made tinctures are made by macerating the herbs using exact water-to-alcohol ratios. This makes a product of very good quality and is generally what we recommend for home use.

On the downside, tinctures do contain alcohol. Although this does not matter for small doses, it certainly does for larger doses. There are two solutions to this. The first is to use glycerin-based extracts (when these extracts are used, the practitioner should check to see that they do not contain alcohol as well). The other solution is to drop the tincture into nearly boiling water. The high temperature will evaporate most of the alcohol. After the mixture has cooled, it may be given to the child.

Doses

The doses listed are for 3-year-olds. For a more in-depth discussion of doses and how they vary with age and constitution, see p. 70.

MAKING TINCTURES

Tinctures can be made at home. Apart from the satisfaction of doing it yourself, there is the advantage that you can be sure that your supplies are organic and that they are completely fresh.

Use an alcohol of at least 30% (60 proof), such as vodka or brandy. (Do not use industrial alcohol, methylated spirits, or rubbing alcohol because these are poisonous.)

Use individual herbs, rather than making a tincture out of an already formulated prescription.

Take 200 g (~7 oz) of dried herbs or 400 g (~14 oz) of fresh herbs, place in a large jar, and steep in 1 L of alcohol.

Let sit for at least 2 weeks.

Press the mix through a wine press or muslin bag, squeezing out as much tincture as possible.

These quantities are applicable for the majority of herbs. Some herbs require a different alcohol/water/herb ratio. For example, valerian *Valeriana officinalis* is best prepared with 60% alcohol, whereas golden seal *Hydrastis canadensis* is normally used with 100 g of herbs to 1 L of liquid. The details, and further descriptions of making your own tinctures, are described in Hoffmann (1992), Tierra (1992), and Chevallier (1996).

Infusions and Decoctions

Some herbs are better given as a warm tea—either an infusion or a decoction. An *infusion* is one in which the herb is placed into the water at just below boiling point and left to stand. In contrast, a *decoction* is one that has been boiled for a few minutes. Infusions are used for aromatic plants such as chamomile *Chamomilla matricaria;* boiling the liquid of these aromatic plants would boil off an important component. Decoctions are often used for roots such as burdock *Arctium lappa,* which require some time to extract the essence from large chunks.

INFUSIONS (USUALLY FOR FLOWERS AND AERIAL PARTS OF PLANTS)
The proportions are as follows:

> 1 tsp dried herb or 2 tsp fresh herb to 1 cup of boiling water
> 20 g (~0.7 oz) dried herb or 30 g (~1 oz) fresh herb to 50 ml of boiling water.

Prepare as directed here:

> Pour the boiling water on the herb, but do not boil.
> Let stand for 10 minutes, then strain and drink.
> Give one third of this (130 ml) over the day in three to four doses for a 3-year-old.

DECOCTIONS (USUALLY FOR ROOTS, TWIGS, BARKS, AND SOME BERRIES)
Add 20 g (~0.7 oz) of dried herb or 40 g (~1.4 oz) of fresh herb to 500 ml of water.
Boil for 10 to 15 minutes. (It is best to break up the herbs or even crush them first.)
The time needed for decoction may be reduced by using a coffee grinder to reduce the herbs to a powder.
Give one third of this (130 ml) over the day in three to four doses for a 3-year-old.

PUTTING INFUSIONS OR DECOCTIONS IN THE BATH
Herbs are readily absorbed through the skin, especially in those younger than 7 years. An effective way to administer herbs to children who would otherwise refuse them is to put the prepared decoction, infusion, or tincture in their bath. Prepare the herbs as usual, with 5 to 10 times more than usual, and pour the preparation in the bath. A thyme bath of this kind is especially useful for babies with whooping cough.

Syrups
Herbs can be preserved in syrups. We make them with sugar, but honey* or glycerin can be substituted. Syrups will last for up to a month, sometimes more, depending on the plant. For example, plantain *Plantago lanceolata,* which contains a plant antibiotic, will last for a year. Syrups made from plants that do not yield an antibiotic may start to grow mold after a week if they are not kept in the refrigerator.

SYRUP PRESCRIPTION 1
Add 350 g of sugar to 0.5 L of liquid from infused herbs or decoction.
Dissolve by warming.

SYRUP PRESCRIPTION 2
Add 1.1 kg of sugar to 0.5 L of water.
Stir and dissolve.
Boil for 2 minutes.
This is a base syrup, and to this you add 1 part tincture to 3 parts of the syrup.

SYRUP PRESCRIPTION 3 (A MORE COMPLEX SYRUP)
Add 2 oz of herbs to 1 quart of water.
Boil down to half its volume.
Strain and add 2 oz of sugar/honey or glycerin.
This is used for barks, twigs, and roots and herbs that can be boiled without losing their properties (not usually used for flowers).

Oils
Simple herbal oils are made as follows:

> Use a cold-pressed good-quality vegetable oil as a base. Olive, almond, sunflower, or safflower oils are best.
> Place the chopped herb (freshly picked or freshly dried) into a clear glass jar. Fill as full

---

*Honey should not be used for children younger than 1 year. See caution on p. 67.

as possible. Then pour over the oil to cover the herbs.

Leave in the sunlight for at least 2 weeks and then strain and bottle.

This method is used for St. John's wort oil among other herbs.

FOR GARLIC AND MULLEIN OIL FOR EARDROPS

Peel and crush one whole bulb of garlic.

Pour over 125 ml of olive oil. Let sit for several days.

Infuse *fresh* mullein flowers *Verbascum thapsus* in oil as described earlier, leaving for at least 2 weeks in sunlight.

Mix 2 parts of the mullein oil to 1 part of the garlic oil. (The amount of garlic may be increased if desired. It depends somewhat on the quality of garlic used and how long it has been allowed to infuse.)

Store in a dropper bottle and use as eardrops.

▪ PERSUADING CHILDREN TO TAKE HERBS

One of the main problems in herbal medicine is getting children to take the medicines prescribed for them. Often, children do not like the taste of medicine and have been brought up to reject any food that is not instantly pleasing. In contrast to earlier generations, many children have never been made to eat something that they do not like.

Another reason why it may be difficult is that children sense that their parents want them to take the herbs and see this as an opportunity to be difficult! There are many solutions.

Sweeten

The oldest and simplest solution is to "sweeten the pill"—simply add sugar. If the child (or parent) reacts badly to sugar, other sweeteners, such as honey,* maple syrup, or fruit sugar, may be used. This method may be used for both teas and tinctures. Tinctures typically may be diluted to a ratio of 1:20, or even more; a teaspoon of honey may

then be stirred in. In addition, the medicine may be mixed in fruit juice to disguise the taste further.

─────────── **Caution** ───────────

Nearly all natural sweeteners contain sugars, which can attack the enamel of the child's teeth if used over a long time. If you are treating a child for a chronic condition that may require months of medication, it is best to find a medicine that does not need sweetening. The alternative is to ensure that the teeth are brushed immediately after taking the sweetened medicine.

Mix with Ice Cream

The tincture may be stirred into ice cream or water ice. Many children get abdominal pains after eating ices and generally we advise against giving cold food to babies and children, so it may seem strange to see this recommendation here—but it seems to work. If you are giving the herbs in ices, it may be helpful to add some warming herbs such as ginger *Zingiber officinalis* or cinnamon *Cinnamomum zeylandica* to the mixture.

Rub Tinctures into the Abdomen or Chest

Applying tinctures topically is a rather messy way to do things, but it requires less cooperation from the child! The principle behind this method is that a child's skin is quite porous, allowing the herbs to be absorbed. Generally, three to five times the amount of tincture is needed if it is administered in this way.

If the child has digestive troubles, the tincture should be applied to the abdomen. If the child has respiratory difficulties, the tincture is massaged into the chest.

---

*Honey is not given to children younger than 1 year because it occasionally is found to have spores of the bacteria that cause botulism, *Clostridium botulinum*. Before 1 year of age, the digestion of some children is not strong enough to destroy the bacteria when they proliferate. Infant botulism is more common when there is constipation and also in infants younger than 6 months. The spores can be sterilized by maintaining the honey at 100° C for 10 minutes.

Rub Essential Oils into the Abdomen or Chest

As with tinctures, topical application of oils is also messy—but very effective. By their nature, essential oils diffuse rapidly through the skin and are therefore absorbed quickly. This method is especially indicated in two situations. The first is when the child flatly refuses to take herbs. The second is in a child with respiratory problems. In the latter case the essential oils seem to be able to penetrate conditions accompanied by a lot of mucus in a way that few other methods can.

Apply Compresses

A variation of the method just described was used widely in the past, in the form of compresses. A towel is soaked in a pan of hot decoction or infusion and then wrung out. While it is still hot and steaming (but not so hot as to burn the skin), it is laid on the affected part of the patient—chest, abdomen, or kidneys.

Use Patches

Yet another variation on topical application is coming back for Chinese herbs in the form of patches. The principle is the same as that for anti-smoking or contraceptive patches.

Essential Oils

Essential oils are distilled essences of plants. As such they are one step more refined than the raw herb, but most have almost the same medicinal effect. They differ in that they stimulate the olfactory senses and thus quickly affect the brain. In this way they are often used for both emotional and physical problems. For example, marjoram herb is commonly used for digestive complaints; in addition to aiding digestion, the oil also helps in the treatment of depression.

DOSAGE

In the past, and indeed in some schools now, essential oils are administered by mouth. We do not

Table 8-1	Dosage of Essential Oils	
AGE		**DOSE IN DROPS**
0-6 months		1-3
6-12 months		1-5
1-4 years		2-5
4-7 years		2-10
7-12 years		2-12
12+ years		3-20

recommend this, especially for children, because essential oils are hundreds of times more concentrated than tinctures. We advise diluting them in a carrier oil and rubbing the oil into the skin, preferably in massage strokes. The doses that we recommend are listed in Table 8-1. The dose refers to total number of drops per treatment, for example, a 6-month-old would have one drop each of three different oils or three drops of the same oil.

As you will notice, there is very little variation in the dose for children younger than 5 years; this is based on the principle that it takes less oil to cover a smaller body. Therefore babies will automatically receive a smaller dose than larger children.

--- **Caution for Essential Oils** ---

- Do not overdose.
- Do not use neat; always dilute.
- Do not take by mouth.

There are widely differing opinions regarding what the best dose is. The doses we give are very safe, and we have also found them effective. Do not be tempted to increase the dose dramatically, especially for babies. One drop of essential oil will smell very strong to a baby, even if it does not to you.

SPECIAL BENEFITS

The great virtue of oils is that they can easily be spread on the skin, with a minimum of fuss, and that they are easily absorbed through the skin. They typically smell quite nice as well. Consequently, essential oils have a special application for children who dislike herbs intensely and for those who are able to wriggle out of taking their herbs. These children are usually quite happy to receive a massage with essential oils.

There is another great virtue: Essential oils penetrate the toughest and thickest mucus, so they have a special use in the treatment of all coughs. In acute coughs they are especially useful because they aid in diminishing the severity of the cough, helping the child expectorate, and hastening the course of the disease.

MEDICAL USES

Essential oils have always been available, at least since Egyptian times, when they were used both cosmetically and for embalming, but the difficulty in extracting them made them very costly. It is only since the middle of the nineteenth century, with the development of new methods of extraction, that their price has been reduced to a level that ordinary people can afford. Only recently have they become freely available. For this reason, our medical knowledge of the oils is not as extensive as that for the more traditional ways of using herbs, which have thousands of years of clinical experience to back up their use.

ADMINISTRATION

In Massage. Essential oils should always be diluted in a carrier oil. We recommend almond, avocado, or grape seed oil because these are easily absorbed, but any vegetable oil will do. Do not use a mineral-based oil; these clog up the delicate skin of a baby. The doses presented in the text are for dilution in 30 ml of a carrier oil.

In the Bath. It is best to dilute the essential oils in a small teaspoon of carrier oil before putting the oils in the bath.

Inhalation. Oils may be added to a bowl of hot water. The child's head is then placed over the bowl and a towel placed on the child's head. This should be used only with great care and only with older children. The child must not be allowed to touch the hot water. For use with babies, the hot bowl can be placed under the crib and the aroma will fill the room.

Diffusers. Many types of diffusers are now commercially available. We advise against using those with a candle because of the obvious dangers. Use those that can be placed on radiators or light bulbs, and follow the instructions of how to use the diffuser you have chosen.

Essential Oils

The following essential oils are briefly described, in alphabetical order, in the *Materia Medica*, together with the herbal uses.

Benzoin *Styrax benzoin*
Bergamot *Citrus bergamia*
Chamomile, German *Chamomilla matricaria*
Clary sage *Salvia sclarea*
Clove *Eugenia caryophyllus*
Cypress *Cupressus sempervirens*
Dill *Anethum graveolens*
Eucalyptus *Eucalyptus globulus*
Fennel *Foeniculum vulgare*
Frankincense *Boswellia carteri*
Geranium *Pelargonium* spp.
Ginger *Zingiber officinalis*
Hyssop *Hyssopus officinalis*
Lavender *Lavandula officinalis*
Lemon *Citrus limonum*
Marjoram *Origanum majorana*
Melissa *Melissa officinalis*
Pepper *Piper nigrum*
Peppermint *Mentha piperata*
Sandalwood *Santalum album*
Thyme *Thymus vulgaris*
Ti-tree *Melaleuca alternifolia*

▪ DOSES OF HERBS

Medicine is an art when it comes to deciding on doses, for people respond to the same herbs very differently. We discuss two doses: The *therapeutic* dose that we consider is the dose range of herbs needed to help when a child is ill. The *safe* dose is the maximum amount that can be taken without incurring any dangerous side effects.

Therapeutic Dose

For an herb to work, it must be given in a therapeutic dose, that is, the amount required to produce a therapeutic result. There are wide variations in people's response to herbs, so there is a corresponding wide range of therapeutic doses.

The subject of dosage is debated. Different herbal practitioners suggest using widely differing doses. The reason for this is to be found in the nature of herbs. A plant is alive, and as such it has energy. It also has material components that contain biomedically active plant drugs. Some practitioners use a large material dose, and others prefer a smaller dose based on the energy of the plant.

STANDARD THERAPEUTIC DOSE

In the *Materia Medica* we frequently refer to the standard dose. For 3-year-olds, this is as follows:

Tincture: 2 to 20 drops
Decoction and infusion: $1/3$ of a teacup

Safe Dose

The safe dose is the amount of herb that can be administered safely. For most of the herbs discussed in this book, the safe dose is much larger than the maximum therapeutic dose. However, you should not exceed the therapeutic dose. Doubling a dose does not mean doubling the effectiveness! If more than the safe dose is administered, significant adverse effects, such as vomiting, diarrhea, and abdominal pain, may occur. Herbs are much safer than most orthodox drugs, but herbs are medicines and there are always dangers when a child is sick. We have not included exact figures for safe doses because these are disputed and vary from herb to herb.

Recommended Dosages

Working with children we have found that giving small doses is very successful. Therefore the doses we recommend throughout this text are at the lower end of the therapeutic range. These doses may be too small or too large for a particular child. There is only one way to find out whether the dose is right, and that is to try it. Always start at the lowest end of the therapeutic range given, and if the dose is not sufficient, it may be increased *gradually*, up to the upper limit. The art of giving herbal medicine is finding the correct amount for the child you are treating.

There may be times when it is appropriate to give a large dose:

1. When the patient does not respond to small doses (Provided you are sure about your diagnosis and have ruled out any possibility of another underlying cause, it is appropriate to increase the dosage.)
2. In acute conditions in which there is no time to waste, and you feel that it is essential to get things moving

Dosage and the Age of the Child

Throughout this text we have given doses of herbs that we recommend for children 3 years old. Table 8-2 lists the guidelines for varying the recommended doses for children of different ages. These are *guidelines*, not strict rules; one cannot halve a drop of tincture! Small variations in dose normally do not affect the outcome.

▪ Case History

This story concerns a middle-age woman who had lived a difficult life. Her husband was a minor official in the diplomatic corps, and she followed him all over the

▪ Table 8-2	Variation of Dosage with Age
AGE	**MULTIPLY 3-YEAR-OLD DOSE BY**
6-12 months	$\times 1/3$
1-2 years	$\times 1/2$
2-4 years	$\times 1$
4-7 years	$\times 1 1/2$
7-14 years	$\times 2$
14+ years	$\times 3$

world, to whatever place he happened to be posted. This was difficult for her because she was a person who made friends only with difficulty.

Not surprisingly, from time to time she suffered from depression and insomnia. Also not surprising is that she took the conventional medicines offered by the embassy doctor. In this case he prescribed diazepam (Valium) to treat her depression and insomnia. The drug did not seem to do much for her. She ended up taking 10 times the recommended dose, and even then the effect was very mild.

At another time, her depression came out in the form of hypothyroidism. She was prescribed thyroxin. Once again, she hardly reacted at all and ended up taking huge doses. Fortunately, she had no more effect discontinuing these powerful drugs than she did in taking them in the first place.

When she came for a consultation, she was once again suffering from insomnia, for which she was recommended a cup of chamomile tea in the evening. This had a startling effect. Within 10 minutes she was yawning and simply could not keep her eyes open. There was a similar, but reverse, effect when she took dandelion tea: She found it so stimulating that she was up all night decorating her dining room. This is the sort of reaction that many people get from drinking coffee, but in her case she was impervious to the effects of coffee, tea, and normal stimulants. The only possible explanation for this unusual behavior is that she simply was not affected by physical substances but was enormously sensitive to the energy of plants.

■ WORKING OUT A PRESCRIPTION

In this book we give numerous prescriptions for the treatment of various illnesses. We consider these good starting points, but you as the practitioner or parent may wish to alter the herbs involved.

When working out a presc ription we believe that it is best done following some basic guidelines. Variations on these guidelines have been used in the Western herbal tradition (advocated especially by the physiomedicalists) and other cultures, such as the Chinese and Japanese, for many years. A prescription prepared on this basis gives very good results.

1. *Be clear about what it is you are trying to treat.* In Chinese medicine this is called the treatment principle. For example, it is common for a person to have a main complaint such as cough, with secondary complaints of poor appetite and poor sleep. It is important to be clear which one you are trying to help first and foremost.

2. *Decide on the main herb to treat the main problem (main herb).* The proportions of the herbs in the formula that treat the main complaint usually outweigh those that treat the secondary problems. In our example of cough with poor appetite and poor sleep, hyssop *Hyssopus officinale* would be the main herb because it is specific for cough and mucus in the lungs

3. *Add any herbs that may help the main herb work (helper herbs).* This is not always necessary. For example, in a cough medicine, white horehound *Marrubium vulgaris* may be added to help loosen mucus and resolve the cough.

4. *Add herbs for secondary problems (assistant herbs).* (These may be the same as 2 or 3.) Often, prescriptions use herbs that not only help secondary problems but also serve to help the main herbs in their task of treating the main problem. For example, in a cough medicine, the addition of aniseed *Pimpinella anisum* not only will support the main herb in eliminating cough but also will improve the appetite. Adding chamomile *Chamomilla matricaria* will strengthen the child's digestive system and help him or her sleep.

5. *Add herbs that reduce any overly strong effect in the prescription (moderators).* These are not always necessary. For example, if the prescription has only very Cold herbs, you will need to add an herb such as ginger to moderate this and to stop griping pains. This is not necessary in this specific example of a child with cough, poor appetite, and poor sleep because the herbs are well balanced.

6. *If necessary, add an additional herb that ensures that the energy of the prescription goes to the*

organ most affected (messenger herb). For example, in general, if you are using a main herb such as golden seal *Hydrastis canadensis* to eliminate mucus, especially in the lungs, add an herb such as coltsfoot *Tussilago farfara* to direct it to the lungs. This is not necessary in our specific example because the main

and helper herbs direct the energy to the lungs.

7. *If necessary, add a harmonizing herb.* Some herbs, notably licorice, have the effect of harmonizing and integrating a prescription. We add this to some of our prescriptions, but it is not always necessary.

9

Materia Medica

The purpose of this very abbreviated *Materia Medica* is to introduce the herbs that we mention in this book and give the reasons why we use them. We provide a summary of the herb's action and indications to enable readers to prepare their own prescriptions. The availability of herbs varies from place to place and from country to country. In Britain we have a particularly rich tradition of using herbs from all over the world, but in other countries there are some herbs that are banned and others that are simply not available. This *Materia Medica* will enable the reader to find substitute herbs.

We regret that limitations of space prevent us from giving as much detail about the herbs as we would like. In particular, we have had to resist the temptation to describe the lovely impression so many of these plants make when viewed growing in the wild. We have also excluded anything that does not have to do with the treatment of children. So, for example, yarrow *Achillea millefolium* and hawthorn *Crataegus monogyna* both have their uses in the treatment of high blood pressure. Hawthorn is also used mainly for heart weakness in adults. Because neither of these problems are common in children, we have not included this information here.

■ NOMENCLATURE

At the time of writing, the botanical names of plants are being revised. For example, some plants are being reclassified into different families in the light of new genetic information. The spelling of other plants changes from time to time. The result is that there is no commonly agreed naming and spelling for many of the herbs. We have taken a pragmatic, rather than scholarly, approach, using the names that are in the catalogues of the herbal suppliers.

■ TERMINOLOGY

We have tried to avoid specialist terms such as *cholagogue* and *diaphoretic*. This may irritate the practitioner, but we hope it will make it easier for parents to understand. There is one term for which we have not found a substitute, and that is *alterative*.

What Is an Alterative?

The term *alterative* denotes a classification of herbs that was in widespread use in the nineteenth and early twentieth centuries. It is based on the idea that the blood could become "impure" or "dirty." When this happened, external signs of the body trying to "throw out the dirt" were evident. These signs included spots, boils, pus formation, and eczema. The patients themselves would be inclined to mood swings, with perhaps depression or outbursts of rage. An alterative is a herb that "cleanses the blood."

This idea has been part of the herbalists tradition for the last 200 years, but after the discovery of antibiotics, attention was focussed more on the immune system than on the condition of the blood. The idea is regaining popularity with the development of leaky gut syndrome, in which there is the idea of impurities leaking into the blood through faulty functioning of the intestines (see Chapter 2).

As the fundamental ideas of medicine evolve, so do the terms; now the term *alterative* is not as useful because it covers two functions. The first is to invigorate and clear the lymph system. This is what we call "softening thick mucus," and many alteratives have a special use for echo patterns. When the lymph system is clearer, fluids circulate better in the body. This explains the secondary function that many alteratives have—that is, being diuretic.

The other function is to stimulate the liver in its detoxifying function. Any impurities in the blood that are not dealt with by the immune system are broken down in the liver. When this function becomes sluggish, a child feels irritable and may have skin problems, too. This explains why alteratives are often used as tonics, as well as for skin problems.

■ HERBS

Achillea millefolium

YARROW
Parts Used. Whole plant.

Actions
- Brings out perspiration in fevers, warms
- Stimulates and tones

Indications
BRINGS OUT PERSPIRATION IN FEVERS, WARMS. Yarrow's special uses are for fevers and when the child is cold. It is helpful in all stages of fever. When the child is cold, it is second to none in warming the child and promoting perspiration.

STIMULATES AND TONES. Yarrow is also a tonic, so it can be used if the child is Weak or Strong and lost all strength from sweating. It can also be used in the few days after the fever has gone down to restore the child's appetite and strength.

As a preventative, it may be combined with hawthorn *Crataegus monogyna* in equal amounts as a general tonic, especially in spring to dispel the tendency to fevers.

OTHER. Yarrow has many other traditional uses as well, among which are the following:

- To provide relief in the first stage of measles, when the symptoms are those of an ordinary fever, and in the middle stage of measles, to bring out the rash
- To stop bleeding (as in nosebleeds) and help poorly healing wounds
- For relief of night cramps
- For treatment of boils and spots

Dose. To bring down a fever in 3-year-old children, make a tea with 1 tsp dried herb to each cup; $\frac{1}{4}$ to $\frac{1}{2}$ cup per dose. Alternatively, use 0.5 to 1 ml of tincture in warm or hot water. Give every 2 hours.

Safe Dose. Standard.

Contraindications. None.

Comments. Yarrow is a very interesting plant biochemically because it has many active components. It seems that many of these components become active only in certain conditions, remaining inactive in other conditions. This is why yarrow can have so many different actions, simultaneously toning and dispersing.

Acorus calamus

SWEET SEDGE (SWEET FLAG)
Parts Used. Roots.

Actions
- Stimulates digestion and the stomach
- Reduces abdominal gas
- Helps teething
- Promotes flow of bile
- Circulates water

Indications
STIMULATES DIGESTION AND THE STOMACH. Sweet sedge stimulates digestion in general and the appetite in particular. It is very effective when

taken with wormwood *Artemisia absinthium* and woodruff *Asperula odorata* in equal amounts, as a motion sickness mixture, but it is very bitter.

REDUCES ABDOMINAL GAS. Sweet sedge is effective for relieving indigestion with colic and flatulence.

HELPS TEETHING. A traditional use for the whole root is for teething babies. It was given to them to suck on. Although quite bitter, when sucked, the aromatic tastes come to the fore, and the whole root soothes painful gums.

PROMOTES FLOW OF BILE. Sweet sedge assists in digestion of rich foods. It can be given to those children who cannot take any fried food, butter, or cream without feeling unwell to help reduce the amount of uneasiness they feel after eating these foods.

CIRCULATES WATER. Sweet sedge has a diuretic effect in some children. This is because it circulates water that has accumulated in the abdomen.

Dose. Standard.

Safe Dose. Standard.

Contraindications. None.

Cautions. Sweet sedge is prohibited in some areas because minute amounts of carcinogen have been detected in some subspecies.

Agrimonia eupatoria

AGRIMONY
Parts Used. Dried flowering tops.

Actions
- Is a tonic and an astringent
- Stimulates the liver and the flow of bile
- Is a diuretic

Indications
IS A TONIC AND AN ASTRINGENT. Agrimony is a tonic for digestion and an astringent, so it is help-

ful in reversing all fluid imbalance conditions. It is used especially for treatment of loose stools and diarrhea in Weak children and those with poor appetites.

STIMULATES THE LIVER AND FLOW OF BILE. Agrimony helps stop diarrhea, but it does not cause constipation. This is because it generally tones and moves digestion by stimulating the flow of bile.

IS A DIURETIC. The toning effect on digestion and its astringent property mean that agrimony helps with water retention, thereby increasing the amount of urine produced.

Dose. Standard.

Safe Dose. Standard.

Contraindications. None.

Allium sativum

GARLIC
Parts Used. Bulb.

Actions
- Helps combat infection—antibiotic and antiviral
- Brings out perspiration in fevers, warms
- Thins and reduces excess catarrh

Indications
HELPS COMBAT INFECTION—ANTIBIOTIC AND ANTIVIRAL. Garlic is used internally to treat all infections. It may also be applied locally to infected wounds.

BRINGS OUT PERSPIRATION IN FEVERS, WARMS. Garlic is more effective in treating Cold infections because it warms the child up and causes a beneficial perspiration.

THINS AND REDUCES EXCESS CATARRH. Garlic has a special affinity for the lungs and upper respiratory tract, where it thins and reduces the quantity of mucus. Very often, garlic is used to treat bronchial conditions and colds. A traditional remedy for whooping cough is to apply crushed garlic to the soles of the feet overnight. The oil is used externally to treat earaches, warts, ringworm infections, and stings.

Dose. The dose is 70 mg of garlic oil. It is normally taken as garlic capsules. Read the instructions on the packet to see how much each capsule contains and to ensure that no unwanted ingredients are present.

Contraindications. Do not use garlic when the child has conjunctivitis because when taken internally, garlic tends to irritate the eyes.

Cautions. Some babies and children have delicate skin, and leaving a garlic plaster in place overnight may cause the skin to blister.

Comments. It is best to use the fresh bulb, but it is much easier to use capsules of the oil.

Althea officinalis

MARSHMALLOW
Parts Used. Leaves (for lung complaints), roots (for digestive complaints).

Actions
- Cools and soothes

Indications
COOLS AND SOOTHES. Marshmallow is one of the best demulcents in that it is soothing to nearly all the mucous membranes. When combined with the appropriate messenger, this herb can be used for inflammation virtually anywhere in the body. Hence it is used for bronchitis when combined with other herbs for the chest, such as plantain *Plantago lanceolata.* It is used for inflammation of the digestive tract when used with digestive herbs, such as golden seal *Hydrastis canadensis.* It is used for cystitis when combined with diuretics, such as maize *Zea mays.* It may also be used as a mouthwash for mouth ulcers and sore or inflamed gums.

The root is also used for inflammation of the digestive tract, especially the stomach and intestines. It may help in constipation when the stools are very dry.

Dose. Larger-than-normal quantities are required for marshmallow to be effective. Give 1 heaped tsp (5 g) of dried herb, or $\frac{1}{4}$ tsp (1 ml) of tincture, in each dose (for a 3-year-old).

Safe Dose. Standard.

Contraindications. None.

Cautions. Do not use any iron utensils with this herb because iron interferes with its action.

Anemone pulsatilla

PASQUE FLOWER
Parts Used. Leaves.

Actions
- Is a tonic for the nerves and cools
- Relaxes spasms and cramps
- Clears rashes
- Reduces mucus

Indications
IS A TONIC FOR THE NERVES AND COOLS. Pasque flower is used mainly as a calming and relaxing herb. It is useful in treating insomnia and hyperactivity, especially the Hot types.

RELAXES SPASMS AND CRAMPS. Pasque flower relieves spasmodic coughs and is particularly recommended when the child is emotional and bursts into tears at the slightest thing. It eases spasmodic pains in the body and tension headache.

CLEARS RASHES. Pasque flower brings out rashes of measles when they are slow to appear.

REDUCES MUCUS. When the Hot type of cough is accompanied by yellow mucus, pasque flower helps reduce both the mucus and the Hot energy.

Dose. The dose is $\frac{1}{3}$ the standard, that is, 1 drop for a 3-year-old.

Safe Dose. Do not exceed the dose listed here.

Contraindications. None (see Cautions).

Cautions. In some patients pasque flower can give rise to quite severe intestinal pains. If this happens, seek the advice of an herbalist. A very safe dose for adults is 2 to 3 drops of tincture, for children it is 1 drop. For babies, put 1 drop in a teacup of water and give half the water. Do not use the fresh plant, for it is poisonous in large doses. Always use the dried herb.

Anethum graveolens

DILL

Parts used. Seeds, essential oil.

Actions
- Warms and tones the digestive system
- Increases the quantity and quality of the mother's milk

Indications

WARMS AND TONES THE DIGESTIVE SYSTEM. Dill is very useful in treating many digestive complaints, especially colic, for which it is usually prepared as a tea. The essential oil is also used as massage oil for babies and children, with the same effect on digestion.

INCREASES THE QUANTITY AND QUALITY OF THE MOTHER'S MILK. For mothers who have difficulty producing enough milk, a tea of dill seeds often makes an enormous difference. The quantity and richness of the milk increases within a few hours.

Dose. Dill is best given in quite large quantities, for example, as a tea, 1 level tsp (5 g) of dried herb to 50 ml of water. Although it has a sweet flavor, many children like to have it sweetened or some extra flavor added.

Safe Dose. Standard.

Contraindications. None.

Comments. There are three similar herbs in the same family: dill, fennel *Foeniculum vulgaris,* and aniseed *Pimpinella anisum.* They all have similar actions. Aniseed is more aromatic, and dill less aromatic than fennel. The more aromatic the herb is, the more effective it is at "dispersing," and therefore better at reducing flatulence. This is one of the guides to choose one herb rather than another.

Angelica archangelica

ANGELICA

Parts Used. Roots, leaves.

Actions
- Expels mucus from the lungs
- Tones the digestive system
- Warms
- Soothes colic

Indications

EXPELS MUCUS FROM THE LUNGS. Angelica is an expectorant and a warming tonic, so it is specific for all Weak and Cold energy patterns of coughs and colds. We use it especially for chronic coughs because both the lungs and the digestion need to be treated.

TONES THE DIGESTIVE SYSTEM. It strengthens the digestive system and appetite, so it is used when convalescing after any infectious illness, especially when there is some residual mucus.

WARMS. Angelica has a gentle warming effect when a child is feeling chilly and withdrawn. It also warms digestion when it is too Cold, enabling the child to take cold foods and drink.

SOOTHES COLIC. Angelica's warming and tonic effect on digestion make it useful for relieving the spasmodic pains of colic.

Dose. Standard.

Safe Dose. Standard.

Contraindications. None.

Anthemis nobilis

ROMAN CHAMOMILE (COMMON CHAMOMILE)
See *Chamomilla matricaria* (German chamomile)

Arctium lappa

BURDOCK
    Parts Used. Roots, leaves, seeds.

Actions

- Nourishes the skin/alterative for lymphatic congestion
- Increases the flow of bile
- Clears the stagnant food pattern
- Is a diuretic
- Reduces rash in measles (seeds only)

Indications

NOURISHES THE SKIN/ALTERATIVE FOR LYMPHATIC CONGESTION. Burdock *root* is used in many skin complaints: eczema, acne, and boils. It improves the skin after chickenpox.

INCREASES THE FLOW OF BILE. Burdock affects the skin by stimulating liver function and promoting the flow of bile, thus helping remove toxins from the blood.

CLEARS THE STAGNANT FOOD PATTERN. Burdock may be used in children with the stagnant food pattern to move digestion. It is also a tonic for weak digestive systems.

IS A DIURETIC. By stimulating the liver and moving digestion, any accumulations of water are also moved, thereby increasing the quantity of urine produced.

REDUCES RASH IN MEASLES. Burdock *seeds* are difficult to find (except of course in the wild, where they are just as easy to find as the root and at phar-

macies selling Chinese herbs). They have a special use for reducing the livid red rash in measles.

Dose. Standard.

Safe Dose. Standard.

Contraindications. None.

Arnica montana

ARNICA (WOLFSBANE)
    Parts Used. Petals.

Actions

- Heals bruises and swellings, especially those caused by injury

Indications

HEALS BRUISES AND SWELLINGS, ESPECIALLY THOSE CAUSED BY INJURY. Used as a tincture, arnica is applied to a compress placed on bruised and swollen areas.

Dose. In homeopathic doses, it is a wonder medicine for treating all types of trauma. There are three situations in which it can make a huge difference to a person's life:

- *Head injury, concussion:* One of the main dangers of head injury comes from the rise in intracranial pressure after the injury. This is similar to the swelling that occurs around a bruise, but because there is nowhere for the fluid to go, it causes the pressure to rise. If Arnica 30C is given every 2 hours, it can often control the pressure so that no damage results.
- *Surgical interventions:* Taking Anica homeopathically, both before an operation and immediately after, can halve the time needed for recuperation and can greatly reduce postoperative pain.
- *Serious back injury:* The same process is at work when the back is badly injured. Lasting paralysis is often not caused by severing of the nerves but rather by local accumulation of

fluid, which causes great pressure locally in the nerves. Timely application of Anica can prevent this.

Safe Dose. The plant is not normally taken internally, except in homeopathic form. The safe dose for homeopathy is 3 tablets a day for 14 days.

Contraindications. Do not apply tincture to broken or sensitive skin.

Cautions. Repeated application may cause skin rash or irritation. Take internally only in homeopathic form—the herbal dose is an irritant to the digestive system, and larger doses may cause heart palpitations.

Ballota nigra

BLACK HOREHOUND
Parts Used. Aerial parts of plant.

Actions
- Reduces vomiting, calms the nerves, and is an astringent

Indications
REDUCES VOMITING, CALMS THE NERVES, AND IS AN ASTRINGENT. Black horehound is used to reduce nausea and vomiting, especially of nervous origin, and to treat motion sickness.

Dose. Standard.

Safe Dose. Standard.

Contraindications. None.

Berberis aquifolium, Mahonia aquifolia

OREGON GRAPE (MOUNTAIN GRAPE, MAHONIA)
Parts Used. Rhizome, root.

Actions
- Stimulates bile and is a gentle laxative
- Is an alterative for lymphatic congestion

- Tones
- Helps eliminate mucus

Indications
STIMULATES BILE AND IS A GENTLE LAXATIVE. Oregon grape is used as a digestive stimulant to the liver. This action produces a moving, mild laxative effect, which makes it useful in treating chronic constipation.

IS AN ALTERATIVE FOR LYMPHATIC CONGESTION. As an alterative for lymphatic congestion, Oregon grape stimulates the liver. It is also used to treat skin conditions.

TONES. While stimulating the movement of digestion, Oregon grape also improves the absorption of food, so is a digestive tonic. It can be used in children with Weak patterns.

HELPS ELIMINATE MUCUS. Oregon grape is especially useful in mucous conditions to clear mucus through the digestion. It is combined with herbs for treatment of chronic cough.

Dose. Standard.

Safe Dose. Standard.

Contraindications. None.

Comments. Some practitioners use Oregon grape interchangeably with golden seal *Hydrastis canadensis,* but Oregon grape has a stronger effect on the liver and is more strongly moving.

Berberis vulgaris

BARBERRY
Parts Used. Bark of root or stem.

Actions
- Stimulates the liver and digestive system
- Promotes the flow of bile

Indications
STIMULATES THE LIVER AND DIGESTIVE SYSTEM. Barberry is mainly used to stimulate liver function

and in children with Weak digestion. Its action is similar to that of Oregon grape *Berberis aquifolium*, although barberry has more effect on stimulating the stomach.

PROMOTES THE FLOW OF BILE. Barberry is a mild laxative through its effect on stimulating the flow of bile.

Dose. Standard.

Safe Dose. Standard.

Contraindications. None.

Boswellia carteri

FRANKINCENSE
Parts Used. Essential oil.

Actions and Indications. Frankincense is very relaxing and calming. It has a special effect in slowing and calming the breathing so that one can take full deep breaths. It is also an antibacterial and antiviral. These two indications together make it an invaluable remedy in treating acute asthma attacks.

Dose. Standard *for essential oils.*

Safe Dose. Standard *for essential oils.*

Contraindications. For external use only. Do not take internally.

Capsicum minimum

CAYENNE
Parts Used. Fruit.

Actions
- Is a strong heating stimulant to the entire system
- Aids digestion

Indications
IS A STRONG HEATING STIMULANT TO THE ENTIRE SYSTEM. Cayenne increases the metabolic rate and, in so doing, increases blood circulation, producing a natural warmth. It is suitable for all Cold conditions, and any condition in which a part of the child is cold, such as a cold sensation on the abdomen or cold hands and feet.

AIDS DIGESTION. Cayenne warms and stimulates digestion, so it is indicated for Cold and Weak children (if they can be persuaded to take it). In other children it is used for the symptoms of colic, flatulence, and indigestion.

Dose. The dose is one fourth the standard.

Safe Dose. Maximum of 5 drops.

Contraindications. In all Hot conditions, for it will heat these children further. Thus it is to be avoided in the Hot type of cough.

Comments. We use it perhaps less than is indicated because many children object to its burning taste.

Chamomilla matricaria

GERMAN CHAMOMILE
Parts Used. Flowers.

Actions
- Calms and tones the digestive system
- Settles overexcitement
- Soothes the pain of teething
- Soothes colic
- Promotes perspiration in fevers

Indications
CALMS AND TONES THE DIGESTIVE SYSTEM. German chamomile helps an enormous range of problems in children and is perhaps the first herb to try for any digestive or emotional complaint.

SETTLES OVEREXCITEMENT. German chamomile is particularly recommended when the child is "overheated," especially when this is accompanied by rage. Thus this herb is good for the Strong child who is red-faced and screaming. German chamomile is the first remedy to try for sleeping problems and general overexcitement.

SOOTHES THE PAIN OF TEETHING. Many of these symptoms accompany teething, so German chamomile the first remedy to try for those sleepless nights. If the tea does not work, homeopathic Chamomilla 6X may work.

SOOTHES COLIC. German chamomile is one of the first remedies to try if the baby or toddler has colic.

PROMOTES PERSPIRATION IN FEVERS. This herb is also good for fevers. This makes it especially useful when a fever is accompanied by the stagnant food pattern.

Dose. Make the tea to a pale straw color and sweeten as desired. For babies 1 tsp (5 ml) of the tea is enough; for children $\frac{1}{2}$ to 1 cup should be given.

Safe Dose. Standard.

Contraindications. None.

Comments. Many practitioners use German chamomile interchangeably with Roman chamomile *Anthemis nobilis.* For children the German chamomile is preferred, especially as a tea, because it tastes better. Roman chamomile is more bitter and is somewhat stronger in its action on the digestive system and mucous membranes.

Essential Oil. The essential oil is a deep blue and has many of the same functions as the herb. It is soothing, calming, and an antiinflammatory. It is used for tension, anxiety, and all digestive problems in children. It is also of great use in earaches when diluted in warm oil and dropped into the ears.

Chelone glabra (Original Name *Celone glabra*)

BALMONY
Parts Used. Whole plant above ground.

Actions
- Increases the secretion of bile, works as a mild laxative
- Stimulates and relaxes

Indications
INCREASES THE SECRETION OF BILE, WORKS AS A MILD LAXATIVE. By increasing the secretion of bile, balmony helps with the digestion of fats. It also has a gentle laxative effect.

STIMULATES AND RELAXES. Balmony is useful in digestive problems accompanied by emotional tension and stagnation, where relaxation and movement are needed more than a pure tonic. Thus it helps colic and indigestion seen in association with a lack of exercise.

Dose. Standard.

Safe Dose. Standard.

Contraindications. None.

Chionanthus virginicus

FRINGE TREE
Parts Used. Bark of roots.

Actions
- Assists digestive function of the liver
- Is a moving tonic
- Is a mild diuretic

Indications
ASSISTS DIGESTIVE FUNCTION OF THE LIVER. Fringe tree is one of the most important remedies for sluggish digestion, especially for difficulty in digesting fats. It may be used for poor appetite and irritability. It is especially beneficial for those who have a red tongue with a yellow coat. Fringe tree is good for children, particularly those older than 7 years, who have stress-related digestive problems. It also helps the digestive system recover when it has been weakened by a bad attack of diarrhea.

IS A MOVING TONIC. Fringe tree's tonic nature arises because it gets the digestion moving, thereby enabling it to work well (as with balmony *Chelone glabra*); it is not a pure tonic. Thus it is not so suitable for pale, Weak children.

IS A MILD DIURETIC. Retained water is eliminated when digestion improves.

Dose. Standard.

Safe Dose. Standard.

Contraindications. Fringe tree promotes the flow of bile and has a laxative effect, so it should not be given to children with acute diarrhea.

Cimicifuga racemosa

BLACK COHOSH
Parts Used. Root.

Actions
- Relaxes spasms and calms

Indications
RELAXES SPASMS AND CALMS. Black cohosh is mainly used for adults, but it may be used to relax spasms in some coughs, whooping cough, and asthma.

Dose. Standard.

Safe Dose. Standard.

Contraindications. None.

Citrus bergamia

BERGAMOT
Parts Used. Essential oil.

Actions
- Regulates digestion
- Promotes perspiration in fevers

Indications
REGULATES DIGESTION. Bergamot can be used to treat loss of appetite, particularly when associated with anxiety and tension. It also helps in overeating.

PROMOTES PERSPIRATION IN FEVERS. Bergamot helps bring down the temperature in fevers.

Dose. Standard *for essential oils.*

Safe Dose. Standard *for essential oils.*

Contraindications. For external use only. Do not take internally.

Citrus limonum

LEMON
Parts Used. Essential oil.

Actions
- Is a bactericidal, thins and reduces excess catarrh

Indications
IS A BACTERICIDAL, THINS AND REDUCES EXCESS CATARRH. Lemon is used in mucous conditions, especially those affecting digestion, such as vomiting mucus, and for poor appetite as a result of excess mucus.

Dose. Standard *for essential oils.*

Safe Dose. Standard *for essential oils.*

Contraindications. For external use only. Do not take internally.

Comments. The oil is taken from the rind. Lemon juice also has anticatarrhal properties. Honey* and lemon drink, taken warm, is good for all coughs and fevers.

Collinsonia canadensis

STONE ROOT
Parts Used. Root.

---

*Honey should not be used for children younger than 1 year. See caution on p. 67.

Actions

- Is a diuretic, promotes perspiration, eases pain in the anus

Indications

IS A DIURETIC, PROMOTES PERSPIRATION, EASES PAIN IN THE ANUS. Stone root strengthens the whole of the lumbar and pelvic region, so it is used mainly in adults. Its use in children is to ease pain in the anus on passing stools and for treatment of bedwetting. It can also be used with other herbs as a tonic for the large intestine.

Dose. Standard.

Safe Dose. Standard.

Contraindications. None.

Crataegus monogyna, C. oxyacantha, C. laevigata

HAWTHORN
Parts Used. Flesh around the berries.

Actions

- Strengthens the heart and circulation
- Calms

Indications

STRENGTHENS THE HEART AND CIRCULATION. The main use for hawthorn in adults is to strengthen the heart. It may also be used in the rare children who have heart weakness.

CALMS. In children, hawthorn is effective for treating insomnia resulting from either overstimulation or weakness. It calms a child who is agitated, and by strengthening the output of the heart, it helps sleep in children with Weak energy.

Dose. Standard.

Safe Dose. Standard.

Contraindications. None.

Comments. The three species of Crataegus have identical properties. *Crataegus* is famed for being "amphoteric," that is, having a balancing effect. If the heart is overactive, this herb calms it down. If the heart is weak, it acts as a tonic. Thus this is a very safe remedy. We see this dual effect in the indications for children—it is good for the Strong type of insomnia, as well as the Weak type.

Another variety of *Crataegus* is used in China to help digestion in babies and toddlers. For this purpose it is made into candy flakes. Our experience is that *C. monogyna* also has this effect, even though it is not commonly used for it.

Cupressus sempervirens

CYPRESS
Parts Used. Essential oil.

Actions and Indications. Cypress has both astringent and antispasmodic properties. It is used as a massage oil for acute asthma attacks because of its antispasmodic properties. It is of special use when there is a lot of diluted watery mucus.

Dose. Standard *for essential oils.*

Safe Dose. Standard *for essential oils.*

Contraindications. For external use only. Do not take internally.

Dioscorea villosa

WILD YAM
Parts Used. Root.

Actions

- Reduces spasms, stimulates liver function

Indications

REDUCES SPASMS, STIMULATES LIVER FUNCTION. Wild yam is mainly used for relaxing muscular spasms. It eases pain in the intestines and is therefore used to treat colic and flatulence when accompanied by griping pains.

Dose. Standard.

Safe Dose. Standard.

Contraindications. None.

Drosera rotundifolia

SUNDEW
Parts Used. Whole plant.

Actions
- Relaxes spasms and cramps, clears mucus from the lungs
- Is an antibacterial

Indications
RELAXES SPASMS AND CRAMPS, CLEARS MUCUS FROM THE LUNGS. Sundew is specific for whooping cough, for which it is often combined with thyme *Thymus vulgaris.*

IS AN ANTIBACTERIAL. Sundew has been shown to have antibiotic effects against *Staphylococcus, Streptococcus,* and *Pneumococcus* bacteria.

Dose. Standard.

Safe Dose. Standard.

Contraindications. None.

Echinacea purpurea/angustifolia

ECHINACEA (RUDBECKIA, CONE FLOWER)
Parts Used. Roots, rhizome.

Actions
- Stimulates the immune system
- Reduces mucus
- Purifies the blood, antiseptic
- Is an antibiotic

Indications
STIMULATES THE IMMUNE SYSTEM. The special use for echinacea is to "rally" the immune system, so it is useful in treating all infections, whether viral or bacterial. If taken when a cold is just appearing, it can avert the cold. Tests have shown that if taken during a cough or any infection, echinacea can shorten the course of the infection. It can be taken as a simple but is often combined with other herbs to reach specific organs (e.g., with coltsfoot *Tussilago farfara* for infection in the lungs). When used in children with Weak patterns, it should be combined with tonics.

REDUCES MUCUS. Echinacea's effect in reducing mucus is most conspicuous in acute chest infections. It is less effective for chronic coughs.

PURIFIES THE BLOOD, ANTISEPTIC. Echinacea is especially useful for conditions in which the body produces pus, such as boils and ulcers. It works by purifying the blood so that the body condition is no longer favorable for the growth of staphylococci. Its effect in purifying the blood makes it useful as an assistant herb in skin eruptions, measles, and chickenpox. It is used both internally and externally as a wash on the affected areas.

IS AN ANTIBIOTIC. In vitro tests have shown that echinacea has an antibiotic effect.

Dose. The dose is 50 mg of the root or $\frac{1}{4}$ tsp (1 ml) of the tincture in water for each dose.

Safe Dose. Standard.

Contraindications. None.

Comments. Echinacea has been promoted by the health industry as a wonder herb and is added to many over-the-counter herb preparations, often unsuitably. There is no evidence that long-term use benefits the body. On the contrary, it seems that long-term use actually weakens the immune system.

Ephedra sinensis

EPHEDRA
Parts Used. Aerial parts of entire plant.

Actions

- Is a strong general stimulant and circulatory stimulant, relaxes spasms and cramps

Indications

IS A STRONG GENERAL STIMULANT AND CIRCULATORY STIMULANT, RELAXES SPASMS AND CRAMPS. Ephedra is little used in childhood complaints, except for treatment of acute asthma and acute allergic response. It has a very powerful effect in relaxing spasms in the lungs, so it can relieve an acute attack of asthma.

Dose. Standard.

Safe Dose. Do not exceed the therapeutic dose.

Contraindications. Do not use in Weak children for more than 2 to 3 days. There are also adult conditions for which ephedra is contraindicated.

Cautions. Ephedra is a very powerful herb and should normally be taken with other herbs to modify its action.

Eucalyptus globulus

EUCALYPTUS
Parts Used. Essential oil.

Actions

- Reduces mucous congestion
- Is an antibacterial and antiviral
- Cools

Indications

REDUCES MUCOUS CONGESTION. Eucalyptus has been used for centuries to relieve the discomfort of colds and to soothe and calm catarrhal coughs. A few drops on a handkerchief are enormously refreshing.

IS AN ANTIBACTERIAL AND ANTIVIRAL. Eucalyptus can be used in a vaporizer so that the disinfecting aroma fills the entire room. Studies in China have shown that doing this reduces the spread of both viral and bacterial infections.

COOLS. Eucalyptus lowers body temperature, so it can be used as a massage oil for all fevers. It can safely be used in children with measles and chickenpox and especially in children with croup, bronchitis, and asthma.

Eugenia caryophyllata

CLOVES
Parts Used. Essential oil.

Actions

- Relieves flatulence, relaxes spasms and cramps
- Calms pain in the gums

Indications

RELIEVES FLATULENCE, RELAXES SPASMS AND CRAMPS. Cloves are especially helpful at relieving the flatulence and colic that arise from eating beans. The flatulence that develops in some babies who take soy formula can likewise be greatly reduced by including clove oil in an abdominal massage.

CALMS PAIN IN THE GUMS. Clove oil (diluted in a carrier oil) applied directly to the gums can help in very severe cases of teething. Neat oil is used in adults, but one should dilute 1 part of essential oil to 5 parts carrier before applying to the gums of babies.

Dose. Standard *for essential oils.*

Safe Dose. Standard *for essential oils.*

Contraindications. None.

Comments. In this book we describe only the use of the essential oil.

Euphorbia pilulifera

PILL-BEARING SPURGE
Parts Used. Flowers, tops of whole plant.

Actions

- Clears mucus from the lungs, relaxes spasms and cramps

Indications

CLEARS MUCUS FROM THE LUNGS, RELAXES SPASMS AND CRAMPS. Pill-bearing spurge relaxes spasms in the chest, so it is used in acute asthma and harsh spasmodic coughs, such as bronchitis and croup. Through relaxation it helps expel mucus from the lungs.

Dose. Standard.

Safe Dose. Three times therapeutic dose.

Contraindications. None.

Cautions. Do not use in overrelaxed conditions.

Filipendula ulmaria

MEADOWSWEET (QUEEN OF THE MEADOW)
Parts Used. Whole plant.

Actions
- Soothes and cools the stomach
- Is an astringent

Indications

SOOTHES AND COOLS THE STOMACH. Meadowsweet, a very cooling herb, is recommended for management of fevers and stomach problems, especially those of a Hot nature. It soothes inflammation, which is experienced as burning in the digestive tract. It is helpful in gastric reflux and projectile vomiting (which are mainly attributable to heat).

IS AN ASTRINGENT. Meadowsweet's astringent action makes it the one of the most effective herbs for treatment of diarrhea in children.

Dose. Standard.

Safe Dose. Standard.

Contraindications. None.

Foeniculum vulgaris

FENNEL
Parts Used. Seeds, essential oil.

Actions
- Aids digestion and soothes colic
- Tones the digestive system
- Clears mucus from the lungs
- Increases milk supply in nursing mothers
- Relaxes spasms and cramps

Indications

AIDS DIGESTION AND SOOTHES COLIC. Fennel is the prime herbal remedy for babies because it gently assists digestion, relieves flatulence, and calms colic.

TONES THE DIGESTIVE SYSTEM. Fennel is the main remedy for children with the Weak digestion pattern, for which it can be combined with licorice *Glycyrrhiza glabra*. Both of these herbs taste quite good and are fairly sweet, but even then, some children will not take them. This is especially true of overstimulated Weak children. For these children, fennel tea may be added to the bath water.

CLEARS MUCUS FROM THE LUNGS. Fennel can be used to expel mucus in coughs. For this it is normally used with other herbs that have a stronger action on the lungs.

INCREASES MILK SUPPLY IN NURSING MOTHERS. In this fennel is similar to dill *Anethum graveolens*, although dill is normally preferred slightly over fennel.

RELAXES SPASMS AND CRAMPS. The essential oil has most of the properties of the seeds when used as massage oil for the abdomen. In this use it is slightly more antispasmodic than the seeds.

Dose. Best given in quite large quantities, for example, as a tea, 1 level tsp (5 g) of dried herb to 50 ml of water. Although it has quite a sweet flavor, many children like to have something sweet added.

Safe Dose. Standard.

Contraindications. None.

Comments. There are three similar herbs in the same family: fennel, dill *Anethum graveolens,* and aniseed *Pimpinella anisum.* They all have similar actions. Aniseed is more aromatic, and dill less aromatic than fennel. The more aromatic the herb is, the more effective it is at reducing flatulence, and this is one of the guides to choose one herb rather than another.

Galium aparine

CLEAVERS
Parts Used. Dried aerial plant, fresh juice.

Actions
- Is a diuretic, astringent
- Is an alterative for lymphatic congestion

Indications
IS A DIURETIC, ASTRINGENT. Cleavers are used in fluid imbalance conditions in which there is a tendency for water accumulation. Sometimes cleavers are used as an astringent and diuretic to "drain" the fluid. Cleavers can be used for children with head colds and runny noses.

IS AN ALTERATIVE FOR LYMPHATIC CONGESTION. Cleavers stimulate the lymph system and decongest it. Therefore cleavers are used for treatment of echo diseases and many skin problems.

Dose. Standard.

Safe Dose. Standard.

Contraindications. None.

Gentiana lutea

GREAT YELLOW GENTIAN
Parts Used. Roots.

Actions
- Tones the stomach and the whole body
- Promotes the flow of bile
- Helps expel intestinal worms

Indications
TONES THE STOMACH AND THE WHOLE BODY. Gentian is a tonic for all Weak conditions, especially after illness, when appetite is poor. Gentian helps stop the Weak pattern of vomiting and is useful in treating all forms of indigestion. When taken before a meal, it can improve a poor appetite. A disadvantage is the bitter taste, which has a cumulative effect, becoming more intense as more herb is taken. What is more, research seems to indicate that the actual sensation of bitterness is an important factor in its action; therefore, if gentian is given in capsules, it seems to be less effective. Surprisingly, there are many children who will actually take the herb!

PROMOTES THE FLOW OF BILE. On its own, gentian may cure mild attacks of the stagnant food pattern, but it is more effective when combined with black root *Leptandra virginica.*

HELPS EXPEL INTESTINAL WORMS. When worms are being treated, the main herbs used are anthelmintics such as wormwood *Artemisia vulgaris* and cathartics such as senna *Cassia angustifolia.* Gentian is used as a tonic to help overcome the weakening effect of the cathartic.

Dose. Standard.

Safe Dose. Standard.

Contraindications. None.

Cautions. Large doses are said to cause vomiting, but it is unlikely that any child would take such a large dose.

Comments. Gentian is a great tonic for the stomach, and unlike ginger, it is slightly cooling. However, in the doses that children are likely to take, this cooling effect is small.

Geranium maculatum

AMERICAN CRANESBILL
Parts Used. Whole plant.

Actions
- Is an astringent

Indications
IS AN ASTRINGENT. American cranesbill may be used for all form of diarrhea, dysentery, and similar conditions, acute and chronic. It is also used to stop bleeding of all types. Its astringent effect makes it useful in treating incontinence and bedwetting. All the geraniums have similar indications, and herb Robert (*Geranium robertiana*) may be substituted.

Dose. Twice the standard dose.

Safe Dose. Standard.

Contraindications. None.

Pelargonium Species

GERANIUM
Parts Used. Essential oil.

Actions and Indications. Geranium is relaxing and invigorating to the skin and lymphatic system. It is used mainly for eczema, especially the wet kind. Some people find the oil relaxing, but others are overstimulated by it.

Dose. Standard *for essential oils.*

Safe Dose. Standard *for essential oils.*

Contraindications. For external use only. Do not take internally.

Comments. The oil known as *geranium oil* is derived from the pot plant of that name, which is in fact a pelargonium. The most commonly used variety for the essential oil is *P. odoratissimum.*

Gingko biloba

GINGKO
Parts Used. Leaves.

Actions
- Is an astringent, clears mucus from the lungs, calms the nerves, tones the lungs

Indications
IS AN ASTRINGENT, CLEARS MUCUS FROM THE LUNGS, CALMS THE NERVES, TONES THE LUNGS. Gingko expels mucus from the chest and is used to stop the symptoms of cough. It is used occasionally in the treatment of some asthmatic conditions if the child is very weak.

Dose. Standard.

Safe Dose. Standard.

Contraindications. None.

Glycyrrhiza glabra

LICORICE
Parts Used. Roots.

Actions
- Is a general tonic and clears mucus from the chest
- Soothes inflammation
- Harmonizes

Indications
IS A GENERAL TONIC AND CLEARS MUCUS FROM THE CHEST. Licorice is used in virtually all major medical traditions around the world as a tonic. In the Western tradition we emphasize its action on the lungs, using it to reduce catarrh and improve respiratory complaints.

SOOTHES INFLAMMATION. We also make great use of licorice's demulcent properties by using it to reduce inflammation, especially in the digestive tract and lungs.

HARMONIZES. Licorice is added to many herbal prescriptions because it has the effect harmonizing the herbs.

Dose. Standard.

Safe Dose. Standard.

Contraindications. None.

Cautions. Licorice is safe for children, but there are some adult conditions for which it should be used with caution. Being demulcent, licorice can aggravate fluid retention.

Grindelia camporum
GUM WEED
Parts Used. Dried leaves, flowering tops.

Actions
- Relaxes the lungs
- Relaxes spasms and cramps, clears mucus from the lungs

Indications
RELAXES THE LUNGS. Gum weed is used to treat asthma, especially spasmodic asthma, and is used when the child is very tight in the chest. It may be used during an asthma attack and also during the time between attacks, when it will have a gradual effect in relieving the tension.

RELAXES SPASMS AND CRAMPS, CLEARS MUCUS FROM THE LUNGS. Gum weed is also used in children with whooping cough to relieve the spasmodic cough. In relieving the spasm it helps loosen mucus in the lungs, so an immediate effect may not be a diminution of the cough but rather a change from a spasmodic cough to one that is more productive.

Dose. Standard.

Safe Dose. Standard.

Contraindications. None.

Humulus lupulus
HOPS
Parts Used. Flowers.

Actions
- Encourages sleep, calms nerves

Indications
ENCOURAGES SLEEP, CALMS NERVES. Hops' main use is for insomnia. Hops can be used in any situation in which a relaxant is needed to soothe the nerves. For example, it may be used in children with tension, irritability, nervous headache, or nervous stomach (when combined with stomach herbs). Even the vapor is helpful, and a hop-filled pillow may help with sleeping problems.

Dose. Standard.

Safe Dose. Standard.

Contraindications. Do not use in children with bedwetting, great lethargy, or depression. Overuse may increase the amount of sleep required.

Cautions. The flowers may cause skin irritation in some people.

Hydrastis canadensis
GOLDEN SEAL
Parts Used. Roots.

Actions
- Is a general tonic and mild stimulant
- Clears mucus from the body
- Is a mild laxative
- Soothes mucous membranes

Indications
IS A GENERAL TONIC AND MILD STIMULANT. Golden seal is an important herb for the digestive system in that it is commonly used and difficult to find a substitute for. It improves digestion and the movement of food through the intestines.

CLEARS MUCUS FROM THE BODY. Golden seal is the herb of choice for long-term conditions characterized by too much mucus; it may be taken over long periods. It is combined with herbs for the chest, such as coltsfoot *Tussilago farfara,* for chronic coughs.

IS A MILD LAXATIVE. Golden seal's laxative effect is more pronounced in Weak patterns, where it provides the energy and stimulation for the digestion to move.

SOOTHES MUCOUS MEMBRANES. A tea made from golden seal is a soothing eyewash, and the tea or tincture can be used as eardrops in children with otitis media.

Dose. Half the standard dose.

Safe Dose. Standard.

Contraindications. None for children, but there are some for adults.

Cautions. At first, golden seal increases the amount of mucus being expelled, so start with small doses.

Comments. Golden seal is an endangered species. Ensure that supplies come from cultivated plants, not from the wild.

Hypericum perfoliatum

ST. JOHN'S WORT
Parts Used. Flowers, leaves.

Actions
- Reduces pain from injury
- Heals deep wounds
- Reduces swellings
- Relaxes breathing, astringent

Indications
REDUCES PAIN FROM INJURY. St. John's wort can be applied externally for injuries. In ointment form, it is a great complement to arnica because arnica brings down the swelling and St. John's wort has a wonderful effect in calming the pain. For example, it instantly soothes the pain caused

by shutting little fingers in the door. It also has a special effect on injuries incurred by falling on the coccyx.

HEALS DEEP WOUNDS. St. John's wort is also useful in wounds that are slow to heal and wounds in which pus has formed—whether these wounds are the result of external trauma or the result of surgery. For this, it may be used internally as tincture or externally as oil. For external use the oil is preferred, but provided the skin is not broken, the tincture may be used (see Cautions).

REDUCES SWELLINGS. St. John's wort is used as a compress in mumps to relieve the ache and pain.

RELAXES BREATHING, ASTRINGENT. The tincture is used for dry coughs and bedwetting. For very tense children, it can be used as a general relaxant.

Dose. Standard.

Safe Dose. Standard.

Contraindications. If the child is very tired, it can have an opposite effect and provoke depression.

Cautions. Do not use the tincture on broken skin because the alcohol content will cause pain. Use the oil.

Comments. At present, St. John's wort is being marketed as a wonder herb for depression. Our experience is that it is helpful in *some* cases, particularly those that are light sensitive. In some people it can make the depression much worse.

Hyssopus officinale

HYSSOP
Parts Used. Whole plant, essential oil.

Actions
- Tones the lungs, soothes coughs, clears mucus from the lungs
- Promotes perspiration in fevers

- Moves digestion
- Calms the nerves

Indications

TONES THE LUNGS, SOOTHES COUGHS, CLEARS MUCUS FROM THE LUNGS. Hyssop is primarily to heal lung ailments, being useful for all lung problems, both chronic mucus and acute infection.

PROMOTES PERSPIRATION IN FEVERS. Hyssop promotes perspiration, so it may be given at all stages of influenza.

MOVES DIGESTION. Hyssop has a mild effect on the digestion, which is an additional help in all coughs with mucus and gives it its secondary use for colic and flatulence.

CALMS THE NERVES. A secondary use of hyssop is to calm the nerves, and it is useful in coughs and asthma linked to anxiety.

Dose. Standard.

Safe Dose. Standard.

Contraindications. None.

Cautions. The essential oil of hyssop should be used only in small quantities for babies because of the risk of causing epileptiform fits.

Comments. The essential oil has similar properties to the whole herb. Being a volatile oil, it is able to penetrate mucous conditions more quickly.

Inula helenium

ELECAMPANE
Parts Used. Roots.

Actions
- Clears mucus from the chest and reduces the production of mucus
- Moves digestion and helps clear the stagnant food pattern
- Is an antibacterial

Indications
CLEARS MUCUS FROM THE CHEST AND REDUCES THE PRODUCTION OF MUCUS. Elecampane is an excellent herb for all lung conditions with mucus, both acute and chronic, such as cough, bronchitis, and asthma. It has a strong effect on both the lungs and digestion, being able to remove mucus from both. This makes it especially useful in treating chronic cough and asthma.

MOVES DIGESTION AND HELPS CLEAR THE STAGNANT FOOD PATTERN. Elecampane has a moving effect on digestion and helps in all cases of stagnant food pattern.

IS AN ANTIBACTERIAL. It is mentioned in Fernie* (1914) that helenin isolated from the extract of elecampane is an antibiotic having a powerful effect against *Bacillus tuberculinum* and the cholera bacillus. We have mentioned earlier (see p. 38) the great advantages of antibiotics isolated from higher orders of plants, rather than lowly fungi, as having effects on specific bacteria. This means that the side effects, if there are any, are minimal.

Dose. Standard.

Safe Dose. Standard.

Contraindications. Not to be used in very large quantities (more than 100 g/day) by anyone who is anemic.

Comments. Elecampane has many similarities to burdock *Arctium lappa*. Elecampane has more of an effect on the lungs compared with burdock, which has more of an effect on the skin.

Iris versicolor

BLUE FLAG
Parts Used. Dried roots.

---

*Fernie WT: *Herbal simples*, ed 3, Bristol, 1914, John Wright.

Actions

- Decongests the lymphatic system and softens thick mucus
- Is a mild laxative
- Is a diuretic
- Stimulates digestion

Indications

DECONGESTS THE LYMPHATIC SYSTEM AND SOFTENS THICK MUCUS. Blue flag is primarily used to treat the echo pattern when there is an accumulation of hard mucus and swollen glands. It has a strong cleansing effect on the lymphatic system. When blue flag is first given, the softening effect on the mucus often causes a productive cough. In small doses it moves the bowels gently. Blue flag is beneficial in many skin conditions because of its stimulating action on the liver and lymphatic system.

IS A MILD LAXATIVE. The softened mucus is often released into the intestines, loosening the stools.

IS A DIURETIC. Once the lymph systems are functioning better, fluid accumulations start to drain, which is what gives its apparent diuretic effect.

STIMULATES DIGESTION. Blue flag is a very helpful herb in those who are sluggish. When the mucus is released, it tends to make these children even more sluggish, but the stimulating effect of *Iris* counteracts this.

Dose. Standard.

Safe Dose. Standard.

Contraindications. None.

Cautions. Do not use on Weak children; wait until their energy has increased. Large amounts may cause diarrhea.

Juglans cinerea

BUTTERNUT
Parts Used. Bark of roots.

Actions

- Moves and tones the bowels
- Reduces mucus
- Clears the stagnant food pattern
- Expels worms

Indications

MOVES AND TONES THE BOWELS. Small doses of butternut work as laxatives and strengthen the bowel muscles. Butternut is suitable for treatment of chronic constipation, especially when a skin disease is also present.

REDUCES MUCUS. Butternut reduces mucus in the system.

CLEARS THE STAGNANT FOOD PATTERN. For this butternut can be used on its own or with herbs such as black root *Leptandra virginica* for the stagnant food pattern of constipation.

EXPELS WORMS. When given in larger doses, butternut is cathartic; the worms are eliminated in the stool. When used for this indication, butternut would normally be combined with another herb, such as wormwood *Artemisia absinthium*.

Dose. Standard.

Safe Dose. Standard, if the child is still constipated. The dose required to move the stools is the safe dose.

Contraindications. Not to be taken by children with the Weak pattern of diarrhea.

Cautions. Large doses are strongly purgative and unsuitable for children.

Lavandula officinalis

LAVENDER
Parts Used. Essential oil.

Actions

- Soothes pain, combats infection, calms
- Soothes burns

Indications

SOOTHES PAIN, COMBATS INFECTION, CALMS. Lavender's relaxing effect makes it especially useful in treating insomnia, irritability, and colic in babies and children. It is good for muscle spasms and bruises (especially useful for children) and for headaches of all sorts.

SOOTHES BURNS. The oil applied immediately to a burn eases the pain and prevents blistering and scarring.

Dose. Standard *for essential oils.*

Safe Dose. Standard *for essential oils.*

Contraindications. For external use only. Do not take internally.

Comments. Lavender oil has a regulating effect and can be added to almost any massage oil.

Leptandra virginica/Veronicastrum virginicum

BLACK ROOT
Parts Used. Dried roots.

Actions
- Clears the stagnant food pattern
- Clears mucus
- Gently moves the bowels
- Relaxes
- Promotes perspiration in fevers
- Purges (in large doses)

Indications

CLEARS THE STAGNANT FOOD PATTERN. Black root regulates digestion in children with the stagnant food pattern and when there is congestion for whatever reason.

CLEARS MUCUS. Black root is especially indicated when there is copious mucus. It is therefore one of the main herbs used to treat whooping cough (when the digestion becomes blocked by excess mucus).

GENTLY MOVES THE BOWELS. Black root has a gentle laxative effect in children with chronic constipation. However, it can also safely be used in small doses for chronic diarrhea, especially when this is related to the stagnant food pattern.

RELAXES. There are some similarities in black root's action to that of golden seal *Hydrastis canadensis.* One important difference is that golden seal is more stimulating to digestion, whereas black root is more relaxing.

PROMOTES PERSPIRATION IN FEVERS. Black root is not the first herb to use in fevers, but this property makes it useful and safe to use in fevers when the stagnant food pattern is also present.

PURGES. Large doses of black root may be used as a slow cathartic. It requires 8 to 12 hours to work.

Dose. Standard.

Safe Dose. Do not give more than is needed to move the bowels.

Contraindications. None, if the dried root is used. The fresh root contains possibly harmful substances.

Cautions. In the first week of treatment, renewed bowel movements may cause flatulence and restlessness at night. The stools may temporarily become rather loose and copious at first because the mucus is voided through the stools. Large doses are a purgative and unsuitable for children.

Comments. For those who do not have access to North American herbs, it is difficult to suggest a substitute. One might use a combination of *Rhamnus cathartica* with yellow dock *Rumex crispus* and chamomile *Chamomilla matricaria* for children with the stagnant food pattern.

Lobelia inflata

LOBELIA
Parts Used. Whole plant.

Actions
- Is a general relaxant
- Clears mucus from the chest
- Encourages perspiration in fevers

Indications

IS A GENERAL RELAXANT. One of the widest-acting relaxants, lobelia is often combined with other herbs to direct its relaxing effect to specific parts of the body.

CLEARS MUCUS FROM THE CHEST. Lobelia is very useful in treating lung conditions because it stimulates the expulsion of mucus and yet relaxes the muscles of the respiratory system. Therefore it is used in cold, harsh coughs such as croup, whooping cough, and asthma. It is also used for congestive respiratory conditions. Lobelia is especially useful in people who need to relax and whose cough or asthma is worse when stressed.

ENCOURAGES PERSPIRATION IN FEVERS. Lobelia is one of the best herbs for coughs with fevers and also promotes beneficial sweating when the fever is very high.

Dose. Standard.

Safe Dose. Standard.

Contraindications. This herb is for Strong patients only (both adults and children). In Weak patients, large doses can weaken them further. In particular, it has the contraindication of nervous prostration or paralysis.

Cautions. In small quantities lobelia may cause a temporary tight (for about half a minute) sensation in the throat, as well as slight nausea, but this soon passes. These effects may be worrisome to people with asthma, but the child should nevertheless be encouraged to continue with the herb. In large quantities it acts as an emetic and induces vomiting.

Comments. This herb is restricted in some countries and can be used only under the supervision of a practitioner. (See the Preface for the reason.) We have found it perfectly safe in the small doses that we give in this book.

Mahonia aquifolia

See *Berberis aquifolium.*

Marrubium vulgaris

HOREHOUND (WHITE HOREHOUND)
Parts Used. Whole plant.

Actions
- Tones the lungs
- Relaxes the chest
- Loosens and clears mucus from deep in the lungs
- Is a bitter digestive tonic

Indications
TONES THE LUNGS. Horehound's tonic action on the lungs means that it is useful for all lung complaints.

RELAXES THE CHEST. Horehound has a special use for dry, harsh coughs because it relaxes the bronchi, thereby loosening the mucus and softening the cough. Typical uses are for acute and chronic bronchitis, whooping cough, and croup. We also find it effective when there is copious moist mucus.

LOOSENS AND CLEARS MUCUS FROM DEEP IN THE LUNGS. After the first effect of clearing the bronchi, the continued use of horehound may loosen thick plugs of mucus that have accumulated deep in the lungs.

IS A BITTER DIGESTIVE TONIC. Horehound is mildly bitter and a mild tonic, which makes it especially useful in treating chronic lung conditions.

Dose. Standard.

Safe Dose. Standard.

Contraindications. None.

Melaleuca alternifolia

TI-TREE, TEA TREE
  Parts Used. Essential oil.

Actions

- Is an antibacterial, antiviral, antifungal, immunostimulant

Indications

IS AN ANTIBACTERIAL, ANTIVIRAL, ANTIFUNGAL, IMMUNOSTIMULANT. Ti-tree is used to treat all infections, especially of the respiratory tract, when it is important to overcome the infection quickly. Its special use is in asthma, in which an attack is likely to be precipitated by an infection, although it can be used for all situations in which the immune system needs a sudden stimulus. Its antifungal properties can help overcome oral thrush in babies.

Dose. Standard *for essential oils.*

Safe Dose. Standard *for essential oils.*

Contraindications. For external use only. Do not take internally.

Melissa officinalis

LEMON BALM
  Parts Used. Whole plant above ground, essential oil.

Actions

- Calms and relaxes the nerves
- Relaxes the digestive tract
- Promotes perspiration in fevers

Indications

CALMS AND RELAXES THE NERVES. Lemon balm helps relieve tension and stress. Traditionally, it is said to strengthen the brain and chase away melancholy.

RELAXES THE DIGESTIVE TRACT. Lemon balm relieves spasm in the digestive tract. It is often used to alleviate digestive problems of nervous origin, such as stomach complaints before examinations.

PROMOTES PERSPIRATION IN FEVERS. Lemon balm is used to promote sweating in fevers.

Dose. Standard.

Safe Dose. Standard.

Contraindications. None.

Comments. The indications of the essential oil are very similar, although being more concentrated and being a volatile oil, which penetrates quickly, it is of use in asthma.

Mentha piperata

PEPPERMINT
  Parts Used. Aerial parts, essential oil.

Actions

- Stimulates digestion
- Relieves nausea and vomiting.
- Promotes perspiration in fevers

Indications

STIMULATES DIGESTION. Peppermint is used to treat many digestive problems because it relaxes the digestive muscles and stimulates digestion. Therefore it is helpful in treating colic, flatulence, and indigestion.

RELIEVES NAUSEA AND VOMITING. Peppermint is useful in treating motion sickness.

PROMOTES PERSPIRATION IN FEVERS. Peppermint is very useful in fevers to cool the child down.

Dose. Standard.

Safe Dose. Standard.

Contraindications. None.

Cautions. Do not use with homeopathic remedies because it nullifies their effect.

Comments. The essential oil has very similar properties.

Myrica cerifera
BAYBERRY
Parts Used. Bark of root.

Actions
- Is an astringent
- Stimulates circulation
- Promotes perspiration in fevers

Indications
IS AN ASTRINGENT. Bayberry is used in many damp conditions in which fluids do not circulate properly, such as loose stools and dribbling from the mouth.

STIMULATES CIRCULATION. At the same time, bayberry stimulates circulation and warms cold hands and feet. It is indicated for babies whose legs have a moist and squashy feel because of slight fluid accumulation.

PROMOTES PERSPIRATION IN FEVERS. Bayberry's warming and diaphoretic properties mean that it can safely be used in Cold infections. It is used by some practitioners for colds, especially where there is very copious clear nasal discharge.

Dose. Standard.

Safe Dose. Standard.

Contraindications. None.

Nepeta cataria
CATMINT (CATNIP)
Parts Used. Whole plant.

Actions
- Promotes perspiration in fevers, cools
- Relaxes digestive spasms and cramps
- Calms nerves
- Is slightly astringent

Indications
PROMOTES PERSPIRATION IN FEVERS, COOLS. Catmint's special use is in fevers because it promotes perspiration without raising the temperature further. It is indicated for Hot fevers to help avert febrile convulsions.

RELAXES DIGESTIVE SPASMS AND CRAMPS. Catmint may be used to treat many digestive problems, including flatulence, colic, and loose stools.

CALMS NERVES. Catmint has further uses for treating headaches, nervousness, cramping pains, and insomnia.

IS SLIGHTLY ASTRINGENT. Catmint's astringent properties make it useful in the treatment of catarrhal congestion in the sinuses and watering noses.

Dose. Standard.

Safe Dose. Standard.

Contraindications. None.

Cautions. The active ingredient of catmint is volatile, so this herb should be taken as a diluted tincture or infusion, never boiled.

Comments. The action of catmint is more cooling and relaxing than that of peppermint *Mentha piperata*.

Origanum majorana
MARJORAM
Parts Used. Essential oil.

Actions
- Sedates, relaxes, opens the chest

Indications
SEDATES, RELAXES, OPENS THE CHEST. Marjoram is used to treat asthma, bronchitis, and colds. Being a relaxant, it is of special use in asthma because it will help ease breathing. Its sedative effects make it useful in insomnia.

Comments. Marjoram herb is rather different, being slightly bitter and benefiting digestion. Its special use is for blood poisoning.

Dose. Standard *for essential oils.*

Safe Dose. Standard *for essential oils.*

Contraindications. For external use only. Do not take internally.

Panax ginseng

GINSENG

Parts Used. Root.

Actions

- Is a strong tonic and stimulant to the entire system

Indications

IS A STRONG TONIC AND STIMULANT TO THE ENTIRE SYSTEM. Ginseng is not much used in children, except in very weak and debilitated conditions, such as after illness, and in undersized children with very thin bones.

Dose. Standard.

Safe Dose. Three times the therapeutic dose.

Contraindications. Strong children should not take this herb because it may affect their growth.

Cautions. Do not overuse.

Comments. There are various subspecies, such as Korean, Chinese, and American, all with slightly different properties. Siberian ginseng *Eleuthero-coccus quinquefolium* is an entirely different plant and is also a strong tonic.

Passiflora incarnata

PASSION FLOWER

Parts Used. Dried whole plant.

Actions

- Relaxes the nervous system, sedates
- Relaxes nervous twitches and muscle spasms

Indications

RELAXES THE NERVOUS SYSTEM, SEDATES. Passion flower is helpful for insomnia after stimulating events such as parties and insomnia from being overtired.

RELAXES NERVOUS TWITCHES AND MUSCLE SPASMS. Passion flower is also used for asthma attacks when there is a strong emotional component and for migraines.

Dose. Standard.

Safe Dose. The safe dose is 8 tsp (50 g) daily.

Contraindications. None.

Cautions. In large doses over a long period, it can cause migraines.

Comments. In small doses, it can safely be given over a long period with no side effects or withdrawal symptoms.

Phytolacca decandra/americana

POKE ROOT

Parts Used. Dried roots.

Actions

- Decongests the lymphatic system and softens thick mucus
- Cools and works as a mild laxative

Indications

DECONGESTS THE LYMPHATIC SYSTEM AND SOFTENS THICK MUCUS. Either alone or in combination with blue flag *Iris versicolor,* poke root is the main herb for the echo pattern when mucus has become thick. It has a strong stimulating effect on the lymphatic system. This, combined with the action of softening the mucus, enables the entire lymphatic system to be decongested. It has a special effect on bringing energy to the throat. Because of this, it is specific for chronic tonsillitis, laryngitis, and mumps. When first taken it causes an increase in mucus discharges and even spots or boils as the mucus resolves. It may also lead to diarrhea because the mucus passes out through the stools.

COOLS AND WORKS AS A MILD LAXATIVE. Poke root is distinguished from *Iris* by being Cooler and by having less effect on the liver. If this herb is used with children who are already Cold, it may be necessary to add a warming herb such as cinnamon *Cinnamomum cassia.*

Dose. The least dose is the same as standard, but the greatest dose is about 7 drops for a 3-year-old.

Safe Dose. The safe dose is 7 to 10 drops. Larger doses may cause nausea or diarrhea.

Contraindications. If the child has a tendency to bedwetting or has only recently become dry, it may cause the bedwetting to return. The reason for this is that this herb diverts the energy to clearing out the lymphatic system, so in these children the slight reduction in overall energy can cause a return of the symptoms.

Cautions. The fresh herb is poisonous; use only when dried.

Pimpinella anisum

ANISEED
Parts Used. Seeds.

Actions
- Tones, warms, and is an antispasmodic for digestion
- Expels mucus from the lungs

Indications
TONES, WARMS, AND IS AN ANTISPASMODIC FOR DIGESTION. Aniseed is very useful in babies and children. The aromatic principle in this herb makes it useful in digestive problems because it is warming and a tonic to the stomach and helps alleviate damp conditions and mucous conditions affecting digestion. Aniseed is very useful in colic and flatulence in babies.

EXPELS MUCUS FROM THE LUNGS. Aniseed has a similar effect on the lungs, warming, toning, and helping expectorate damp mucus.

Dose. Best given in relatively large quantities, for example, up to 1.5 ml tincture (with the alcohol evaporated off) or as a tea, 1 level tsp (5 g) of dried herb to 50 ml of water. Although it has quite a sweet flavor, many children like to have extra sweetening added.

Safe Dose. Standard.

Contraindications. None.

Comments. There are three similar herbs in the same family: Fennel *Foeniculum vulgaris,* dill *Anethum graveolens,* and aniseed. They all have similar actions. Aniseed is more aromatic, and dill less aromatic than fennel. The more aromatic the herb is, the more effective it is at reducing flatulence, and this is one of the guides to choose one herb rather than another.

Piper nigrum

BLACK PEPPER
Parts Used. Essential oil.

Actions
- Is warming, a stimulant, and an antispasmodic

Indications
IS WARMING, A STIMULANT, AND AN ANTISPASMODIC. Black pepper is used to treat digestive problems, especially Cold, sluggish ones. Occasionally, it may be used to treat colic.

Dose. Standard *for essential oils.*

Safe Dose. Standard *for essential oils.*

Contraindications. For external use only. Do not take internally.

Comments. Pepper sprinkled on the food has a similar effect, although obviously it is used for older children and not at all for babies!

Plantago lanceolata

RIBWORT PLANTAIN
Parts Used. Leaves, aerial parts.

Actions
- Cools, clears mucus from the lungs
- Soothes inflammation, astringent
- Is a diuretic

Indications
COOLS, CLEARS MUCUS FROM THE LUNGS. Ribwort plantain is a cooling herb taken internally for Hot conditions, especially inflammation in the lungs or urinary tract. It may be used in Hot, dry coughs as a gentle expectorant that soothes inflammation.

SOOTHES INFLAMMATION, ASTRINGENT. In children, ribwort plantain helps earaches (otitis media). For this indication, the tincture is diluted with an equal volume of warm water and dropped into the ear at hourly intervals. (Do not use if the eardrum is perforated.)

IS A DIURETIC. Ribwort plantain clears any fluid in the lungs and generally increases the flow of urine.

Dose. For urinary or lung problems, use in larger quantities. For children the dose is $1/2$ tsp (3 g) of dried herb, as a tea, every 2 hours.

Safe Dose. Standard.

Contraindications. None.

Comments. Common or round-leaved plantain *Plantago major* has similar demulcent effects, but some report it to be slightly less effective. Both have been found to contain antibiotics.

Populus tremuloides

WHITE POPLAR
Parts Used. Bark.

Actions
- Is a tonic for the intestines, general tonic
- Improves the circulation of water

Indications
IS A TONIC FOR THE INTESTINES, GENERAL TONIC. White poplar is used in many Weak energy conditions because of its tonic effect on digestion. It also will gradually improve the appetite.

IMPROVES THE CIRCULATION OF WATER. As the intestines work better, excess water is absorbed from the stools, thus firming up loose stools and increasing the output of urine. Thus it is useful for treating the Weak pattern of diarrhea without the risk of causing constipation.

Dose. Standard.

Safe Dose. Standard.

Contraindications. None.

Potentilla tormentilla

TORMENTIL
Parts Used. Whole plant, including roots.

Actions
- Is an astringent
- Functions as a cleanser

Indications
IS AN ASTRINGENT. Tormentil is one of the strongest, yet safest, astringents, which is beneficial in treating all forms of diarrhea and other discharges, such as nosebleeds.

FUNCTIONS AS A CLEANSER. Tormentil is also recommended for cleansing, treating skin eruptions and boils, and aiding in the healing of wounds and burns. It may be used to gargle with to soothe sore and ulcerated throats, although there are very few parents who will let their children reach this state of illness without administering antibiotics.

Dose. Standard.

Safe Dose. Standard.

Contraindications. None.

Cautions. Large doses may lead to vomiting.

Prunus serotina

WILD CHERRY
Parts Used. Bark (the leaves are poisonous).

Actions
- Suppresses the cough reflex, sedative
- Is an astringent
- Stimulates digestion

Indications
SUPPRESSES THE COUGH REFLEX, SEDATIVE. Wild cherry is used to treat many coughs because it sedates the cough reflex. This may be necessary in the short term (e.g., if the child is exhausted and needs sleep) but is not recommended for the long term. A secondary use is as first aid in the acute stage of asthma, when it can often bring relief.

IS AN ASTRINGENT. Wild cherry is slightly astringent and is therefore effective at drying up excessive watery discharges and watery coughs.

STIMULATES DIGESTION. Wild cherry has a mild tonic action on digestion.

Dose. Standard.

Safe Dose. The safe dose is 20 drops tincture.

Contraindications. None.

Comments. Wild cherry is best given as a syrup, which has an agreeable taste.

Rhamnus cathartica

BUCKTHORN
Parts Used. Berries.

Actions and Indications. Buckthorn is native to Europe. Its action is very similar to that of *Rhamnus purshiana*, only milder. This makes it especially suitable for children.

Dose. Small doses (5 to 20 drops of tincture daily). Adjust the dose to suit the child; usually, it can be gradually reduced with time.

Safe Dose. The safe dose is 5 ml tincture. Do not exceed the dose needed to move the bowels.

Contraindications. None.

Rumex crispus

YELLOW DOCK
Parts Used. Roots.

Actions
- Is a laxative and stimulates the flow of bile
- Is an alterative for lymphatic congestion
- Moves digestion
- Improves the appetite

Indications
IS A LAXATIVE AND STIMULATES THE FLOW OF BILE. Yellow dock may be used as a laxative, which works by stimulating digestion and increasing the flow of bile.

IS AN ALTERATIVE FOR LYMPHATIC CONGESTION. Yellow dock is used in conditions in which there is stagnation. It is combined with other herbs to decongest and cleanse the lymph and blood. Yellow dock is very useful in treating many skin complaints, including eczema.

MOVES DIGESTION. As yellow dock gradually moves the digestion, it improves the appetite and improves the assimilation of food.

IMPROVES THE APPETITE. This makes yellow dock especially useful for pale and Weak children with a poor appetite.

Dose. Standard. The medicine will probably need to be sweetened. Black strap molasses is especially suitable because it also provides additional tonic action.

Safe Dose. Standard. Do not exceed the dose needed to move the bowels.

Contraindications. None.

Rhamnus purshiana

CASCARA (CALIFORNIAN BUCKTHORN)
Parts Used. Bark.

Actions
- Is a laxative
- Tones the intestines

Indications
IS A LAXATIVE. In the past, cascara's main use was as a purgative. Now we use smaller doses as a gentle laxative.

TONES THE INTESTINES. Small doses over a long period tone the muscles of the intestines and encourage regular bowel movements.

Dose. Small doses (5 to 20 drops of tincture daily). Adjust the dose to suit the child; usually, it can be gradually reduced with time.

Safe Dose. The safe dose is 5 ml tincture. Do not exceed the dose needed to move the bowels.

Contraindications. Diarrhea.

Cautions. The safe dose is safe if constipation is still present. Once the bowels have started to move

frequently, any dose above this is potentially unsafe. Large doses (20 times standard) are a violent purgative.

Salvia sclarea

CLARY SAGE
Parts Used. Essential oil.

Actions
- Is a tonic, relaxant, especially for the muscles

Indications
IS A TONIC, RELAXANT, ESPECIALLY FOR THE MUSCLES. Clary sage is used when convalescing after influenza and fevers. It is also used to relieve tension and stress and to reduce the spasms of asthma and cramps in the digestive tract.

Dose. Standard *for essential oils.*

Safe Dose. Standard *for essential oils.*

Contraindications. None.

Sambucus nigra

ELDER
Parts Used. Flowers.

Actions
- Promotes perspiration in fevers
- Cools
- Clears mucus from the lungs

Indications
PROMOTES PERSPIRATION IN FEVERS. The flowers promote perspiration in the early stages of influenza, especially when combined with peppermint *Mentha piperata.* Both are conveniently preserved in syrup.

COOLS. Elderflower is especially helpful in fevers of the Hot type, where the child is bright red and restless. It is also very refreshing on a hot day when the heat is beginning to make everyone irritable.

CLEARS MUCUS FROM THE LUNGS. Elder helps relieve mucus that collects in the upper respiratory tract (before the cough has gone down deep into the chest). It is useful for treating sinusitis and coughs.

Dose. Standard.

Safe Dose. Standard.

Contraindications. None.

Cautions. None for the flowers or berries.

Comments. We have listed only one of the many uses for this plant. The berries, the leaves, and the bark are all used medicinally.

Sanguinaria canadensis

BLOODROOT
Parts Used. Roots.

Actions
- Calms harsh coughs
- Clears mucus from the lungs
- Warms

Indications
CALMS HARSH COUGHS. Bloodroot relaxes the bronchial muscles. It is used to treat harsh coughs such as croup, whooping cough, bronchitis, and asthma.

CLEARS MUCUS FROM THE LUNGS. Bloodroot stimulates the lungs to expel mucus.

WARMS. Bloodroot is gradually warming, so is useful in Cold conditions, especially those that affect the lungs. There is no tonic action to blood root, so it should be used only in children with Strong conditions.

Dose. Half the standard dose.

Safe Dose. Twice the therapeutic dose.

Contraindications. None.

Cautions. In larger doses bloodroot is likely to cause vomiting and diarrhea.

Santalum album

SANDALWOOD
Parts Used. Essential oil.

Actions and Indications. Sandalwood's use in children is for dry, persisting, irritating coughs. It is mildly antiseptic. It can be used as a massage oil or be inhaled to calm the tickling cough.

Dose. Standard *for essential oils.*

Safe Dose. Standard *for essential oils.*

Contraindications. For external use only. Do not take internally.

Schizandra sinensis

SCHIZANDRA
Parts Used. Fruit.

Actions
- Tones, is an astringent, calms

Indications
TONES, IS AN ASTRINGENT, CALMS. Schizandra is used only occasionally for children's conditions, namely for very Weak, debilitated children who have thin bones. When combined with other herbs, it may be used for the symptoms of insomnia, low energy, and asthma.

Dose. Standard.

Safe Dose. Standard.

Contraindications. None.

Scrophularia nodosa

FIGWORT
Parts Used. Whole plant.

Actions
- Is an alterative for lymphatic congestion, mild diuretic, mild laxative, stimulant

Indications
IS AN ALTERATIVE FOR LYMPHATIC CONGESTION, MILD DIURETIC, MILD LAXATIVE, STIMULANT. Figwort is used to treat skin problems, especially those accompanied by swollen lymph nodes and sluggish lymph circulation. It may also be used in all echo patterns as a substitute for queen's delight *Stillingia sylvatica.*

Dose. Standard.

Safe Dose. Standard.

Contraindications. None.

Stillingia sylvatica
QUEEN'S DELIGHT
Parts Used. Root.

Actions
- Decongests the lymphatic system
- Is an alterative for lymphatic congestion
- Mildly stimulates the system
- Relaxes muscular spasms

Indications
DECONGESTS THE LYMPH SYSTEM. Queen's delight is used as one of the main herbs in echo patterns to soften hard mucus and decongest the lymphatic system. Thus it is useful for chronic bronchitis when the child has enough energy and most of the mucus has been cleared.

IS AN ALTERATIVE FOR LYMPHATIC CONGESTION. Queen's delight plays an important role in treating chronic skin conditions, especially if wet and oozing.

MILDLY STIMULATES THE SYSTEM. Queen's delight is mildly stimulating, so it may be used when there is either weakness or sluggishness.

RELAXES MUSCULAR SPASMS. Queen's delight has a mild relaxing effect on the muscles. This, combined with the softening of thick mucus, makes it useful in the treatment of growing pains.

Dose. Standard, but do not exceed the standard dose.

Safe Dose. The safe dose is 1.5 ml tincture. More than this may cause vomiting and diarrhea.

Contraindications. None.

Cautions. Queen's delight causes vomiting and diarrhea in large doses.

Styrax benzoin
BENZOIN
Parts Used. Essential oil.

Actions and Indications. Benzoin clears mucus from the system and is soothing. It is warming, so it is of special use in Cold types of cough and is also of use in colic. It has the great virtue of both calming the child and stimulating the body and digestion.

Dose. Standard *for essential oils.*

Safe Dose. Standard *for essential oils.*

Contraindications. For external use only. Do not take internally.

Taraxacum officinale
DANDELION
Parts Used. Roots.

Actions
- Stimulates digestion
- Is a diuretic
- Is a mild laxative

Indications
STIMULATES DIGESTION. Dandelion is a strong stimulant to the digestive system, so those with a

Weak or slow digestion feel a boost of energy from taking it.

IS A DIURETIC. A strong diuretic, dandelion helps clear fluid accumulations in the fluid imbalance patterns. It may be used as a tonic, but it works more by virtue of stimulating digestion and removing excess fluids rather than by being a pure tonic.

IS A MILD LAXATIVE. Dandelion's laxative effect is more pronounced in the Weak patterns. It may also be used in chronic loose stools when caused by Weak energy.

Dose. Standard.

Safe Dose. Standard.

Contraindications. None.

Thymus vulgaris

THYME
Parts Used. Leaves, flowering tops.

Actions
- Calms convulsive coughs and is expectorant
- Warms the lungs and digestion
- Is a tonic
- Helps the throat
- Is an antiseptic
- Relieves spasms and cramps
- Is an astringent
- Expels worms

Indications
CALMS CONVULSIVE COUGHS AND IS EXPECTORANT. Thyme has always been valued in the treatment of whooping cough and is used in many cough medicines because it reduces spasms and helps rid the lungs of mucus.

WARMS THE LUNGS AND DIGESTION. Thyme warms the lungs, so is helpful in all Cold type of coughs. It also warms digestion, thereby providing support to

cure the cough. Thyme also treats indigestion and may be used to treat diarrhea.

IS A TONIC. If the infusion is left to brew for a 15 minutes or more, the tea becomes quite bitter, but the resultant drink is a stronger digestive tonic.

HELPS THE THROAT. A tea of thyme will help throat problems, such as laryngitis and tonsillitis. It is even more effective if gargled.

IS AN ANTISEPTIC. Thyme contains a high percentage of volatile oils that are antiseptic, hence its use in bacterial infections of the lungs.

RELIEVES SPASMS AND CRAMPS. The essential oil may be used as a component in a massage oil to relieve growing pains.

IS AN ASTRINGENT. Thyme is an astringent, and this is put to use occasionally in bedwetting.

EXPELS WORMS. Thyme may be used with other herbs to eliminate threadworms.

Dose. For children, make a simple infusion of $\frac{1}{2}$ to 1 level tsp (3 to 5 g) of dried herb to 1 cup of water and sweetened with honey. For babies or toddlers, administer thyme as a bath.

Safe Dose. Standard.

Contraindications. None.

Comments. The essential oil has very similar properties, although being a volatile oil, it can be inhaled and has a quick effect on the lungs when there is much mucus.

Tilia europoea

LIME FLOWER
Parts Used. Flowers.

Actions
- Calms nerves, relaxes spasms and cramps

- Calms a nervous stomach
- Promotes perspiration in fevers

Indications

CALMS NERVES, RELAXES SPASMS AND CRAMPS. Lime flower is an all-purpose calming herb made into a tea that is popular in many parts of Europe. It calms and strengthen the nerves and settles the stomach, so it can be used to treat headaches, insomnia, and irritability, especially in sensitive children.

CALMS A NERVOUS STOMACH. Lime flower is also recommended to calm general nervousness, specifically nervous stomachs.

PROMOTES PERSPIRATION IN FEVERS. Lime flower's action in promoting perspiration in fevers makes it suitable for a distressed and anxious child with a Hot fever.

Dose. Standard.

Safe Dose. Standard.

Contraindications. None.

Trifolium pratensis

RED CLOVER
Parts Used. Flowers.

Actions
- Is an alterative for lymphatic congestion
- Clears mucus from the lungs, relaxes spasms and cramps

Indications
IS AN ALTERATIVE FOR LYMPHATIC CONGESTION. Red clover is used mainly as a remedy for skin problems.

CLEARS MUCUS FROM THE LUNGS, RELAXES SPASMS AND CRAMPS. Secondary uses of red clover include treating sore throat, coughs, and whooping cough.

Dose. Standard.

Safe Dose. Standard.

Contraindications. None.

Tussilago farfara

COLTSFOOT
Parts Used. Whole plant.

Actions
- Clears mucus from the chest, soothes inflammation
- Tones the lungs

Indications
CLEARS MUCUS FROM THE CHEST, SOOTHES INFLAMMATION. Tussilago means "cough-dispeller," and it is the herb of choice for all coughs because it also eliminates mucus from the respiratory tract. It is a soothing expectorant and antispasmodic, so it is especially helpful when there is the need to soothe the cough when harsh, dry, and irritable. It helps "break" the cough and remove mucus from the lungs, making the cough more productive.

TONES THE LUNGS. Coltsfoot's tonic effect on the lungs make it useful in the long-term treatment of asthma. It can safely be given when the child is weak because it soothes the bronchi. It is often used in combination with horehound *Marrubium vulgaris* and licorice *Glycyrrhiza glabra.*

Dose. Standard.

Safe Dose. Standard.

Contraindications. None.

Urtica dioica

NETTLES
Parts Used. Aerial parts.

Actions
- Is an alterative for lymphatic congestion
- Is an astringent

- Is a diuretic
- Stimulates circulation

Indications

IS AN ALTERATIVE FOR LYMPHATIC CONGESTION. Nettles is used to treat many skin diseases, especially eczema, and other itching conditions.

IS AN ASTRINGENT. Nettles stops bleeding, so it is good for nosebleeds and bleeding from wounds.

IS A DIURETIC. Nettles is used to "cleanse" the system by eliminating toxins through the urine.

STIMULATES CIRCULATION. Nettles is used as a spring tonic to get the system "moving." It is rich in minerals, including iron, and stimulates circulation.

Dose. Standard.

Safe Dose. Standard.

Contraindications. None.

Valeriana officinalis

VALERIAN
Parts Used. Roots.

Actions
- Calms the nerves
- Aids digestion
- Relaxes spasms and cramps

Indications
CALMS THE NERVES. This herb has a great reputation as a relaxant. It relaxes without tiring; in fact, in many users the relaxation quickly gives way to a feeling of vigor and clarity of thought. Valerian is used for conditions arising out of tension and anxiety, such as nervous headaches and migraines. It is used in many cases of insomnia, especially that resulting from anxiety or tension.

AIDS DIGESTION. Valerian aids digestion and often relieves flatulence, especially when associated with tension, anxiety, and suppressed emotions.

RELAXES SPASMS AND CRAMPS. Valerian relaxes spasms and cramps throughout the body, including feverish fits in babies. It can be used to treat colic.

Dose. Standard.

Safe Dose. Standard.

Contraindications. None.

Cautions. Valerian is safe in medicinal doses, but in very large doses, it may cause palpitations and increase agitation. What is more important clinically is that when stressed patients (usually adults) take this for the first time, they can wake up the next morning feeling drugged. This is not because valerian is a narcotic but rather because of the effects of suddenly relaxing.

Verbascum thapsus

MULLEIN
Parts Used. Dried leaves and flowers.

Actions
- Clears mucus from the chest
- Moistens and is mildly relaxing
- Cools inflamed mucous membranes

Indications
CLEARS MUCUS FROM THE CHEST. Mullein is very useful in nearly all respiratory conditions. It acts on the mucous membranes to help loosen and expel accumulated mucus.

MOISTENS AND IS MILDLY RELAXING. Mullein is especially useful in treating hard dry coughs.

COOLS INFLAMED MUCOUS MEMBRANES. Mullein cools and soothes inflammation in bronchitis.

Dose. Standard.

Safe Dose. Standard.

Contraindications. None.

Cautions. If using the leaves, take care to strain out the tiny hairs on the underside of the leaves because these can be a little irritating.

Comments. The oil is used to treat earaches.

Veronicastrum virginica

See *Leptandra virginica*.

Viola odorata

VIOLET
Parts Used. Leaves, flowers.

Actions
- Clears mucus from the lungs, cools
- Is an alterative for lymphatic congestion

Indications
CLEARS MUCUS FROM THE LUNGS, COOLS. Violet is used to treat coughs and bronchitis when there is a need to cool and soothe the lungs.

IS AN ALTERATIVE FOR LYMPHATIC CONGESTION. Violet is often used as in the treatment of eczema, and it may also be used for the echo pattern.

Dose. Standard.

Safe Dose. Standard.

Contraindications. None.

Xanthoxylum americanum (Also Known as *Zanthoxylum americanum*)

PRICKLY ASH
Parts Used. Bark of roots.

Actions
- Stimulates circulation
- Tones the digestive system

- Promotes perspiration in fevers

Indications
STIMULATES CIRCULATION. Prickly ash is mainly used as a stimulant to the peripheral circulation to reduce cramps and warm cold hands and feet.

TONES THE DIGESTIVE SYSTEM. Prickly ash stimulates the stomach and is used in children with poor or weak digestion who have a swollen abdomen, flatulence, a pale face, and lethargy.

PROMOTES PERSPIRATION IN FEVERS. Prickly ash can help warm up a feverish but "chilly" child and is effective in the later stages when the child lacks adequate strength to overcome the last of the illness.

Dose. Standard.

Safe Dose. Standard.

Contraindications. Do not use if the child is very Hot because it may increase the heat further.

Zingiber officinale

GINGER
Parts Used. Fresh roots, essential oil.

Actions
- Warms the body and stimulates digestion
- Promotes perspiration in fevers
- Clears mucus from the chest

Indications
WARMS THE BODY AND STIMULATES DIGESTION. Ginger is used for Cold and Weak conditions in children (and elderly persons), especially when digestion is weak. It is very warm and soothing and therefore aids Cold children who dislike cold foods—both physically cold foods and foods with Cold energy, such as cucumbers and lettuce. It stimulates digestion and aids in the treatment of colic, indigestion, flatulence, and nausea.

The simplest way to give ginger to the very young is to add a little of the fresh root to food.

Simmer it in the milk for bottle-fed babies or grate a little into the baby food for weaned babies.

PROMOTES PERSPIRATION IN FEVERS. Ginger is used to promote perspiration in Cold fevers.

CLEARS MUCUS FROM THE CHEST. Ginger is also of use in cold and wet types of cough because it helps clear mucus from the chest. For this indication, it may be combined with lemon juice and honey (for those older than 1 year).

Dose. Standard.

Safe Dose. Standard. Do not exceed the dose needed to warm the child up.

Contraindications. None.

Cautions. If taken in large doses over long periods (10 times standard), ginger can cause inflammation and weakness. Do not use if the child is already Hot because it will increase the heat.

Comment. If children refuse to take ginger, they may be warmed by putting a few drops of the essential oil in the bath. The oil has very similar properties to the root.

■ HOMEOPATHY

Homeopathy sprang out of herbal medicine in the eighteenth century. In a reaction against the rising use of poisons in medicine, the famous founder of this system of medicine, Dr.Hahnemann, started using smaller and smaller doses. Eventually, he found he could use preparations that had less than one molecule of the original poison per pill. To his astonishment, he found that in certain circumstances these were as effective as any other medicine, without any danger of poisoning the patient. To those who do not believe in energy and that the material world is all that there is, his findings are still regarded as erroneous, despite two centuries of astoundingly successful clinical use and numerous double-blind studies.

The Basis for Prescribing

Homeopathy is prescribed on a slightly different basis from other medicines. It is based on the principle that "like cures like." The remedy is chosen on the basis of a match to a "symptom picture," that is, a collection of symptoms that occur when the poison is given in material doses. In clinical practice this means choosing the remedy that best fits a particular child.*

Preparation of Remedies

The remedies are prepared diluting in stages. Typically, a tincture is taken and diluted 10 times. It is then shaken vigorously (succussed). This process is repeated many times. If the process is repeated 6 times, the remedy is called 6X, the 6 referring to the number of dilutions or succussions and the X referring to the factor of 10 in dilution. A similar series of remedies is obtained by diluting by a factor of 100 each time. If this is performed (say) 30 times, the resultant remedy is known as 30C, the C referring to the 100-time dilution at each stage.

Combining Remedies

Opinions are divided regarding the suitability of combining remedies. Some believe that only one remedy should be given at a time, whereas others have found effective ways of combining them. One such combination is a child's remedy known as *ABC*, which contains aconite, belladonna, and chamomilla. This combination is used as a catch-all in fevers.

---

*For the purposes of this book we have simplified the principles of prescribing. There are in fact many different schools of homeopathy, and each one emphasizes different aspects of the person. Some, for example, stress the importance of the child's constitutional type, others give more importance to the emotional reaction of a child, and yet others concentrate on hereditary dispositions.

Homeopathic Remedies

This is not a book about homeopathy, so we have chosen just a few remedies that are often useful when treating children. For more information, we refer you to the bibliography. Here we present abbreviated symptom pictures of the following remedies.

- Aconite
- Arnica
- Arsenicum album
- Belladonna
- Chamomilla
- Gelsemium
- Mercurius solubilis

Remedy	Symptom Picture
Aconite	Sudden fevers, fear, shock, contracted pupils, shivering, white face, cold, and very little or no perspiration. In our classification, it corresponds approximately to the Strong Cold condition.
Arnica	Used mainly for trauma, such as concussion, wounds, and injury. If the child has been hurt so badly to require treatment at a hospital, this can be given on the way. If the child has to undergo surgery, this may be given both before and after to assist in recovery. In high potencies it has the effect of releasing any shock that may have become stuck in the child.
Arsenicum album	The remedy of choice for diarrhea and food poisoning; burning pain in the throat, stomach, anus, and rectum; diarrhea with cramping pains; anxieties; and exhaustion. Also used as a tonic, after any illness, and sometimes used at the first signs of a cold to boost the energy to throw out the cold.
Belladonna	Longer fevers, heat, red face, no sweating, throwing off the blankets, dilated pupils, sensitivity to light, and throbbing headaches.
	The child is very restless and uncomfortable (compared with the aconite child who is more frightened). In our classification it corresponds approximately to the Strong Hot condition.
Chamomilla	One cheek red, irritable, impatient and angry, swollen abdomen, possible teething, bilious, colic, and foul-smelling stools. In our classification it corresponds approximately to fevers with the further development of the stagnant food pattern.
Gelsemium	Fever is not so high, but lots of watery or mucous discharges; dusky, red complexion. Child looks and feels heavy and is somewhat lethargic. In fevers, this child is difficult to console but is grumpy rather than frightened or restless. In our classification it corresponds approximately to the heat with damp condition, which is described in more detail under coughs.
Mercurius solubilis	Fever with profuse greasy sweat. Despite sweating, the child does not cool down. The child is restless and a bit anxious. Also used when any mucous discharges are sticky and yellow.

▪ MASSAGE

Massage is one of the oldest and most instinctive forms of healing, and although it is pleasant, it is surprisingly powerful. This is especially true of the Chinese forms of massage, which are based on the energy channels in the body (sometimes called *meridians*). Massage can be used to treat a wide range of conditions, and it is an established therapy in Chinese state hospitals. Massage is especially favored in China for the treatment of children because it can be so gentle and because the physical contact benefits both the child and parent.

Massage is a natural complement to the administration of essential oils and is especially suited to children who dislike all but the simplest food and those who are very cuddly. It is less suited to the boisterous, impetuous, restless children.

Many people in the West are unfamiliar with the techniques of massage. For this reason, simpler and more effective strokes have been included here. They are completely safe (provided they are not done too vigorously), are suitable for babies and children, and can be combined with any other type of therapy, including orthodox medicine.

How to Perform Massage

- Calm yourself and the child as much as possible before starting. This is often difficult with an ill, restless, or irritable child, but it is worth making the effort. Spend a little time doing slow breathing exercises or a similar relaxation technique.
- If you can, choose calm and peaceful surroundings, without bright lights, loud music, or other distractions. Turn the television off if possible.
- Lubricate the area to be massaged with oil. Almost any oil is suitable, and almond oil is a good general choice. Even better is to include essential oils appropriate to the child's condition.
- Massage gently but firmly, being responsive and aware of the child's reaction. Speak calmly and gently. If the child becomes agitated, stop and relax, then start again.
- While massaging, imagine a healing force coming from your hands and fingertips to benefit the child. Do not let your wrists become stiff—keep them flexible, allowing the healing energy to flow through.
- Imagine that the massage strokes direct the child's energy to where healing is needed. For example, try to draw Hot energy away from the head in the spinal stroke massage, or imagine stimulating movement in the bowels in the down sacrum stroke.
- If you are treating your own child, count the number of strokes you are doing and time the number of minutes that you spend doing the massage. A good treatment takes between 10 and 20 minutes.

Frequency

The frequency of performing massage depends on the situation and is similar to the frequency with which you would administer herbs. In a child with an acute condition such as fever, it is helpful to give a massage every 2 hours. In a child with a chronic cough, two or three times a day is enough.

Response to Massage

The response to massage is variable and depends both on the person giving the massage and the person receiving it. Some people have a natural gift for healing massage, and some children are especially responsive to this therapy. In this happy combination, the effect of massage is almost instantaneous. A much more common response is that the energy is definitely changed after 15 to 20 minutes of massage, and after that healing starts to take place.

Individual Massage Techniques

All of the massage strokes included in this book are listed here. They are in "top-to-toe" order, beginning with the head and face, then chest and back, arms and hands, and finally legs and feet.

ACROSS FOREHEAD (Figure 9-1)
1. Hold the child's head facing you, with both hands.
2. Using your thumbs, gently stroke across the forehead, outward from the center.
3. Repeat 50 times.

Indications. Fevers, headaches.

Comments. This is especially indicated when the child has a headache with a hot head. Sometimes, the headache starts to subside after just a few gentle strokes.

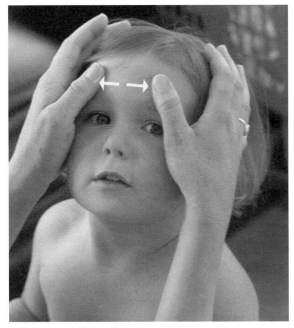

Figure 9-1 Across forehead.

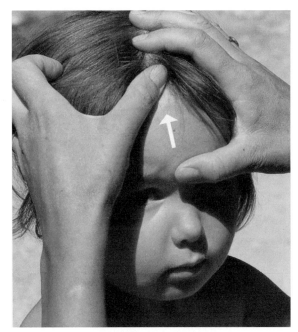

Figure 9-2 Up forehead.

UP FOREHEAD (Figure 9-2)
1. Hold the child's head facing you, with both hands.
2. Stroke upward with alternate thumbs, from the bridge of the nose to the hair line.
3. Repeat 50 times.

Indications. Fevers, headaches.

Comments. This has a similar effect to the previous massage. It is also especially useful in strong fevers when you want to take the heat away from the head. This massage starts the energy flowing over the top of the head, so the next massage, which follows naturally, is the spinal stroke massage.

CHEST (Figure 9-3)
1. Sit the child on your knee, facing you, and hold him or her firmly under the arms.
2. Use your thumbs to massage the chest between the nipples, gently stroking away from the midline toward each nipple.
3. Massage for 3 to 4 minutes.

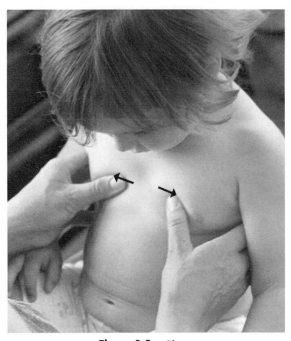

Figure 9-3 Chest.

Indications. Coughs, asthma.

Comments. This massage should be done gently, and effects are somewhat slower to take place. It is of more use in strengthening the lungs in long-term conditions because it brings energy to the lungs.

SHOULDER (Figure 9-4)
1. Sit the child on your knee, either facing toward you or away.
2. Find the highest point of the shoulder, midway between the tip of the shoulder and the spine.
3. Press down both sides with a vibrating movement for a minute or more.

Indications. Acute cough, asthma.

Comments. This massage can sometimes avert an asthma attack.

SCAPULAR (Figure 9-5)
1. Sit the child on your knee, facing away from you, and hold him or her firmly under the arms.
2. With your thumbs, massage the back between the shoulder blades.
3. Stroke firmly, starting from near the top of the back and then progressing down to between the bases of the shoulder blades (scapulae).
4. Repeat 50 to 100 times.

Indications. Coughs, asthma, wheezing, general weakness.

Comments. This is one of the best massages for an asthma attack and can be done quite firmly. The response normally is immediate opening of the chest. This massage used long term will strengthen the lungs.

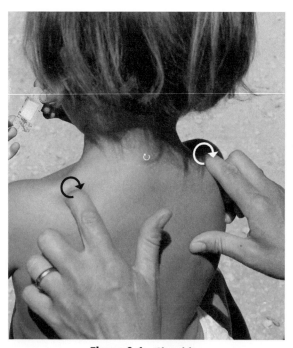

Figure 9-4   Shoulder.

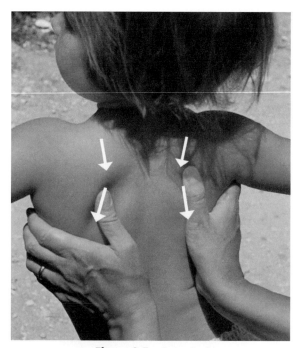

Figure 9-5   Scapular.

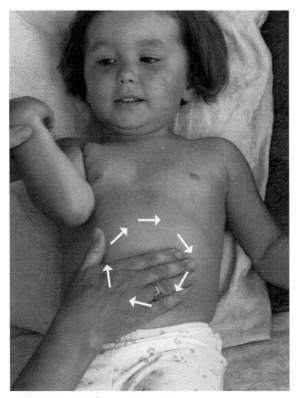

Figure 9-6 Abdomen.

ABDOMEN (Figure 9-6)
1. Have the child lie comfortably, chest up.
2. Gently massage in a large circle round the abdomen, using your fingertips. For constipation, rotate clockwise to encourage peristalsis in the large intestine. For diarrhea, rotate counterclockwise to slow down peristalsis. For general conditions, do half the massages round one way, and half round the other.
3. Repeat 50 to 100 times.

Indications. Stagnant food pattern, constipation, colic and abdominal pain, insomnia caused by abdominal pain, Weak digestion.

Comments. Children with Weak digestion usually love this massage and describe the feeling of

warmth coming from the fingertips. In contrast, children with the stagnant food pattern can become very restless and fidgety, and it may even cause the abdomen to become painful as the stagnation starts to move.

HEEL ON UPPER ABDOMEN
1. Use the heel of your hand to massage the upper part of the abdomen between the base of the rib cage and the navel.
2. Gently push about 50 times.

Indications. Indigestion, Weak digestion, insomnia related to Weak digestion, lack of appetite.

Comments. This massage is more of a tonic. The pushing should be very gentle, with the thought of Warm energy coming out of the heel of the hand.

HEEL ON LOWER ABDOMEN
1. Use the heel of your hand to massage the lower part of the abdomen, below the navel.
2. Gently push about 50 times.

Indications. Indigestion, Weak digestion, insomnia related to Weak digestion, lack of appetite, general weakness, bedwetting, cystitis, and other urinary problems.

Comments. See comment for heel on upper abdomen. Massaging lower down helps the lower part of the body, which accounts for its help in treating urinary problems.

SMOOTH DIGESTION (Figure 9-7)
1. Have the child lie comfortably, chest up.
2. Gently massage the point midway between the navel and the lower tip of the breastbone (sternum) using your index and middle fingers.
3. Gently vibrate for 1 to 2 minutes.

Indications. Stagnant food pattern, indigestion, Weak digestion, general weakness, lack of appetite.

Comments. The vibrating action gently stimulates the digestive system. For children with Weak

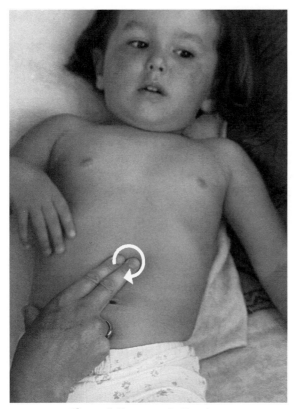

Figure 9-7   Smooth digestion.

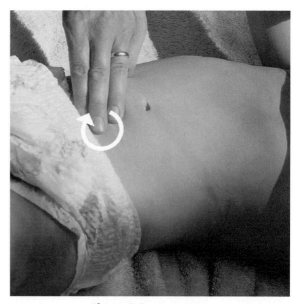

Figure 9-8   Intestines.

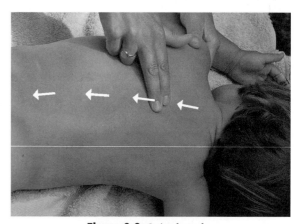

Figure 9-9   Spinal stroke.

digestion, this can be very pleasant, but for children with the stagnant food pattern, it can cause quite severe discomfort.

INTESTINES (Figure 9-8)
1. Have the child lie comfortably, chest up.
2. Gently massage the point midway between the navel and the top of the pubic bone, using your index and middle fingers.
3. Gently vibrate for 1 to 2 minutes.

Indications. General weakness, urinary problems.

Comments. The vibrating action gently stimulates the digestive system. Being lower down, it is also of help in bringing energy to the urinary system.

SPINAL STROKE (Figure 9-9)
1. Have the child lie face down.
2. With your index and middle fingers, massage gently down the spine from the base of the head to the tip of the "tail" just above the buttocks, taking 2 to 3 seconds.
3. Repeat 100 times.

Indications. Fevers, headaches.

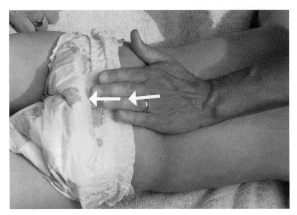

Figure 9-10 Down sacrum.

Comments. This is one of the first massages to do if the child has a fever with a hot head because it draws excess energy away from the head.

DOWN SACRUM (Figure 9-10)
1. Using the heel of your hand, massage firmly down the sacrum to the tip of the "tail" just above the buttocks.
2. Repeat 50 to 100 times.

Indications. Constipation.

Comments. This massage can be done quite firmly and has a strong downward energy. In some children the effect can be dramatic if there are a lot of retained feces.

UP SACRUM (Figure 9-11)
1. Using the heel of your hand, massage firmly up the sacrum from the tip of the "tail" to a level just above the buttocks.
2. Repeat 50 to 100 times.

Indications. Diarrhea.

Comments. This massage can be used for both acute and chronic diarrhea and can be combined with many other therapies.

THUMB TO ELBOW (Figure 9-12)
1. Hold the child's hand in your left hand (if you are right-handed) and gently stroke up

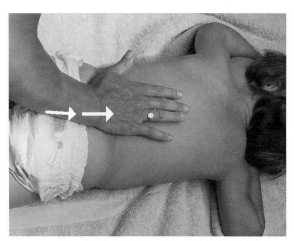

Figure 9-11 Up sacrum.

the forearm from the base of the thumb to the inside of the elbow, using your index and middle fingers (see Elbow to Little Finger).
2. Repeat 30 to 50 times and then repeat on other side.

Indications. Weak digestion, chills, diarrhea; especially effective in children younger than 3 years.

Comments. The effect of this massage depends on the flow of energy in the channels, for the site of massage is far away from the digestive organs, on which is has a strong effect. The massage is done toward the trunk, with the thought of pushing energy into the body.

ELBOW TO LITTLE FINGER
1. Hold the child's hand in your left hand (if you are right-handed) and gently stroke down the forearm from the inside of the elbow to the little finger, using your index and middle fingers.
2. Repeat 30 to 50 times and then repeat on other side.

Indications. Fevers, hot head, panics; especially effective in children younger than 3 years.

Comments. This massage also depends for its action on the flow of energy in the channels. The

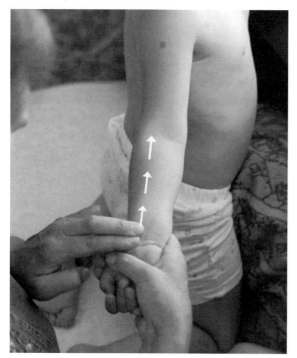

Figure 9-12   Thumb to elbow.

massage is done away from the trunk, with the thought of drawing excess energy and congestion from the head.

STOMACH CHANNEL (Figure 9-13)
1. Hold the child's leg in your left hand (if you are right-handed) and massage up the front of the shin, on the muscle one fingerbreadth (the child's fingerbreadth) to the outside of the shin bone.
2. Massage for 1 to 3 minutes and then repeat on other side.

Indications. Indigestion, vomiting, diarrhea, general weakness.

Comments. The stomach channel connects with the stomach and all the other digestive organs, so this massage is particularly useful for children with Weak digestion. As in the thumb to elbow massage, the thought is of pushing the energy into the body, so the massage is done toward the trunk.

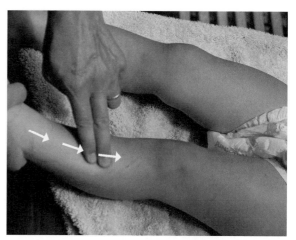

Figure 9-13   Stomach channel.

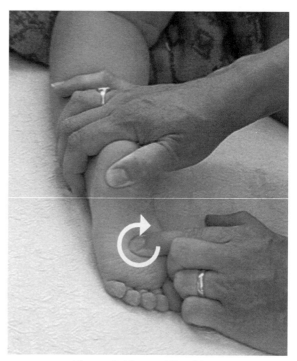

Figure 9-14   Middle of foot.

MIDDLE OF FOOT (Figure 9-14)
1. Find the point on the sole of the foot, on the midline, one third of the way from toes to heel.

2. Grasp the child's foot with your left hand (if you are right-handed) and massage the point with your thumb or index finger for 1 to 2 minutes.
3. Repeat on other foot.

Indications. Fevers, hot head, red or sore eyes.

Comments. This massage works by drawing energy away from the upper part of the body and in "grounding" the child. In overexcited children this sometimes has a marvelous calming effect.

Treatment of Illnesses

10

Constipation

Constipation can be very distressing. Not passing stools for several days on end causes children to become more and more grumpy and lethargic. In addition, they start to have abdominal pains and disturbed sleep. Constipation is a very common accompaniment to many other conditions. Occasionally, merely treating the constipation on its own is enough to cure a long-standing disease such as asthma.

Herbs Versus Over-the-Counter Laxatives

Over-the-counter laxatives are usually very powerful ones—ones that come under the category of drastic purgatives. Even though they often contain herbal derivatives, the herbs used (e.g., senna *Cassia angustifolia*) are not often used by herbalists for children. They are invaluable for occasional use, when there is a severe blockage, but they are not appropriate for longer-term conditions for which gentler herbs are more appropriate.

What Is Constipation?

We consider constipation to be present in either of the following conditions:

- The stools are hard and difficult to pass.
- There are frequently days when the child does not pass a stool.

This latter definition sounds rather strict, and it implies one day without passing a stool constitutes constipation. The reason for this tight definition is not some freudian hang-up, but it is because of the importance we attach to digestion. If a child is not evacuating regularly, the digestive system cannot be working as well as it could.

Danger Signs

Constipation is usually straightforward and easily treated with herbs and diet. However, an organic cause is possible, and constipation may indicate the presence of a more serious disease. If any doubt exists or in children with severe constipation, a thorough examination should be performed. Constipation in a newborn may indicate a congenital problems such as Hirschsprung's disease, or it may indicate appendicitis if accompanied by abdominal pain, lack of appetite, and a tight abdomen that is painful to touch. Blood or blood and mucus in the stools accompanied by severe abdominal pain must always be investigated.

There are rather different patterns for children younger than 3 years and those older. Babies and toddlers tend to have simple patterns. When they are constipated, the entire system becomes blocked, not just one part of the intestines. When they are older, different parts of the intestines have differentiated in their function and it is often necessary to make a more careful diagnosis. Obviously, the 3-year transition is not precise. It is not the stroke of midnight on their third birthday that the patterns change. Some children need a more careful diagnosis at the age of 2 years, and others still have baby patterns at 4 years. We start by describing the symptoms and treatments for children younger than 3 and then proceed to those who are older.

▢ PATTERNS FOR CHILDREN YOUNGER THAN 3 YEARS

For children younger than 3 years, the main distinction one needs to make is between the stagnant food pattern and Weak digestion.

Symptoms and Signs*

STAGNANT FOOD PATTERN

The stagnant food pattern is easy to recognize. When the child first comes to see you, you will notice the following:

- Sturdy
- Red cheeks
- Often irritable

On questioning and examining, you will find the following:

- Stools smell sour or smell terrible.
- When the stools come, they may be hard or may be loose.
- Abdomen is like a drum.

Variation: Stagnant Food Pattern with Pain on Passing. The symptoms of a stagnant food pattern with pain are essentially the same as those seen with the typical stagnant food pattern. The exceptions are as follows:

- Child holds onto stools.
- Child cries out when passing stools.

Causes. The causes for the stagnant food pattern are discussed in detail in Chapter 2. They are as follows:

- Overfeeding
- Irregular feeding
- Unsuitable food

---

*Facial color reveals a lot about a child's energy. See p. 54 for a discussion of facial colors and variations among racial groups.

Here we give a brief reminder of these causes:

OVEREATING. All parents are happy to see their child eat a lot. There is a deep-seated instinct that relates a large appetite to a state of health—we even call it a *healthy appetite*. Consequently, many mothers encourage their children to continue eating even after they are full. This pattern is more common after the children have been weaned, but it can even occur in breast-fed children if the mother has a copious supply of milk.

IRREGULAR FEEDING. The digestive system works best if food is eaten at regular times, and the stomach works best if it is allowed time to empty before being refilled. The exact pattern of feeding is not important. Different families and different countries have widely varying feeding patterns. The important thing is that the pattern is regular and that there are no snacks between meals. An easy trap to fall into if you have a small child is to provide a snack when your child is unhappy or tired. This may start off as a one-time treat, but it can easily develop into a habit of the child snacking all the time and not really eating proper meals. This opens the way for the stagnant food pattern.

UNSUITABLE FOOD. Eating unsuitable foods means different things at different ages. In babies who are bottle fed, this means that they cannot easily digest the milk they are receiving. For example, many children have cow's milk intolerance; others cannot easily digest soya milk. In toddlers younger than 3 years, unsuitable food can be food that they simply cannot digest, but more often it means that the food is too rich for them—it may be too fatty or too high in protein. It may also mean that the range of foods that they are eating is too great. Toddlers should be eating very simple food.

Causes for the Variation of Stagnant Food Pattern with Pain on Passing. The main symptoms and signs are the same. The chief difference is that there is pain on passing stools, probably from irritation of the anus. This is one of the main factors in the constipation starting in the first place.

The child experiences pain every time while passing stools and in response, learns to hold the stools until the last possible moment. To begin with, there is often a time in the day when the bowels would move. At this time the child may whimper and strain as he or she makes a huge effort to keep the stools in. After some days of this, the child cannot retain the stools and cries out when they are passed. In this case it is actually the retention of stools that leads to the stagnant food pattern.

WEAK DIGESTION
We describe here one main pattern with two variations. The main pattern we call *simple;* the reason for simple constipation is that the child is exhausted and does not have enough energy in his or her the system for digestion to work well. There is not enough energy for the intestines to move. It is called *simple,* for the lack of energy shows itself in many different ways. The first variation is Weak children with nervous energy. The second variation is another apparently Strong pattern, in which the child has all the appearance of being Strong, but the energy in the digestion is Weak.

When a child with the simple Weak pattern comes into the clinic, you will notice the following:

- Pasty face
- Dull eyes
- Quiet voice
- Clinging to mother

In severe cases the head is large compared with the body, and the bones stick out (an example is given in Figure 7-6, p. 59).

On questioning and examining, you will find the following:

- Poor appetite
- Passage of stools every 5 days or even longer
- Ability to go without passing stools for a long time without exhibiting many signs of distress
- Easily tired

When you feel the child, you will notice the following:

- Thin and weak arms and legs (or occasionally may be puffy and flabby)
- Thin abdomen

Causes. The causes for this pattern are explained in some detail in Chapter 2. Here we recapitulate the major points:

- Long labor
- Exhaustion of the mother
- Any long illness
- Excessive immunizations
- Unstructured nursing
- Poor-quality food

Variation 1: Weak with Nervous Energy. The physical symptoms and signs are the same; in particular, these children eat very little. It is the behavior that is different. These children have the following characteristics:

- Like to be the center of attention
- Are on the go all the time
- Go to bed late
- Always seem to get what they want

CAUSES. The causes for the basic energy are the same. The reasons why the child develops the nervous energy are discussed in Chapter 2.

Variation 2: Apparently Strong. This one is the opposite way round. The appearance of the child is strong. In particular, they may have the following characteristics:

- Sturdy
- Strong arms and legs
- Strong bones

In these children, it is just the digestion that is weak, so you will see the following:

- Poor appetite

- Very limited range of foods
- Weak energy in the abdomen

CAUSES. The apparently Strong pattern is seen in children who eat regular meals and have a set bedtime, but even so they have a desire for stimulation. These children often spend a lot of time in their heads, preferring reading and computer activities to physical activities. Their energy is concentrated in the head, so there is not enough for the digestion.

■ TREATMENT

Dosages*

Doses are given for 3-year-olds (Table 10-1). The tinctures are given three times a day in about 25 to 50 ml of warm water. The medicine may be sweetened. The doses we suggest are *suggestions only.* Each child may need something different.

STAGNANT FOOD PATTERN
Sample Prescription

Black root *Leptandra virginica*	4 drops tincture
Cascara sagrada *Rhamnus purshiana*	2 drops tincture
Yellow dock *Rumex crispus*	2 drops tincture
Aniseed *Pimpinella anisum*	2 drops tincture

If the child experiences griping pains when this starts to work, increase the amount of aniseed, or add the following:

Ginger *Zingiber officinalis*	2 drops tincture

If there is a lot of mucus (e.g., nasal discharge, cough), replace cascara *Rhamnus purshiana* with the following:

Butternut *Juglans cinerea*	2 drops tincture

To relieve pain associated with passing stools, add the following:

Stone root *Collinsonia canadensis*	3 drops tincture

---

*For more detailed information, see Chapter 8.

Table 10-1

AGE	MULTIPLY 3-YEAR-OLD DOSE BY
6-12 months	$\times \frac{1}{3}$
1-2 years	$\times \frac{1}{2}$
2-4 years	$\times 1$
4-7 years	$\times 1\frac{1}{2}$
7-14 years	$\times 2$
14+ years	$\times 3$

Explanation. Black root is specific for the stagnant food pattern. It gently stimulates digestion by acting on the liver while being overall a slight relaxant. Cascara given in small doses is a gently moving tonic for the bowels and supplements the action of black root. Yellow dock is a mild tonic laxative and gently moves digestion; butternut has a similar action to cascara but is more effective when a lot of is mucus present. Aniseed is included to prevent the pains of flatulence, which are likely to occur when the stools start to move. Even despite this, the child may have griping pains, in which case ginger may be added. Stone root is specific for weakness in the rectum with pain on passing stools. (Stone root should not be given on its own because it is a strong tonic. When pain occurs with the passing of stools, the energy has been withdrawn from the rectum only. Only the rectum needs to be toned; the rest of the digestive system needs to get moving.)

Results of Treatment. As mentioned, the results of treatment are inclined to be rather sudden. It is rather like untying the neck of a balloon. Once the stools have started to flow, they may come out very quickly and in large quantities. It is a good idea to warn the parents of this and also to advise them to stop taking the herbs if they begin to pass more than two or three stools a day. The herbs may be resumed at a smaller dosage and taken until the abdomen is no longer swollen. This may take a week or two.

Warning. The dosage needs to be controlled carefully. If it is not large enough, then not much will happen. If it is too large and the child has uncontrollable diarrhea for several days, there is a danger of the diarrhea taking hold and the child becoming seriously ill through dehydration. After this, it may be necessary to give a mild tonic to the digestion, such as the following:

Barberry *Berberis vulgaris*	4 drops tincture
Fringe tree *Chionanthus virginicus*	4 drops tincture
Fennel *Foeniculum officinale*	2 drops tincture

In the unlikely event that the stools are still loose and a bit watery after 7 to 10 days, replace berberis with the following:

Peruvian bark *Cinchona calisaya*	3 drops tincture

Explanation. Barberry is a bitter tonic and helps digestion. It promotes the flow of bile and is therefore also gently moving. Fringe tree helps move digestion gently, maintaining regular bowel activity, and also helps with absorption. Fennel is a general tonic for Weak digestion. Peruvian bark is used specifically when the body has lost a lot of fluid. It is particularly useful if the stools continue to be a little loose and do not firm up after a few days.

Advice. The parents must be advised of the necessity of children having regular food, suitable food, and not too much. If they cannot provide this for their children, the constipation may recur. See Chapter 2 for a more in-depth discussion.

WEAK DIGESTION
Prescription 1

Barberry *Berberis vulgaris*	4 drops tincture
Fennel *Foeniculum officinale*	2 drops tincture
Licorice *Glycyrrhiza glabra*	2 drops tincture

Prescription 2

Buckthorn *Rhamnus cathartica*	2 drops tincture
Aniseed *Pimpinella anisum*	2 drops tincture
Honey	1 tsp

Note that the honey should be pasteurized for children younger than 1 year. See note on p. 67.

Variation: Weak with Nervous Energy. The prescription is exactly the same. The main differ-

ence is that there will be great difficulty in getting the child to take the medicines.

Variation: Apparently Strong. Once again, the prescription is the same, although to improve the appetite, one could add the following:

Gentian *Gentiana lutea*	2 drops tincture

Variation: Pain on Passing Stool. Once again, the previous herb may be used to alleviate this symptom:

Stone root *Collinsonia canadensis*	2 drops tincture

Variation: Squashy Legs. Squashy legs is a symptom we referred to in Chapter 2. It means that the legs are somewhat fatter than you would expect and that they are softer to the touch than you would expect. This is because of the poor circulation of fluids in the legs. Once the constipation has started to move, add the following:

Poplar bark *Populus tremuloides*	2 drops tincture

Explanation. *Prescription 1* is for the weaker children. Berberis is a bitter tonic that strengthens the whole body gradually while also gently moving digestion. Fennel is also a tonic and is included (in preference to aniseed) to prevent any griping sensations. Licorice tones the body and also helps move the bowels. Poplar bark, taken over a long time, helps tone the bowels, especially the small intestine.

Prescription 2 is for slightly stronger children. Buckthorn is a close relative of cascara and has a similar action, although it is gentler. When taken in small doses, it is also a tonic to the bowels and provides the all-important moving function. Aniseed is slightly more dispersing and less tonic than fennel. Honey helps lubricate the bowels. Stone root is a tonic for the large intestine and rectum. Poplar is a tonic specific for water retention. It is often prescribed to treat diarrhea but may also be used to clear constipation.

Results. There is a temptation to use large doses to produce quick results, but this is a mistake. You may get the quick result of the child passing stools, but it is not the best thing for the child. The results that one is really looking for are an increase in the child's energy. This is something that can happen only gradually over a period of some weeks, possibly even 2 months. This means that in the first week, little effect from taking the herbs may be noticed and it may take some persuasion to get the parents to continue taking the herbs. Only after about 2 weeks will some improvement in the bowels be seen, and even then there may still be significant delays. If no change at all is seen after this time, the dosage should be increased. In addition, it may be helpful to point out to the parents that the intestines are made up of muscles and that if these muscles are weak, it simply takes time to build up their strength.

■ PATTERNS FOR CHILDREN OLDER THAN 3 YEARS

At 3 or 4 years of age, the different parts of the digestive system start to function more independently. It is possible for one part to work well while another part is blocked. When this happens, the symptoms are more specific and it may be necessary to use more specific remedies. A traditional differentiation is as follows:

- Sluggish liver
- Weak or Cold small intestine
- Lazy large intestine

The sluggish liver pattern leads to constipation because there is insufficient bile secretion for digestion of food and for lubrication. The intestines may be become weak through overall weakness, or they may become stagnant because of Cold accumulating; the large intestine may become lazy for a variety of reasons.

Where the Discomfort Is Felt

Liver	Below the ribs; the sensation of heaviness, or a weight, going from one side to the other
Small intestine	General aching pain all around the umbilicus, sometimes even a cramping pain (if there is Cold)
Large intestine	Pain and sometimes bloating below the umbilicus

Symptoms Pointing to the Different Patterns

LIVER

- A feeling of heaviness, obstruction, or pain is felt in a line just below the diaphragm.
- The child is irritable.
- The face appears yellowish.
- There is a strong relation with fatty foods, either dislikes fatty foods or consumes too much of them.

SMALL INTESTINE

- The abdomen feels heavy and may ache.
- There is a strong relation with cold foods such as ice cream and cold carbonated drinks (the child may dislike or consume too much).
- The middle of the abdomen may feel cold to touch.

LARGE INTESTINE

- The child has lower abdominal pain.
- Passing stools is difficult.
- The child may forget to go to the toilet.
- The child may be unaware of passing stools, so has occasional "accidents."
- The child may walk on tiptoe or have some feet problems.

Causes

LIVER

- The child consumes excessively fatty foods, such as burgers and chips or creamy cakes, which put a strain on the liver, as does excess sugar intake.
- The child drinks a lot of fluid with meals. One needs enough fluid with the meal to moisten the food to digest it, but if a child drinks too much fluid, especially carbonated drinks, the stomach

fluids become diluted and the stomach and the liver are strained. This may weaken the stomach, or it may give rise to constipation.

- The child does not exercise enough. A basic minimum of exercise is essential to keep the energy moving in the body. Below a certain minimum, the child can easily become constipated. This is especially likely if the child slouches in front of the TV after eating, which constricts the abdomen.
- The child is emotionally upset or brooding. In this case constipation results from the child holding onto feelings and taking them internally. It is especially associated with feelings of resentment, anger, and revenge. Very occasionally, this pattern appears in children as young as 3 years, when they are angry at the arrival of a younger sibling. It is common in teenagers, in whom a state of being angry is the norm.

SMALL INTESTINE

- The child eats Cold food and/or too much raw food and eats irregular meals. Cold food (physically cold food and food with Cold energy, such as salads and cucumbers) and raw food are somewhat difficult for children to digest and may be passed from the stomach to the small intestines still slightly Cold and not sufficiently digested. When this happens, the intestines become a little weak and do not function properly. The same happens when the child eats irregular meals.
- The child does mental work or watches TV while eating. When the mind is busy, all the energy leaves the body and goes to the head. It especially leaves the digestive system. This means that if a child is concentrating while eating, there is not enough energy for digestion and the intestines become very sluggish.

LARGE INTESTINE

- The child does too much mental work, reading, or dreaming. This cause is similar to the previous one, but refers to too much mental work altogether. The child's energy goes up into its head and does not come down into its body. This can also happen when a child has had an experience that he or she wishes to forget. Sometimes the child lives so much in his or her head that the energy does not reach the feet properly, resulting in orthopedic problems.

- The child has anxieties about going to the toilet or anxieties in general. This is the classic Freudian "anal retention." A child may hold onto stools as part of a larger picture of anxiety. He or she holds onto stools just like everything else in life, for fear of things slipping away or for fear of being criticized.

- The child has a case of mild aluminium poisoning. Aluminium in excess has a paralyzing effect on the intestines. This can lead to a vicious circle because the normal way of eliminating aluminium from the body is through the large intestine. If a child is already constipated and is taking in very small doses of aluminium (e.g., from the cooking pot, from food wrapped or served in aluminium), the levels of aluminum accumulate, resulting in the constipation becoming more and more entrenched. Eventually, this can lead to paralysis of the large intestine with compacted stools.

◼ TREATMENT

Liver

Many of these herbs are ones that promote the flow of bile.

PRESCRIPTION 1

Yellow dock *Rumex crispus*	5 drops tincture
Lemon balm *Melissa officinalis*	3 drops tincture
Dandelion root *Taraxacum officinalis*	3 drops tincture
Aniseed *Pimpinella anisum*	2 drops tincture

If the constipation is severe, add the following:

Cascara *Rhamnus purshiana*	3 drops tincture

If there are severe spasms, add the following:

Wild yam *Dioscorea villosa*	3 drops tincture

PRESCRIPTION 2

Yellow dock *Rumex crispus*	5 drops tincture
Balmony *Chelone glabra*	3 drops tincture
Lemon balm *Melissa officinalis*	3 drops tincture

Explanation. Yellow dock increases the secretion of bile and is specific for this condition. Once the bile flows, digestion starts to move. Lemon balm relieves spasm in the digestive tract and helps relieve tension and stress. It is often used for digestive problems. Dandelion root is a strong stimulant to digestion and should be increased if the child is wan and pasty. Aniseed is included to relieve any flatulence and colic that might arise when the bowels start to move. Cascara is a strong laxative and can be added if the main prescription is not moving enough. Wild yam can be included if there are severe spasms and colic—more than can be controlled by aniseed. Balmony regulates the digestive system, and because it increases the flow of bile, it is also specific for this condition.

VARIATION: CONSTIPATION FROM EMOTIONAL CAUSES

When the constipation comes mainly from emotional causes and brooding, one needs to include herbs to relax the child:

Lobelia *Lobelia inflata*	5 drops tincture
Wild yam *Dioscorea villosa*	4 drops tincture
Yellow dock *Rumex crispus*	3 drops tincture
Balmony *Chelone glabra*	3 drops tincture

Explanation. Lobelia is a strong relaxant. In some children, just relaxing is enough to enable them to pass stools. Wild yam relieves spasms. Yellow dock is gently moving and a mild toner (to balance the dispersing effect of the other herbs). Balmony helps regulate digestion when tension is present.

Small Intestine

PRESCRIPTION 1

Yellow dock *Rumex crispus*	5 drops tincture
Ginger *Zingiber officinalis*	3 drops tincture
Barberry *Berberis officinalis*	3 drops tincture
Wormwood *Artemisia absinthium*	2 drops tincture

PRESCRIPTION 2 (WHEN THERE ARE A LOT OF SPASMS)

Butternut *Juglans cinerea*	5 drops tincture
Wild yam *Dioscorea villosa*	3 drops tincture

Cayenne *Capsicum minimum*	2 drops tincture
Sweet sedge *Acorus calamus*	3 drops tincture

Explanation. The small intestine pattern tends to be related to weak intestines, so all the herbs are mild tonics. In addition, yellow dock and barberry both move digestion gently. Ginger is included because most children with this pattern have a Cold digestion and a Cold stomach. Wormwood is a bitter tonic and also moves the intestines and helps relieve spasms. If the child hates the taste of the prescription, try omitting wormwood.

The second prescription has somewhat stronger herbs, with less tonic effect. Butternut is more strongly moving. Wild yam is stronger in relieving spasms. Cayenne is more strongly heating than Ginger and more strongly stimulating. The tonic in the prescription is sweet sedge. The proportions we have suggested are useful for a start. If it is too dispersing a prescription and the child becomes too tired, increase the cayenne and sweet sedge. If the prescription is not moving enough, increase the butternut.

Large Intestine

PRESCRIPTION 1

Sweet sedge *Acorus calamus*	5 drops tincture
Yellow dock *Rumex crispus*	3 drops tincture
Licorice *Glycyrrhiza glabra*	3 drops tincture
Fennel *Foeniculum vulgare*	3 drops tincture

PRESCRIPTION 2

Cascara *Rhamnus purshiana*	5 drops tincture
Wormwood *Artemisia absinthium*	2 drops tincture
Aniseed *Pimpinella anisum*	3 drops tincture
Licorice *Glycyrrhiza glabra*	3 drops tincture

Explanation. Sweet sedge has a specific effect on strengthening and gently moving the energy in the lower abdomen. Yellow dock is included again for the large intestine pattern (as well as the liver pattern) because it is a general tonic for digestion. Fennel is included to relieve flatulence and colic when the bowels start to move. It has a similar action to aniseed, but it has a stronger tonic effect and less effect on flatulence and colic. Licorice is an overall tonic for the entire body and is also a gentle laxative.

The second prescription is more moving. Cascara is a strong laxative. Wormwood is a tonic to the entire digestive system. Licorice is an overall tonic for the whole body and is also a gentle laxative. Aniseed is included again to relieve flatulence and colic when the bowels start to move.

Administration. Give these herbs in warm water at least three times a day. Slightly better results will be noticed if they are given before meals.

Results. The results in the first few days are variable. Sometimes there is a sudden release of tension, and stools are passed. Sometimes nothing happens. What one is looking for is a longer-term effect. After a week or so, there should be a slight improvement, but one should not expect a cure in this time. If there is no change after 2 weeks, increase the dose or reexamine the prescription. The herbs should be given for at least a month, possibly 2 months.

Advice. A number of simple remedies can help constipation:

- Eat a good-quality diet with organic fruit and vegetables.
- Consider the possibility that there is a food intolerance, such as intolerance to wheat.
- Make sure the child is drinking enough water. Some children do not seem to feel thirsty, and others get so absorbed in what they are doing that they forget to drink. This is particularly important in hot weather.
- A teaspoon of honey dissolved in hot water taken first thing in the morning is helpful for the older children (i.e., those older than 1 year; see note on p. 67).
- Give a few teaspoons of prune juice each day.
- Give syrup of figs. (Always read the label on the bottle. Some proprietary blends contain all sorts of weird chemicals, as well as drastic purgatives).

- For toddlers and older children, make sure that they are getting enough exercise. The bowels will not move if the other parts of the body do not move. Sometimes just going for a walk is enough to cure the problem.
- Try and make a time of at least 5 minutes each day (preferably after breakfast) when the child sits on the toilet. Sometimes merely sitting there is enough to get the bowels moving.

THE USE OF SENNA CASSIA ANGUSTIFOLIA. This chapter is remarkable in its omission of senna, one of the few remaining herbal medicines in the orthodox pharmacopoeia. The reason for this omission is that its continued use is not advised, for it has the reputation of causing irritation of the lining of the bowels. It does have a place as a drastic purgative. It should be used with great caution in babies and young children because of the danger of provoking uncontrollable diarrhea, and hence creating a worse situation.

THE USE OF RHUBARB RHEUM PALMATUM. Rhubarb is best used as a drastic purgative, when quick results are needed. Some practitioners use small quantities to move the bowels gently, but we prefer to use other herbs. It is normally given with herbs such as ginger *Zingiber officinalis* and fennel *Foeniculum vulgare* to allay the griping caused by its extremely Cold energy.

Other Treatments

BULK LAXATIVES

At 7 years of age, the digestive system is much maturer and the normal laxatives given to adults can be used. At this age it may be beneficial to give children high-fiber foods such as wholemeal bread. One can also use bulk laxatives (fiber that passes through the system undigested). Commercial brands that are quite satisfactory are available, but we prefer to use the following:

Psyllium husks (1)　　　　　　　　　　2 tsp in water

Make sure that the child drinks at least 250 ml ($\frac{1}{2}$ pint) of water with it. The water makes the psyllium husks swell and gives bulk to the feces. (Note that these should not normally be used in children younger than age 3 years.)

CASTOR OIL RUB

A teaspoon of castor oil is massaged into the abdomen. Use a gentle clockwise motion. Some of the castor oil is absorbed into the gut and gently moves the intestines. This is especially good for breast-fed babies and in other situations in which it is difficult to give herbs by mouth. The effect is much less violent than taking castor oil by mouth, something that we do not advise for children.

MASSAGES

The following massages can be helpful in relieving constipation (see figures in Chapter 9). They should be done at least once a day to begin with, although once the bowels are functioning, this frequency can be reduced. This normally means that the parents will have to perform the massages. Massages with essential oils are especially useful when treating the Weak pattern because these children are likely to be very fussy and refuse to take herbs by mouth. For these children, a daily massage with essential oils may be the way to build up the energy and thereby cure the problem.

General Abdominal Massage. Gently massage around the abdomen in a clockwise direction. You can use the palm of your hand, or you can make a point with your first two fingers. You may use a simple massage oil, such as almond oil, combine the essential oils, or use castor oil. Go round and round for about 2 to 4 minutes. If you can do this two or three times a day, it can be very effective. Our experience has been that younger children become bored and restless once the novelty has worn off but that older children respond well to it.

Heel on Upper Abdomen. Use the heel of your hand to massage the upper part of the abdomen (see Heel on Lower Abdomen) between the base of the rib cage and the navel, gently pushing about 50 times. This treatment is indicated for indigestion, weak digestion, insomnia related to weak digestion, and lack of appetite.

Heel on Lower Abdomen. Use the heel of your hand to massage the lower part of the abdomen, below the navel, gently pushing about 50 times. This treatment is indicated for general weakness, bedwetting, cystitis, and other urinary problems, as well as the indications for Heel on Upper Abdomen.

Stomach Passage. Let the child lie down comfortably with the chest up. Gently massage the point midway between the navel and the lower tip of the breastbone (sternum) using your index and middle fingers. Gently vibrate for 1 to 2 minutes. The vibrating action gently stimulates the whole of the digestive system. This treatment is indicated for the stagnant food pattern, indigestion, weak digestion, general weakness, and lack of appetite.

Intestines Point. As for Stomach Passage, but massage the point midway between the navel and the top of the pubic bone. This treatment is indicated for general weakness and urinary problems.

Down Sacrum. Using the heel of your hand, massage firmly down the sacrum from just above the buttocks to the tip of the "tail." Repeat 50 to 100 times. This treatment is indicated for constipation.

Results. The results vary according to the condition and to the child. Sometimes the stools are waiting there ready to come out and just need a gentle massage to release them. In other cases, especially in the Weak patterns, massage needs to be given every day for several weeks to build up the energy and to get the bowels moving regularly.

■ ESSENTIAL OILS

Essential oils can help relieve constipation, although their use is secondary (as opposed to their use in coughs, where they are almost indispensable). We advise using them as additions to massage oil. The following have a reputation of helping constipation:

- Rosemary *Rosmarinus officinalis*
- Marjoram *Origanum marjorana*

Add 2 to 3 drops of the oils of each to 25 ml (1 oz) of massage oil.

Explanation

The main effects of these oils is to enliven the digestive system and to relieve any spasms and colic. They do not have a direct effect on moving the bowels, but they definitely add to the effect of the massage. For the weak pattern, add fennel *Foeniculum vulgaris*.

11

Chronic Diarrhea

Parents sometimes bring their children in just for the symptom of diarrhea, and it is common for children who are brought in for another complaint to have the additional symptom of chronic diarrhea. Digestion is so important for babies and toddlers that the diarrhea must be addressed if the child is to get well. It often happens that merely by curing the diarrhea, the balance of the body is so much improved that the illness resolves without further treatment.

What Is Diarrhea?

Where should one draw the line between unformed stools and diarrhea? There are no hard and fast rules. What is normal for one child may be abnormal for another. Bearing this in mind, we consider that there are two criteria for determining that a child has diarrhea:

- The stools are loose.
- The stools are loose and frequent.

If the stools are loose and frequent, it is simple diarrhea. If the stools only come once every other day, but are loose when they come, this is called diarrhea alternating with constipation. As for frequency, this varies with age (Box 11-1). If the frequency of bowel movements is more than that shown in Box 11-1, for most children it is considered abnormal and is classified as diarrhea.

If any child under your care has any of the symptoms listed in the following box, a thorough examination is necessary.

Box 11-1

A Guide to the Number of Times a Day That a Child Passes Stools, without Being Pathologic

AGE	NUMBER OF BOWEL MOVEMENTS PER DAY
0-6 months	6
6 months-1 year	4
1-4 years	3
4+ years	2

◼ PATTERNS

There are three main patterns of diarrhea:

- Stagnant food pattern
- Weak digestion
- Weak digestion with nervous energy

The stagnant food pattern is seen in Strong, energetic children and comes about because they eat more than they can easily digest. In a state of health, these children are enthusiastic and great fun to be with, but when they have diarrhea and the food is fermenting inside them, they become very irritable and difficult.

The Weak digestion pattern is a common pattern, and one in which there is not enough energy to digest food properly. This often means that these children seek sugary food, or sometimes fruit juice, because this is all that they feel they can digest. In fact, these sugary foods are usually the worst thing for them.

The weak digestion with nervous energy pattern has the same basic cause. The difference is in the presentation of children with this pattern. They appear to have boundless energy, but when you start to make inquiries, you realize that the energy they appear to have could not possibly come from the amount of food they are eating. Each of these patterns is discussed in greater detail in Chapter 2.

◼ CAUSES

A cause for diarrhea irrespective of pattern is the use of antibiotics. Digestion is a complicated process that takes place with the assistance of beneficial bacteria in the intestines. When a child takes a course of antibiotics, the beneficial bacteria are killed along with the malignant ones. This considerably weakens the digestive system and can lead to diarrhea.

Stagnant Food Pattern

A detailed explanation of the causes of this pattern was given in Part 1 (see Chapter 2), so we only give summary here. The basic causes are as follows:

- Overfeeding
- Irregular feeding
- Unsuitable food

There may be a trigger factor that causes the pattern to develop into diarrhea. Possible trigger factors include the following:

- Aftereffects of gastroenteritis
- Teething
- Infections
- Immunizations

OVEREATING

All parents are happy to see their child eat a lot. There is a deep-seated instinct that relates a large appetite to a state of health—we even call it a *healthy appetite.* Consequently, many mothers encourage their children to continue eating even after they are full. This pattern is more common after the children have been weaned, but it can occur in breast-fed children if the mother has a copious supply of milk.

IRREGULAR FEEDING

The digestive system works best if food is eaten at regular times, and the stomach works best if it is allowed time to empty before being refilled. The exact pattern of feeding is not important. Different families and different countries have widely varying feeding patterns. The important thing is that the pattern is regular and that there are no snacks between meals. An easy trap to fall into if you have a small child is to provide a snack when your child is unhappy or tired. This may start off as a one-time treat, but it can easily develop into a habit of the child snacking all the time and not really eating proper meals. This opens the way for the stagnant food pattern.

UNSUITABLE FOOD

Eating unsuitable foods means different things at different ages. In babies who are bottle fed, this means that they cannot easily digest the milk they are receiving. For example, many children have cow's milk intolerance; others cannot easily digest soya milk. In toddlers younger than 3 years, unsuitable food can be food that they simply cannot digest, but more often it means that the food is too rich for them—it may be too fatty or too high in protein. It may also mean that the range of foods that they are eating is too great. Toddlers should be eating very simple food.

FINDING THE FOOD INTOLERANCE

Food intolerances most likely to cause diarrhea are intolerance to cow's milk and gluten. Included in this category is celiac disease, that is, diarrhea related to gluten. This used to be a cause for death until quite recently, but now most doctors are on the lookout for it. However, many subacute cases of diarrhea have their origin in gluten intolerance.

> Food intolerance is a major cause of diarrhea. See Chapter 15 for the most likely foods.

Finding the food intolerance is obviously important in curing the problem. This is discussed in more detail in Chapter 15.

TRIGGER FACTORS

Often, the child has a tendency to one of the basic patterns but manages to remain fairly healthy until something happens to tip the balance, giving rise to the symptom of diarrhea. Once the diarrhea has started, the child never has the energy to get back to a state of health. Following are some common triggers.

Aftereffects of Gastroenteritis. When a child starts to interact with other children, it is easy for him or her to catch the "bug" that is going round the nursery or school. If the stagnant food pattern already exists, the child is predisposed to catching the bug. After the child is more or less better, the stools may remain loose for a long time.

Teething. Teething puts a stress on the entire digestive system. If the stagnant food pattern is present, this extra stress can tip the balance and give rise to the full-blown symptoms described in Chapter 2.

Infection. As the child tries to fight off infection, there is a temporary lowering of energy. If the stagnant food pattern is almost there, the reduction in energy available for digestion can give rise to diarrhea.

Immunization. The effect of immunization is similar to that of acquiring an infection: There is a temporary lowering of energy. If the stagnant food pattern is almost there, the reduction in energy available for digestion can lead to diarrhea.

Weak Digestion

There are many causes in life of weak digestion. Common causes are as follows:

- Long and difficult birth
- Any long or severe illness
- Immunizations
- A bad attack of diarrhea that has weakened the child
- Difficulty in finding food that suits the child
- Too much mental stimulation
- Too much fruit juice
- Too much ice cream or ice-cold food
- Food straight from the fridge

Most of these causes for Weak energy were covered in some detail in Chapter 2. The causes that have not been covered are too much ice-cold food and drink. Many children love ice creams and ice-cold drinks and food. It seems to have a soothing effect on the stomach. However, if they take too much, the energy required in the stomach to warm up the ice-cold food or drink may take all the energy that is available for digestion. The food cannot be digested properly, and the child may get diarrhea.

▪ SYMPTOMS AND SIGNS*

Stagnant Food Pattern

- The stools are foul smelling and often green. In mild cases they may only smell sour.

---

*Facial color reveals a lot about a child's energy. See p. 54 for a discussion of facial colors and variations among racial groups.

- Abdominal distention and pain may be present.
- Before passing the stool, the child may be in pain and may cry out.
- The breath smells foul.
- The days of diarrhea may be interspersed with days of constipation.
- The child is typically Strong, with red cheeks and a greenish tinge around the mouth if the stools are passed up to two times a day. If stools are passed more frequently, the child is more likely to be green round the mouth without red cheeks.
- Nasal discharge is often present.

Weak Digestion

Weak digestion can range from mild to serious.

- Stools are loose and do not smell. They may be watery or contain undigested food and water. There may be white lumps of curdled milk in the diaper, or the stools may consist of food particles and other waste products.
- In severe cases diarrhea may occur every time food or milk is taken.
- Facial color is pale.
- The child likes to sleep during the day.
- The child has no appetite.
- The spirit is weak, and the child may appear exhausted.
- The child has only a slight thirst and then for warm drinks.

WEAK DIGESTION WITH NERVOUS ENERGY
- Stools are loose and do not smell.
- Facial color is pale.
- The child's appetite is poor, and he or she is picky about food.
- The child often drinks a lot of juice.
- The child appears to have a lot of energy, runs around a lot, does not complain of the cold, and does not seem to need to sleep much.
- Often, the parents are exhausted.
- The child may be attention seeking.

An explanation for these symptoms is given in Chapter 2.

▪ TREATMENT

The doses we give are for children aged 3 years (Table 11-1).* The doses we suggest are *suggestions only.* Each child may need something different.

Stagnant Food Pattern

PRESCRIPTION 1
For loose, foul-smelling stools, alternating with constipation and not more frequent than twice a day, use the following:

Black root *Leptandra virginica*	4 drops tincture
Agrimony *Agrimonia eupatoria*	2 drops tincture

If the child has an insatiable appetite, add the following:

Meadowsweet *Filipendula ulmaria*	2 drops tincture

Explanation. Black root is specific for the stagnant food pattern. Often, one does not need to use anything else. It must be remembered that in large doses, black root is a purgative, and even in small doses, it can be helpful in relieving constipation related to the stagnant food pattern. Surprisingly, in small doses it can also be used for diarrhea, for its action is regulating. Agrimony, which may or may not be necessary, is an astringent and will help dry up the loose stools.

▪ Table 11-1	
AGE	**MULTIPLY 3-YEAR-OLD DOSE BY**
6-12 months	× $\frac{1}{3}$
1-2 years	× $\frac{1}{2}$
2-4 years	× 1
4-7 years	× $1\frac{1}{2}$
7-14 years	× 2
14+ years	× 3

*For more detailed information about dosages, see Chapter 8.

If the child has an insatiable appetite, it will be difficult to prevent overeating. This means that even if the diarrhea is cured, it will soon return because of this overeating. In these cases meadowsweet can help cool down the overactive stomach, as well as reduce the diarrhea.

Results. Some odd reactions may be noted in the first day or two of treatment. If there has been significant constipation alternating with diarrhea, the diarrhea may worsen at first if the herbs are administered at the end of a constipation cycle. Apart from this, there may not be any significant reduction in the diarrhea for a week or two. If there is no change after this time, then before increasing the dosage, ask the parents in detail about the diet and whether they have managed to change it.

If the child has had diarrhea for any length of time (some months), the villi in the intestines will be injured. It takes time for these to regrow, so the herbs often need to be taken for a month or two. In addition, they should be taken for 2 to 3 weeks after the main symptoms have disappeared to consolidate the treatment.

PRESCRIPTION 2

For loose stools that come more frequently than twice a day or for watery, foul-smelling stools, try the following:

Black root *Leptandra virginica*	4 drops tincture
Agrimony *Agrimonia eupatoria*	2 drops tincture
Cranesbill *Geranium maculatum*	2 drops tincture

If the child has an insatiable appetite, add the following:

Meadowsweet *Filipendula ulmaria*	2 drops tincture

Explanation. Once again, black root is the main herb, this time with the addition of agrimony and American cranesbill as astringents. This will help dry up the liquid in the stools. Geranium is often used for this, but many other astringents work just as well.

Results. Aggravation of the diarrhea is uncommon. Rather, it should gradually get better. Once again, do not expect rapid changes. The main change at first is that the stools should smell slightly better. If there is no improvement after 2 weeks, check that the changes in diet have been made and then increase the dosage.

Advice. The child should avoid the following:

Cold food
Ice-cold food and drinks
Fruit juice

In addition, make sure that the food is regular and that the child reduces the quantity of food eaten. Without doing this, there is no hope of curing the symptom. This may present problems because children are usually strong willed and demanding, and they like getting their own way. You can reassure the parents by pointing out that they need to persist for only 5 days. After that, new habits will have been formed.

Problems in Changing the Diet. There are very real problems in changing the diet, but if it is changed, the stools usually get better eventually, even without treatment. This means that if they are no better after a month, even with herbs, the child's diet needs to be examined again: the quantity, the regularity, and whether there is any food intolerance. We have found it particularly difficult to persuade some parents that their children's digestion can cope only with relatively small amounts of food. For example, it took us many months of weekly visits to persuade one patient that a whole egg was too much for his 2-year-old to eat at one sitting. (This is discussed in more detail in Chapter 3.)

Weak Digestion

There are two classes of herbs to be included. One is astringents, which stop the diarrhea, and the other is tonics, which build up the energy. Among astringents are the following:

Agrimony *Agrimonia eupatoria*
Bistort *Polygonum bistoria*

Cranesbill *Geranium maculatum*
Tormentil *Potentilla tormentilla*
Oak bark *Quercus robur*

Among tonics are the following:

Fennel *Foeniculum vulgare*
Bayberry *Myrica cerifera*
Peruvian bark *Cinchona calisaya*
Ginger *Zingiber officinalis*
Cinnamon *Cinnamomum zeylandicum*

A typical prescription for mildly loose stools is as follows:

Agrimony *Agrimonia eupatoria*	4 drops tincture
Fennel *Foeniculum vulgare*	3 drops tincture

For very loose stools, the following prescription may be tried:

Bistort *Polygonum bistorta*	4 drops tincture
Cranesbill *Geranium maculatum*	3 drops tincture
Oak bark *Quercus robur*	3 drops tincture
Fennel *Foeniculum vulgare*	4 drops tincture

If there is great exhaustion, add the following:

Cinnamon *Cinnamomum zeylandicum*	4 drops tincture

If the problem has arisen from taking too much Cold food and drink or if the child has signs of Cold energy, add the following:

Ginger *Zingiber officinalis*	3 drops tincture

If there is a lot of dribbling from the mouth, the following may be added:

Bayberry *Myrica cerifera*	3 drops tincture

EXPLANATION

The astringents will help dry up the stools. Agrimony is a tonic and an astringent, and fennel assists it by being a tonic. For very loose stools, agrimony is replaced by the three herbs bistort, cranesbill, and oak bark, which, when combined, have a stronger effect in drying the stools. In cases of great weakness, cinnamon is a great tonic that is also astringent and warming. When the whole digestive system has become very Cold, ginger will help warm it up. Bayberry is an astringent tonic that works more on the upper part of the digestive system, so it is suitable to add when there is dribbling from the mouth.

RESULTS

Some change should be noticed within a day or two as the astringents start to work. If there is no change after 7 to 10 days, increase the dosage and start to ask questions about the diet. After some weeks of improved stools, it is safe to start reducing the quantities of astringents. The tonics should be continued for much longer—until the appetite has improved.

WEAK DIGESTION WITH NERVOUS ENERGY

The choice of herbs is the same as for the previous pattern. The main difference is that there may be even more problems in persuading the child to take the herbs. The more pleasant-tasting ones such as fennel and agrimony are more acceptable. If the child refuses to take the herbs, then massage with essential oils is the next thing to try.

ADVICE, FOR ALL PATTERNS

- Avoid the following:
  Cold food
  Ice-cold food and drinks
  Fruit juice
- Eat good-quality organic food.
- In the case of long-standing diarrhea, take a good-quality food supplement.
- Look for possible food allergies.
- For the child with low-energy patterns, reduce the amount of liquid intake. In particular, all fruit juice should be avoided. This too may present problems, especially for difficult children who manage to wriggle their way out of things they do not want to do. Bear in mind that there is no hope of curing the condition if the child is drinking too much liquid.
- If the child is taking (or has recently taken) antibiotics, give a teaspoon of live yogurt each

day. This will help reestablish the intestinal flora that have been killed by the antibiotic.

MASSAGES

Massages on their own can be of great help in curing chronic diarrhea, especially in children with Weak patterns. As with all long-term problems, do not expect immediate results. The diarrhea is not going to stop after just a day or two if it has been present for months. Look for gradual improvement over a few weeks (in the Weak child). If there have been no changes by that time, then massage may not be appropriate. It is helpful to combine the massage oil with the essential oils given here. (See Chapter 9 for descriptions and illustrations of the massages.)

General Abdominal Massage. Gently massage around the abdomen, in a counterclockwise direction. You can use the palm of your hand, or you can make a point with your first two fingers. You may use a simple massage oil, such as almond oil, or combine it with the essential oils. Go round and round for about 2 to 4 minutes. If you can do this two or three times a day, it can be very effective. Our experience has been that younger children become bored and restless once the novelty has worn off but that older children respond well to it.

Heel on Upper Abdomen. Use the heel of your hand to massage the upper part of the abdomen between the base of the rib cage and the navel, gently pushing about 50 times. This treatment is indicated for indigestion, weak digestion, insomnia related to weak digestion, and lack of appetite.

Heel on Lower Abdomen. Use the heel of your hand to massage the lower part of the abdomen, below the navel, gently pushing about 50 times. This treatment is indicated for general weakness, bedwetting, cystitis, and other urinary problems, as well as the indications for Heel on Upper Abdomen.

Stomach Passage. Let the child lie down comfortably with the chest up. Gently massage the point midway between the navel and the lower tip of the breastbone (sternum) using your index and middle fingers. Gently vibrate for 1 to 2 minutes. The vibrating action gently stimulates the whole of the digestive system. This treatment is indicated for the stagnant food pattern, indigestion, weak digestion, general weakness, and lack of appetite.

Intestines Point. As for Stomach Passage, but massage the point midway between the navel and the top of the pubic bone. This treatment is indicated for general weakness and urinary problems.

Up Sacrum. Using the heel of your hand, massage firmly up the sacrum from the tip of the "tail" to a level just above the buttocks. Repeat 50 to 100 times. This treatment is indicated for diarrhea.

▪ ESSENTIAL OILS

Essential oils can help relieve diarrhea, although their use is secondary (as opposed to their use in coughs, where they are almost indispensable). We advise using them as additions to massage oil. The following have a reputation of helping diarrhea:

Lavender *Lavandula officinalis*	2 drops
German chamomile *Chamomilla matricaria*	2 drops
Fennel *Foeniculum vulgare*	3 drops

If following a viral attack, add the following:

Eucalyptus *Eucalyptus globulus*	3 drops

If the child has strong abdominal pain, add the following:

Ginger *Zingiber officinalis*	2 drops

Add 2 to 3 drops of the oils of each to 25 ml (1 oz) of massage oil.

Explanation

Lavender is very relaxing and calming. Chamomile is a tonic for the digestive system and is also relaxing. In addition, it helps relieve colic. Fennel is a tonic for the digestive system. Eucalyptus has a good reputation for curing all types of diarrhea, including bacterial. Ginger is very warming to the digestive system and will help relieve colic.

Results

If you are skilled in massage, doing the massage every day, without even including the essential oils, is often enough. If the essential oils are included as well, the outcome is achieved even quicker. Massage may be one of the best ways to treat Weak children who refuse to take herbs by mouth.

General Comment

The great majority of children with chronic diarrhea have it because what they are eating does not suit them in one way or another. There are two conclusions that can be drawn from this: First, if they continue taking unsuitable food (or drink), then they will not respond to herbal treatment. Second, many of the children will get better even without the use of herbs if they start to consume food and drinks that suit them.

12

Infantile Colic

Infantile colic causes great distress. During an attack, the child is obviously in great pain. This naturally affects the mother, who in turn becomes distressed to the point of desperation. The mother's anxiety communicates itself and further feeds the child's distress, thereby creating a vicious circle. It is a condition that is very common but for which there is very little satisfactory orthodox treatment. By contrast, many wonderful herbs can help.

What Is Infantile Colic?

Infantile colic is severe abdominal pain in babies that comes and goes. Typically, the onset is sudden, and it may last for a few minutes to 20 minutes, only to resolve as quickly as it arrived. The problem is functional, not anatomic, and is caused by intestinal spasms. The spasms may come once or many times a day. Often, they are noticed a short time after feeding, although they can appear suddenly in the middle of the night.

■ PATTERNS

The symptoms of infantile colic are fairly uniform, but there are some small variations. These variations conceal significant differences in the underlying causes and great differences in the corresponding treatments. A summary of the patterns follows:

- Internal Cold
- Stagnant food pattern
- Shock
- Birth trauma

■ CAUSES

The causes of infantile colic are directly related to the patterns.

Cold

Infantile colic may result from Cold energy lodging in the abdomen. It is thought that this Cold energy causes muscles to spasm and obstructs the normal flow of energy. This is analogous to the muscular spasm of rheumatism that is felt when the back is exposed to cold. In rheumatism the cold comes from outside, but in colic, the internal muscular spasm comes from internal Cold energy. This pattern is also seen when the child consumes too many beans or bean products, such as soy milk. The digestive system is not Warm enough to digest the beans, resulting in intestinal gas.

Common sources for Cold getting into such a young body are as follows:

- Ice-cold milk
- Cold-energy food such as melons, yogurt, and bananas
- Cold-energy medicines such as acetaminophen (Tylenol; Calpol), aspirin, and antibiotics
- Anesthetics used during childbirth
- Immunizations, especially the polio immunization

In less developed places, the Cold can come simply from having the abdomen exposed to a cold wind.

Blocked Food

Blocked food may be a problem seen after the child eats too much raw or fibrous food or eats at irregular times, preventing the stomach from having adequate time to empty before additional food is eaten. One way or another, food that is only partly digested is passed through the small intestines, which react by going into spasm.

This pattern is very similar to the stagnant food pattern that appears again and again as one of the causes underlying many of the conditions described in this book. The difference here is that the child is not nearly as Hot, so the food does not ferment in the same way. The result is that the face is white, the child suffers much more from Cold problems, and the child responds well to warming herbs such as ginger.

Shock

If the baby is involved in a terrifying event, such as a car accident, or even if the mother experienced a shock while that baby is in the womb, it can cause the entire digestive system to spasm. The mechanism for this is not entirely clear, but it is similar to the nausea that one can experience on seeing a revolting sight.

Birth Trauma

If the head is badly distorted because of a difficult or very rapid birth, the craniosacral rhythms, which are so important for the functioning of the body, can be disrupted. This can affect the rhythms of the digestive tract in particular, causing colic.

▪ TYPICAL SYMPTOMS FOR ALL PATTERNS*

- The child screams in pain and cannot be consoled.
- The pain is so great that the child arches the back.
- Sweating may be associated with periods of pain.

---

*Facial color reveals a lot about a child's energy. See p. 54 for a discussion of facial colors and variations among racial groups.

- The face is white but turns red or even purple during attacks.
- Often, the abdomen feels cold.
- Often, pain comes after eating.
- When the pain has resolved, the child is cheerful again.

▪ SYMPTOMS ACCORDING TO PATTERN

The main way to distinguish between the patterns is by asking about the history. The following distinctive symptoms are sometimes seen.

Internal Cold

- The child's hands and feet may be cold.
- The child typically has a pale face.
- The abdomen may be cold to the touch.

Blocked Food Pattern

- The abdomen is very swollen because of the accumulated food.

Shock

- The face is blue or gray, or there is blue between the eyes.

Birth Trauma

- The baby has to bang his or her head or has to be bounced up and down vigorously to go to sleep.

▪ TREATMENT

Although the different patterns have almost identical symptoms, their treatments are quite different.

Cold

PRESCRIPTION 1 FOR MILD COLIC

Chamomile tea	1 tsp to 1 cup of boiling
Chamomilla matricaria	water, sweetened and
	given in a bottle

PRESCRIPTION 2 FOR STRONGER COLIC

Ginger *Zingiber officinalis*   See next paragraph
Cloves *Eugenia caryophyllata*   for dosages
Dill *Anethum graveolens*
Caraway seeds *Carum carvi*

The best way to take this prescription is to prepare a tea from equal quantities of the herbs. Use 1 tsp to a small cup. Several teaspoons of the tea are given as many times as needed. Some babies like to drink large quantities of the tea from a bottle. If it is given during the time of colic, it may relieve the symptoms at once.

VARIATION: FOR COLIC WITH FLATULENCE
Add the following to the tea:

Wild yam *Dioscorea villosa*   3 drops tincture

Explanation. Ginger is a warming and soothing tonic for the digestive system. Cloves are warm and disperse flatulence. Dill and caraway are similar in action, and both are soothing and warming to the digestive system. Wild yam is specific for flatulent colic. If only one or two of the herbs are available, then use those, but the result will be better if all herbs are used.

Results. This prescription may soothe the colic straight away. If this prescription is given regularly and if the following advice is adhered to, the colic should resolve within a few weeks.

Advice. If the mother is nursing, she should not eat cold foods or Cold-energy foods such as cucumbers, salads, or green peppers. She should also avoid foods likely to cause flatulence in the baby, such as beans and cabbage. If the baby is being bottle fed, make sure the milk is warm enough and try different formulas. Many children find that cow's milk and formulas made from cow's milk are too Cold in energy.

Blocked Food

Treatment is the same as for Cold, with the addition of the following:

Black root *Leptandra virginica*   2 drops tincture

Two drops of the tincture may be added to one of the teas listed previously for the Cold pattern. Black root is specific for the blocked food pattern.

Results. The main tea should soothe the colic to some extent within half an hour, but it may not clear it completely. With the addition of black root, the basic cause, the blocked food, starts to be expelled, so sometimes the colic worsens a little initially. Normally, when the blocked food pattern is treated, there is evacuation of rather foul-smelling stools over the next 2 to 3 days. After a week or so of taking this prescription, the baby should be much better.

Advice. The advice is the same as for the previous pattern. Make sure that the child has suitable food, a regular feeding pattern, and not too much food; otherwise, the colic will return. This is discussed in detail in Chapter 2.

Shock

As in many shock conditions, the best remedies are to be found outside herbal medicine. In particular we recommend the following:

Homeopathic Arnica   6X every 4 hours for 3 doses
                         for shock less than 3 days
                         ago
                         12C, 1 dose mornings and
                         evenings for 3 doses for
                         shock more than 3 days ago
                         but less than 2 week ago

If the shock was more than 2 weeks ago, three doses of the 12C potency may be effective, but we advise seeking the help of a homeopathic practitioner.

DR. BACH RESCUE REMEDY
Prepare in the standard way and give the child a few sips frequently. If the baby is nursing, a few drops can be dropped onto the mother's nipple before or during feeding.

Results. The results are sometimes rather dramatic, especially if the shock has been there for some months. The sudden relaxation after such a long time of tension leads to the discharge of toxins. It is not unusual for the child to have very loose painful stools for about a week. Sometimes the anus becomes very inflamed when this happens. Once this process has come to an end, the child feels very much better and the colic should resolve. If it still remains after 2 weeks, it is likely that one of the other patterns is present as well.

Birth Trauma

The treatment of choice is craniosacral osteopathy. In addition, if there is significant bruising or a history of hematoma, the homeopathic remedy Nat. Sulph. is often of benefit. Seek the help of a homeopathic practitioner for prescription details because this remedy should be given only if other imbalances have already been corrected. The unskilled use of this remedy can sometimes cause very fierce headaches. Herbal remedies for bruising and head damage are also available, but the treatment of such traumatic injuries is beyond the scope of this book.

Advice for All Patterns

The mother may need help too. A common pattern is for the mother to become very distressed by her baby's colic. This distress communicates itself to the baby and worsens the colic. If the mother can be helped to overcome her anxiety and stress, the baby will benefit as well.

In addition, in all types of colic, the following should be done:

- Avoid bananas, avocado, yogurt, and ice-cold food.
- Always warm food and drink. Never give straight from the fridge.
- Avoid high-fiber foods.
- Avoid beans and bean products (including soy milk).
- Keep the abdomen well covered.
- Try to give regular meals.

- When weaning onto solids, introduce only one new food each week.

▪ OTHER TREATMENTS
Massage

Massage the abdomen with or without oils.

DETAILS OF MASSAGE
The massages are the same as for constipation and diarrhea. See Chapters 10 and 11 for details.

- Heel on upper abdomen
- Heel on lower abdomen
- Stomach passage
- Intestines point

Do the massages at least three times a day. They may also be done when the child is in pain. The abdominal massages need to be done gently. As you do them, think of a Warm energy coming out of your hand.

If the child has a tendency toward constipation, try the following massage:

- Down sacrum

If the child has a tendency toward diarrhea, try the following:

- Up sacrum

Results. In some children the massages produce very quick results, relieving the pain within about 10 minutes. In others the results are slower but are cumulative. In these children the massages start to have a noticeable effect after about 3 or 4 days.

▪ ESSENTIAL OILS

Essential oils are very helpful in relieving colic. The oils penetrate through the skin directly to the site of the trouble. Use these oils with the aforementioned massages.

Cold Pattern

Ginger *Zingiber officinalis*   2 drops
Fennel *Foeniculum vulgare*   2 drops *or*
Dill *Anethum graveolens*   2 drops

Add the essential oils to 30 ml (1 oz) of massage oil.

Blocked Food Pattern

German chamomile *Chamomilla matricaria*   2 drops

Add the essential oil to 30 ml almond oil and use as massage oil.

Explanation. Ginger is very warming and is good for the Cold type of colic. Fennel and dill are warming and help move flatulence that is stuck. Chamomile helps reduce spasms and is a tonic for the digestive system.

Note: Some essential oils nullify the effect of homeopathic remedies.

13

Regurgitation and Continued Vomiting

Vomiting was once a major problem affecting adults and children alike. Part of the reason for this was the relative scarcity and variety of foods. Children simply had to eat what was put in front of them, whether they liked it or not. Today all sorts of foods are available at all times of the year. We are well aware of the ecologic and social disaster of growing cash crops in places where they were never grown before, but it does mean that children can now have food that is easy to digest. Vomiting is thus a relatively uncommon presenting symptom. This is not to say that children do not vomit any more. Of course they do; but what has happened is that the symptoms of vomiting are usually not serious enough to threaten the child's health.*

Now, the urgency in treating comes not from the threat to health from the vomiting itself but rather from the orthodox treatments that may be given. At present, one of the standard procedures in orthodox medicine is to reduce the strength of the stomach muscles surgically. The stomach muscles are literally cut to weaken them. Likewise, strong medicines, with inevitable side effects, are used to treat the relatively mild symptom of gastric reflux. The use of gentle herbs can often avoid the need for more invasive treatments.

---

*It is normal for children to vomit from overeating from time to time because they easily get carried away by the excitement of eating. The problem needs attention only if it happens time and time again.

Sudden Vomiting

Sudden vomiting may be something mild such as an epidemic of diarrhea and vomiting that goes around a play group, or it may be something much more serious. Appendicitis, acute blockage of the intestines, roundworms, urinary tract infections, and meningitis may all present with vomiting and require treatment. If in doubt, seek the advice of a qualified practitioner.

Danger Signs Requiring Immediate Investigation

- Vomiting of blood (may look like coffee grounds)
- Vomiting of bile
- Projectile vomiting (heat)
- Dehydration
- Fever
- Great pain
- Great lethargy

In this chapter we consider only continued vomiting, that is, fairly stable vomiting in a child whose health and life are not under immediate threat. The main danger signs are as follows:

Danger Signs for Continued Vomiting

- The child is becoming increasingly weak.
- The child is progressively losing weight.
- The child has severe nausea.

If a child has any of these symptoms, a thorough examination is necessary.

What Is Vomiting?

We use the term *vomiting* to mean something coming from the stomach out of the mouth. This term thus includes regurgitation, gastric reflux, spitting up, projectile vomiting, and others.

▦ CAUSES AND PATTERNS

First and foremost in the causes of vomiting is food intolerance. Repeated vomiting is often caused by an inability to digest food; it is the body's way of simply rejecting something that is unsuitable. In particular, one should watch for signs of intolerance to cow's milk and gluten. A fuller discussion is given in Chapter 15.

The following patterns are often seen:

- Stagnant food pattern
- Weak digestion
- Mucus
- Projectile vomiting (heat)
- Emotional/nervous

▦ SYMPTOMS AND SIGNS*

Stagnant Food Pattern (Mainly Younger Than 3 Years)

The child with stagnant food pattern usually eats well—may be too well—for a few weeks, then the appetite decreases, and the child has a bout of vomiting. After a good clear-out, the child feels like eating again.

The typical symptoms and signs are as follows:

- Curdled milk or undigested food is vomited.
- The vomit has a sour smell, and the breath may smell bad.
- The child has abdominal pain that improves after vomiting.
- The child is quite irritable and clingy.
- The child may lose his or her appetite before vomiting.

---

*Facial color reveals a lot about a child's energy. See p. 54 for a discussion of facial colors and variations among racial groups.

- The child may have a fever related to fermenting food.

The characteristic signs of the stagnant food pattern will also be apparent:

- Red cheeks
- Green nasal discharge
- Smelly and irregular stools

Explanation. The child's digestive system is blocked lower down by the accumulation of food. The stomach is working well, but when it is time for the food to be passed to the duodenum, there is no room for it, so inevitably it comes up instead of going down. The stomach is reasonably strong, so the child may continue retching for a while after the stomach is empty. Because the stomach is working reasonably well, the vomit contains partially digested food. All of the other symptoms and signs are what you would expect to see with the stagnant food pattern (see Chapter 2).

Causes. This condition usually arises from eating too much or eating when overexcited. Eating slouched in front of the TV also contributes to its onset. Vomiting can also occur if the child eats inappropriate foods (e.g., too much muesli in a toddler or too many burgers and chips in older children).

Weak Digestion

Children with weak digestion are usually thin and have Weak energy and poor appetites. They have pale faces and often appear blue above the mouth. The digestive system is already Cold from weakness, but strangely these children often eat a lot of Cold-energy damp foods (e.g., lettuce, tomatoes), which you would think they would dislike. This type of diet makes things worse.

The typical signs and symptoms are as follows:

- Vomit contains undigested food (or milk in babies).
- The face is pale.
- The skin above the lips appears blue.

- Sometimes, the eyes lack the sparkle expected in children.
- The child is oversensitive to cold weather.
- The arms and legs easily get cold.
- The child has a poor appetite.
- The child tends to go to sleep during feedings.
- The child tends to be tired during the day.
- The stools may be loose and contain undigested food.
- The child may have occasional constipation.

Discussion. Here the blockage that is preventing the food from going down arises because the intestines are not functioning at all. What little movement the intestines have does not synchronize with the movement of the stomach. When the child vomits, he or she does not have the same energy as in the previous pattern. The energy in the stomach is relatively Weak, so the food is barely digested at all, even though it may have been in the stomach for hours. All of the other symptoms and signs are what you would expect in a child with weak digestion, with the energy being low (see Chapter 2).

Causes. Some common factors that cause the child to become short of energy follow:

- A long, traumatic birth
- Use of anesthetics during childbirth
- Immunizations
- Long-term illness

The problem may be compounded by the child drinking a lot of fruit juice or eating too much ice cream. Sometimes the problem arises because the mother was anemic during pregnancy, or the mother, for some reason, is completely exhausted and does not have enough energy to devote to the child. Some other factors that may influence this pattern are given in Chapter 2.

Mucus

The main characteristic in this pattern is that the child is full of mucus. This pattern may overlap with the previous pattern, or it may be on its own.

There are Stronger children with a lot of mucus, Weaker ones with somewhat less, and still other children halfway between.

SYMPTOMS AND SIGNS
The main distinguishing features of this syndrome are as follows:

- Vomit contains mucus or water. This may look like food mixed with water or watery milk if the child is being breast-fed.
- Vomit may become yellow or green during prolonged attacks.
- Undigested food may be vomited as well.
- The child is usually fairly Strong.
- The child feels heavy when picked up.*
- The child may have a poor appetite, which is surprising in one so heavy.
- Stools are often a bit loose and glistening (from the mucus).
- Sometimes the child passes mucus-containing stools.
- Other signs of mucus include a runny nose, blocked ears, and so forth.
- The tongue often has a greasy coat on it.

A common pattern is that the child vomits about once a week and then feels better. The mucus gradually builds up again. As it does, the child becomes more irritable and the appetite declines until the next bout of vomiting.

Explanation. The digestive system is slightly weak, and the whole body is filled with mucus. This means that the mucus gradually accumulates in the stomach. The presence of this mucus in the stomach upsets digestion, often reducing their appetites. When they vomit, the food is mixed with mucus, sometimes watery, sometimes foamy, sometimes thick.

Causes. In these children the digestive system appears to be weak because of their poor

---

*Subjectively, these children seem to feel heavier than they really are.

appetite, but in reality the problem is caused by the digestive system being clogged with mucus. It is usually caused by a combination of the following:

- History of illness treated with antibiotics
- An echo pattern, especially from an immunization such as whooping cough or polio
- Too many dairy products, fruit, or any other Cold-energy damp food
- A hereditary disposition to mucus

VARIATION: COUGH

Frequently, these children have a chronic cough as well. If there is so much mucus that it collects in the stomach, it is common to find mucus in the lungs as well.

VARIATION: SPITTING UP

Spitting up refers to the small amount of milk that trickles out of the baby's mouth after a feeding. The baby is usually happy and cheerful after feeding, and with a special smile (and after burping the baby), some milk trickles out of the baby's mouth onto mom's new dress. When the baby is breastfed, it may be the mother herself who has a Cold energy or a lot of mucus. Spitting up is quite normal when it happens from time to time and should be treated only if it is really a significant problem (e.g., when more than half the food is vomited or the vomiting continues for more than half the baby's waking hours).

Projectile Vomiting (Heat)

With extreme forms of projectile vomiting, the child vomits violently and suddenly, with such force that the vomit may travel 2 to 3 m (6 to 9 feet). There are intermediate stages that are not quite so violent, but one gets an impression of force behind the vomiting. Projectile vomiting happens because the stomach has gone into "overdrive" and the peristalsis is much too strong. It is nearly always associated with heat concentrating in the stomach.

> **Note:** Projectile vomiting is a main symptom of pyloric stenosis. The condition is serious and may need surgical intervention. This is not always necessary. We have seen children successfully treated with herbs, as well as with acupuncture and with osteopathy.

SYMPTOMS AND SIGNS

- The child vomits soon after eating. The vomit has a foul smell and may appear yellow.
- After vomiting, the child feels better and may ask for more food.
- Projectile vomiting, or at least strong vomiting, has occurred.
- The child tends to be quite Strong but thin and wiry.
- The child has a good appetite (sometimes voracious).
- The child has increased thirst.
- The child is irritable and restless.
- The child is clingy.
- The child sleeps lightly and wakes up frequently at night.
- The body is hot (does not feel the cold)
- The face is red.

Discussion. Even though these children vomit soon after eating, the food is already partially digested. During the periods when they are not vomiting, their appetite is large, sometimes enormous. This is because the stomach is so active. All of the other signs are those of heat in the system (see Chapter 2). The pattern may occur suddenly (i.e., soon after the cause) if there is a sudden attack of heat, or it may come and go in waves of a few days interspersed with periods of no vomiting.

Causes. This pattern usually arises soon after something that causes heat to build up in the body. The common causes follow:

- The child's diet includes too many oily, fatty, greasy, and spicy foods. One sees this especially in families whose diet is normally hot and spicy.

- The heat can also be passed to the child from the mother. In this case you will notice that the mother also has a red face.
- The child has an echo pattern from an immunization or a febrile disease in which the body temperature was very high.

Emotional/Nervous

It is normal for children to vomit very occasionally when they get overexcited. There are also some children who can make themselves vomit merely by thinking about it, and do so to avoid some unpleasant event. It is pathologic when it happens frequently.

- Child vomits when upset or under pressure (e.g., before an examination).
- The child vomits when very excited.
- The child is sensitive and high strung.
- Often, the child has a weak constitution.
- The bones are thin.
- The tongue may have a red tip.

Discussion. This happens in sensitive children and those who easily become overexcited. Often, they are somewhat thin and do not have powerful bodies. On the other hand, they often have very vivid imaginations.

Causes. The main cause is constitutional: The children are just born that way. Supplementary causes are those that lead to a weak digestive system (see Chapter 2).

■ TREATMENT

Stagnant Food Pattern

In mild cases, a very simple herb can help:

Peppermint *Mentha piperata*	1 tsp in 1 cup of water, possibly sweetened, taken as a tea (babies can take as much as they like in a bottle)

Summary of What the Vomit Is Like in the Different Patterns	
Stagnant food pattern	Vomit is partly digested and therefore smells rather bad.
Weak	Undigested food comes back, sometimes in small amounts and sometimes many hours later.
Mucus	Vomit is mixed with water. Sometimes the child vomits the contents of the stomach and then continues vomiting a watery fluid.
Projectile vomiting (Heat)	The child vomits soon after eating, with great strength. Often, the child feels like returning to the table after a few minutes.
Nervous/emotional	The child vomits when excited or nervous. Food is usually undigested.

In more severe cases, the following prescription will help:

Gentian *Gentiana lutea*	3 drops tincture
Black root *Leptandra virginica*	3 drops tincture

Gentian is an excellent herb to treat vomiting, and black root helps clear the stagnant food pattern. If the other symptoms of stagnant food pattern (e.g., foul-smelling stools) are very strong but the vomiting is not excessive, you may reduce the gentian and increase the black root. Other herbs may be added according to additional symptoms.

If the child is constipated (has a bowel movement less than every 2 days), add the following:

Yellow dock *Rumex crispus*	3 drops tincture
Cascara *Rhamnus purshiana*	3 drops tincture

If the constipation is severe, treat the problem more as constipation than as vomiting; see Chapter 10.

If the child has a voracious appetite, add the following:

Meadowsweet *Filipendula ulmaria*   3 drops tincture

Explanation. Vomiting occurs mainly because there is nowhere for the food to go when peristalsis starts. The duodenum and intestines are blocked, so the food comes up instead. Thus the treatment is aimed at clearing the blockage lower down. Black root is our favored specific herb for the stagnant food pattern. When the stomach is weak, black root may initially cause nausea. This should not happen if the child is Strong, but it does sometimes occur, in which case black root is simply omitted and yellow dock and cascara are used. Yellow dock is used for children who are constipated because it increases the flow of bile. Cascara helps clear the intestines lower down. If the child has a huge appetite, overeating may result in a recurrence of the vomiting after the stagnation has been cleared. Meadowsweet can help reduce appetite.

Results. As always when treating the stagnant food pattern, there may be a sudden rush of stools. If this happens, the medicine should be discontinued until the child has a bowel movement only once or twice a day. Even if the child does not have sudden evacuations, foul-smelling stools are likely during the first few days. If there is no reaction of this kind, the dosage should be increased. After about 1 week, the bowel movements should regulate and the condition should be more or less righted. The child should continue taking the herbs for another week after the symptoms have improved.

Advice. The normal advice for the stagnant food pattern applies here, namely reduce the quantity of food, ensure a regular feeding pattern, and make sure that the food is suitable. This is covered in detail in Chapter 2.

Weak Digestion

In mild cases of weak digestion, start with the following:

Chamomile *Chamomilla matricaria*	1 tsp in 1 cup of water, possibly sweetened, taken as tea (babies can take as much as they like in a bottle)

In more severe and long-lasting cases, the following will help:

Gentian *Gentiana lutea*	4 drops tincture
Sweet sedge *Acorus calamus*	3 drops tincture
Fennel *Foeniculum vulgare*	2 drops tincture
Ginger *Zingiber officinalis*	2 drops tincture

Explanation. Gentian and fennel are two of the best tonics for treating the stomach and the digestive system generally. Calamus is a tonic that will help the middle and lower parts of the digestive system. Ginger is also a tonic and will help warm the Cold.

Results. The main problem will be getting the child to take the herbs. If the child's appetite is already poor and the child does not want to take anything except sweet fruit juice, he or she probably will not want to take the gentian. However, it is always worth a try, and it is worth sweetening heavily. You may have better results with ginger and fennel.

An alternative is to cook the child's food with fresh ginger root and also with fennel seeds. For example, include rice combined with ginger and cookies made with fennel seeds.

Mucus

| Gentian *Gentiana lutea* | 4 drops tincture |
| Golden seal *Hydrastis canadensis* | 3 drops tincture |

Explanation. Gentian is one of the main herbs for the stomach, and golden seal is specific for clearing mucus from the system.

Results. At first the amount of mucus in the system may appear to increase. In addition, mucus will be voided through the stools, so stools may be loose. After the first week or two, these aggravations should die down and the child should gradually improve. If no changes of this kind are seen, the dosage should be increased until some changes are seen. The amount of time for a complete cure varies and depends on how Strong the child is and how much mucus there was there in the first place.

When digestion is stagnant, vomiting may increase slightly at first. If this persists for more than a few doses, the prescription will need to be changed. The next herbs to try are yellow dock *Rumex crispus* and possibly even butternut *Juglans cinerea*. Yellow dock moves digestion in the middle region (it is thought to do this by promoting the flow of bile), and butternut helps clear the bowels, particularly when a lot of mucus is present.

VARIATION: COUGH

Add herbs for cough, such as the following:

Elecampane *Inula helenium*	2 drops tincture
Coltsfoot *Tussilago farfara*	2 drops tincture

Explanation. The herbs given here are indicated when vomiting is the main symptom and cough secondary. If cough is the main symptom and vomiting is secondary, change the proportions of the herbs (consult Chapter 17).

Results. The first symptom to subside will probably be the cough. Otherwise the results will be similar to vomiting without cough.

VARIATION: SPITTING UP

Spitting up is almost a halfway house between weak digestion and mucus. The first step in treatment is to ensure that the child is not eating Cold-energy foods, either directly in the form of yogurt or cow's milk or indirectly from the mother's diet (via her milk).

If the baby is breast-fed, it may be better to give the herbs to the mother, for then both the mother and child will feel better. If the baby is bottle fed, obviously only the baby needs the herbs.

For the baby, use the following herbs:

Ginger *Zingiber officinalis*	2 drops tincture
Prickly ash *Zanthoxylum americanum*	2 drops tincture

For the mother, use the following:

Dill *Anethum graveolens*	1 tsp of the seeds taken as a tea three or more times a day
or	
Fennel *Foeniculum vulgare*	Same as above

Both of these increase and enrich the supply of mother's milk. Alternatively, the mother may take the following prescription:

Ginger *Zingiber officinalis*	10 to 20 drops tincture
Prickly ash *Zanthoxylum americanum*	10 to 20 drops tincture

Results. Some improvement should be noticed after about a week. The herbs may need to be continued for a few months.

Advice. Make sure that the baby stays awake throughout the feeding and for about 10 minutes afterward. This will help the child digest the food/milk.

Diet. The mother should avoid cold foods and Cold-energy foods (e.g., lettuce, tomatoes). Stews are particularly recommended.

Projectile Vomiting (Heat)

A suitable prescription to start with follows:

Meadowsweet *Filipendula ulmaria*	4 drops tincture
Marshmallow leaves *Althea officinalis*	4 drops tincture

Explanation. Meadowsweet and marshmallow cool the stomach. We suggest using the leaves of marshmallow rather than the root, for the root has much more mucilage and these children often have too much mucus to begin with. If the children are very Dry, then use the root.

Another possible way of looking at the action of these herbs is that they calm the excessive activity of the stomach and help synchronize its action with the pyloric sphincter and the duodenum.

Results. There should be a gradual improvement over the next 3 to 4 weeks (do not expect immediate results). Not only should the vomiting improve, but also the other signs, such as restlessness and red face, that show the child is too Hot should resolve. If there is no change after this time, one must use another approach.

A possible herb to be used is pasque flower *Anemone pulsatilla*, given in minute, almost homeopathic doses (e.g., 1 drop in 25 to 50 ml and taken in three doses over the day). Small doses are important because large doses irritate the stomach. The purpose of this herb is to bring the Heat from the inside to the outside.

Emotional/Nervous

In the short term, the following herbs will be of benefit. They may be given before an exciting event such as a party or an examination, and they are also of use after the episode of vomiting.

Lime flowers *Tilea europea*	5 g of herb to 1 cup of water
German chamomile *Chamomilla matricaria*	5 g of herb to 1 cup of water
Vervain *Verbena officinalis*	5 g of herb to 1 cup of water
Lemon balm *Melissa officinalis*	5 g of herb to 1 cup of water

Administration. Choose one or two of these herbs and give as a tea. In many places tea bags are available, which make preparation much simpler. We have chose German chamomile, which has a milder effect but a much more pleasant taste than Roman chamomile *Anthemis nobilis*.

Explanation. These herbs are all calming to the nervous system, with a particular effect on the stomach. Usually, one gives only one of the herbs. Determining which herb to use is based on the child's behavior.

- *Lime flowers* for nervous, jumpy children who are perhaps a bit oversensitive

- *Chamomile* for red-faced children who also may have tantrums
- *Vervain* for children who go on and on about the same thing and have difficulty in stopping what they are doing
- *Lemon balm* for very tense, high-strung children

Results. All of these herbs are relatively short acting and should have an effect in calming the child enough to cope with a difficult situation. If they are not effective, the next remedies to try are the Bach flower remedies.

After that, there is a homeopathic remedy that is specific for this situation: Gelsemium. As with all homeopathic remedies, this is best given under the supervision of a homeopathic practitioner because reactions can occur, particularly the expulsion of thick mucus (from the nose, the lungs, and other orifices).

BETWEEN BOUTS OF NERVOUS VOMITING

Another class of herbs should be used between exciting events to build up the strength of the stomach and the nervous system. These include the following:

Gentian *Gentiana lutea*	3 drops tincture
Passion flower *Passiflora incarnata*	3 drops tincture

If the child's overall constitution is weak, one may add the following great tonic:

Ginseng *Panax ginseng*	2 drops tincture

Explanation. Gentian is a well-established tonic to the digestive system and to the stomach in particular. Passion flower is a tonic to the nervous system and may be used long term. Ginseng is a great tonic to the whole constitution. It affects the entire body and the rate of growth, so it is not normally given to children, unless they are very Weak, have very thin bones, and are small for their age.

Results. The herbs should be given for 6 months to 1 year, or even longer in some children. Note that the herbs we have given are *suggestions only.* If you are giving herbs over a long period, they should be adapted to the individual. During that time you will probably need to vary the prescription as the child changes.

■ ESSENTIAL OILS

Essential oils may be used on their own by being rubbed into the abdomen. They may be made more effective by massaging them, using the massages described in Chapters 10 and 11. The following oils will be of help.

German chamomile *Chamomilla matricaria*	3 drops
Lavender *Lavandula officinalis*	3 drops

If mucus is present, add the following:

Lemon *Citrus limonum*	3 drops

If the child is Hot, add the following:

Peppermint *Mentha piperata*	3 drops

If the child is Cold, add the following

Pepper *Piper nigrum*	3 drops
or	
Ginger *Zingiber officinalis*	3 drops

Add the essential oils to 30 ml almond oil and use as massage oil (or simply rub into the abdomen).

Explanation. The combination of German chamomile and lavender is an all-purpose combination. Chamomile is good for most types of vomiting, including that related to the stagnant food pattern. Lavender is not specific for vomiting, but it is so calming to the nerves that it takes care of other types of vomiting. Lemon has a strong effect in cutting through and dissolving mucus, and peppermint is a gentle tonic for the stomach that is also cooling. For the Cold types, both pepper and ginger are obviously heating.

■ MASSAGE

The massages given in Chapters 10 and 11 are suitable. The massages for constipation are almost the same as those for diarrhea, with the exception of the direction of rotation on the abdomen. For constipation massage in a clockwise direction, but for diarrhea massage counterclockwise. If neither constipation nor diarrhea is present, give half the strokes clockwise and half counterclockwise.

14

Poor Appetite

A reduction in appetite is a symptom seen in association with a wide range of illnesses. Anything that affects the digestive system or the overall energy is likely to reduce the appetite. This is important to remember, because if a child has a poor appetite as the main symptom, an examination should be carried out to ensure that nothing else is significantly wrong.

What we cover here are two circumstances when there is something functional wrong with the appetite but nothing organically wrong. We confine ourselves to the following two common situations:

- After an infection
- Habitual

Danger Sign

Unexplained weight loss

■ AFTER AN INFECTION

In the past it was common to have long and very debilitating illnesses. In *The Old Curiosity Shop* by Charles Dickens, there is a description of a raging fever with delirium for 3 weeks. After an illness of this kind, a child would be totally exhausted and would be too weak to eat very much. Tonics for the digestive system would greatly speed the rate of recovery.

Illnesses of this intensity are fortunately uncommon, so there is little need for this sort of tonic. Moreover, there is a much wider range of foods available now, and there are vitamin and mineral supplements to assist in recovery.

However, there is a situation in which herbs can be of great benefit: When a child has had a febrile disease and sweated profusely over 2 or 3 days, the whole digestive system occasionally shuts down. The child is not deeply exhausted but seems as though in a state of shock. In these circumstances herbs can be of enormous benefit in restarting movement in the digestive system. Another time herbal treatments can be of great value is when a child has been adversely affected by anesthetics used in surgery. The anesthetics used often depress the digestive system.

In the situations we are referring to, one will see the following symptoms and signs:

- The face is pale, possibly with red blotches.
- There is a dull, vacant look in the child's eyes; older children may stare blankly at the wall.
- The child may be described as very floppy (young children have to be carried; older ones sit without moving).
- The child will not take food or drink.
- The child is *not* emaciated, and the eyes are *not* sunken.

It seems as though the child is in a state of shock and is not quite all there. It is very alarming to see, for it seems as though the child has lost the will to live. In fact, the condition is rarely serious, and it only needs a "kick start" for the digestive system to work. Such a kick start is provided by the following prescription*:

---

*Dosages are for 3-year-olds.

| Gentian *Gentiana lutea* | 4 drops tincture |
| Fennel *Foeniculum vulgare* | 2 drops tincture |

Alternatives to gentian are as follows:

Sweet sedge *Acorus calamus*	4 drops tincture
or	
Wormwood *Artemisia absinthium*	4 drops tincture

Explanation

Gentian is the main herb. It has been shown that the bitter taste of gentian has a strong effect on the stomach and digestive system. Fennel is an assistant. Sweet sedge and wormwood have similar effects.

Administration

Put the tinctures in a small amount of warm sweetened water. Do not use too much water, or it will be difficult to administer. For young children, squirt the mixture into the child's mouth with a dropper. Older children may be persuaded to take a gulp of medicine.

Other Remedies

There are two homeopathic remedies of special use after an operation:

> Opium 6X (or 6C) when the child appears drugged
> Nux. vom. 6X (or 6C) when the child has nausea or even vomiting

These may be taken every 2 hours after an operation for a total of six doses. If possible, consult a homeopathic practitioner for advice.

▪ HABITUAL

We now turn to the treatment of the common symptom of poor appetite. We call it habitual in the sense that the condition we are talking about is not dangerous in itself. There is no organic disease.

It is just that the child does not eat very much. It is unlikely that parents will take their children to an herbalist merely for this symptom, but it is nevertheless a common symptom in the later stages of treatment for another disease. For example, we have treated patients with a wide range of diseases, from bedwetting to asthma, who have been healed of their main symptom, but who, in our opinion, are not completely cured because their appetite is still very poor. If the appetite remains poor, it is easy for the original symptoms to recur.

Causes of Poor Appetite

The basic reasons for a poor appetite is that the digestive energy is Weak or that there is something blocking digestion. The blockage may be the accumulation of mucus, the long-term consumption of poor-quality food, or possibly something that has affected the entire system, such as immunizations. The child may even have a mild food allergy (see Chapter 15).

Causes of Habitual Poor Appetite

- Weak energy
- Mucus
- Immunizations
- Poor-quality food

Developing Good Eating Habits

In the past it was considered important that children develop good eating habits, and it was believed that they needed to be taught these. It was considered important for children to be able to eat anything that was put in front of them, regardless of whether they liked it or not. Sometimes the methods used were heavy handed, but in days when food was scarce, developing habits of this kind was a basic survival skill.

There is less need for habits of this kind today, and parents are also less willing to impose their will on their children—sometimes even the most basic eating habits are not taught. If the child is healthy and has a good appetite, this may not be of much consequence. On the other hand, if a child has been ill and a poor appetite is part of the problem, proper eating habits are key for the child's health.

IMPORTANCE OF MEALTIMES

Life is very exciting for children. They have the whole world to discover. Many of the things that we adults take for granted, such as the light switch on the wall, hold endless fascination for children. Most children up to the age of 12 years have an endless curiosity. This is even more true now than in the past because there are so many new things—from computers to cellular phones—to stimulate the mind. In these circumstances it is no wonder that children are not as interested in food. As far as they are concerned, there simply is not time enough to waste on eating.

This is where the adults can teach the children. When a child spends time on mental activities, such as watching TV and playing computer games, all the energy leaves the digestive system and goes to the head, which can lead to a poor appetite. This child needs to spend time unwinding and getting the energy back into the stomach. This may take some time, and for many children it means turning the TV off and reducing other sources of stimulation as much as possible. The traditional way of doing this seems to us to be very sensible: The child should sit down for 20 to 30 minutes at mealtimes, preferably with other members of the family. Even if the child does not eat anything, he or she should sit at the table for this length of time

This is of course very time consuming and can be exhausting initially if the child is not used to sitting still, but for most children with a poor appetite, a habit of this kind is essential. They will never eat well unless they allow time for it.

A common complaint of parents is that they have tried sitting their children down in this way and that it simply does not work. Everyone becomes exhausted, and still the children do not eat anything. This is where herbs that help the digestive system are of benefit. It is unlikely that the appetite will really improve with herbs alone, though, if the child does not sit down at mealtimes.

■ SYMPTOMS AND SIGNS*

There are three main patterns of poor appetite:

- Weak digestion
- Weak digestion with nervous energy
- Thick mucus

Weak Digestion

- The face is pale and may have a slight yellow tinge.
- The child appears rather droopy.
- The child is often shy.
- The child does not appear very forceful.
- The appetite is poor, and the child is very picky and choosy about food.
- Most calories may be obtained from fruit juice.
- Constipation is common; the child may occasionally have loose stools.
- The child cries easily.
- The arms and legs are thin, or they may be rather squashy—without good tone.
- The child tires easily.

Weak Digestion with Nervous Energy

The main symptoms and signs are the same as for Weak digestion, except that you will find the following as well:

- The child never tires and is always on the go.
- The child never wants to go to bed at night.
- The child likes to be the center of attention.

Thick Mucus

- The face appears gray and may be a little puffy.
- The child appears sturdy.
- The child's appetite varies—he or she may eat a lot but is choosy about food.
- Weight may be put on easily.
- The child occasionally vomits water.

---

*Facial color reveals a lot about a child's energy. See p. 54 for a discussion of facial colors and variations among racial groups.

- The child has a tendency to develop a productive cough.
- Nasal discharge is common.
- The child may have swollen glands.

▣ TREATMENT

The prescriptions we give here are merely sample prescriptions, intended to give a starting point. The dosages we give are for children aged 3 years (Table 14-1). They should be modified for each individual.*

Weak Digestion

Fennel *Foeniculum vulgare*	4 drops tincture
Sweet sedge *Acorus calamus*	2 drops tincture
Licorice *Glycyrrhiza glabra*	2 drops tincture

If the child is constipated, add the following:

Yellow dock *Rumex crispus*	4 drops tincture

If the stools are loose, add the following:

Agrimony *Agrimonia eupatorium*	4 drops tincture

Explanation. Fennel is a general tonic for the digestive system. Sweet sedge is a bitter tonic and improves the appetite. Some children find it too bitter, but many have no problem taking it. Licorice is another sweet tonic, and it influences the entire body. Yellow dock and agrimony are

▣ **Table 14-1**	
AGE	**MULTIPLY 3-YEAR-OLD DOSE BY**
6-12 months	$\times \frac{1}{3}$
1-2 years	$\times \frac{1}{2}$
2-4 years	$\times 1$
4-7 years	$\times 1\frac{1}{2}$
7-14 years	$\times 2$
14+ years	$\times 3$

*For more detailed information about dosages, see Chapter 8.

both tonics, the former being a laxative and the latter an astringent.

Another herb that can be of use is gentian *Gentiana lutea*. This is of great help in stimulating the digestive system and to build up the body as a whole. The disadvantage is that it is *very* bitter. It is always worth trying to include some in the prescription, even if it is much less than the normal dose.

Results. Patience is needed. It may be necessary to continue taking the herbs for as long as 6 months or 1 year, which is why it is important to find a prescription that the child is willing to take. No parent can face having to battle over medicine three times a day for a year. During this time, the appetite should gradually improve. Often, the progress is so slow that it is hardly noticeable, so it is helpful to discuss the details of what the child is actually eating about once a month. Some parents even like to keep little notebooks on the subject.

Weak Digestion with Nervous Energy

The same prescription is suitable, but it may be difficult to get the child to take the herbs. In this case it may be appropriate to use massage with essential oils (see later discussion).

Thick Mucus

Blue flag *Iris versicolor*	3 drops tincture
Poke root *Phytolacca decandra*	3 drops tincture
Black root *Leptandra virginica*	2 drops tincture
Sweet sedge *Acorus calamus*	2 drops tincture

Alternatives to blue flag and poke root are as follows:

Queen's delight *Stillingia sylvatica*	3 drops tincture
Figwort *Scrophularia nodosa*	3 drops tincture

Explanation. Blue flag and poke root soften the hard mucus in the system and release it into the intestines. Only small quantities of these herbs should be given at first; then the proportions may be gradually increased. If too large of quantities are given initially, the child may become nauseous and have diarrhea.

The proportions of the herbs are important and may need to be adjusted to the individual, for the action of black root is to clear relatively soft mucus from the digestive system. At first the child may even have mild diarrhea as the mucus is expelled through the bowels. Sweet sedge is included to stimulate the digestive system, which may become rather sluggish with expelling all the mucus.

■ FAVORABLE TIMES TO TREAT

Changing a habit of a lifetime is always difficult. The easiest time to make such an attempt is when many other aspects of life are also changing. This happens naturally when a child first goes to school or moves from one school to another. It also happens at the great transitions at 7 years and 14 years (see Chapter 6). This means that these times are ideal for changes in eating habits and corresponding changes in health. Therefore the best time to treat a long-standing poor appetite is immediately before these transitions take place. If the child is due to go to school at the age of 5 years, start treating 6 to 9 months before. The other great ages to treat are at 6 and 12 years so that there is time for the child to accumulate enough energy to ensure that the next transition goes in a favorable direction.

■ ESSENTIAL OILS

Fennel *Foeniculum vulgare*	5 drops essential oil
Ginger *Zingiber officinalis*	5 drops essential oil
Bergamot *Citrus bergamia*	5 drops essential oil

If a lot of mucus is present, add the following:

Lemon *Citrus limonum*	5 drops essential oil

Add the drops of each oil to 30 ml of base oil for the massage.

■ MASSAGE

The massages described in Chapters 10 and 11 are suitable for children with poor appetites as well. The massages for constipation are almost the same as those for diarrhea, with the exception of the direction of rotation on the abdomen. For constipation, massage in a clockwise direction; for diarrhea, massage counterclockwise. If neither constipation nor diarrhea is present, the number of clockwise strokes should be the same as the number of counterclockwise strokes.

15

Food Allergies

◼ OVERVIEW

In this chapter we describe a new approach to treating allergies. The subject is complex and vast, so in a book of this kind we only have space for covering the main principles.

Food allergies are a relatively recent phenomenon. In the past the phenomenon of allergies was known, but it was uncommon. Now it is so common that one is frequently asked, "Do you have any allergies?"

This dramatic increase in food allergies is partly attributable to the greater variety of food now available. Fifty years ago people ate only organic food grown locally. Most of us now eat food from all over the world—food that is mass produced and grown with fertilizers and sprayed with pesticides,* some of which remain in the food. The soil it is grown from is poor in nutrients, which in turn produces crops deficient in essential minerals and vitamins. The harvested crop is cleaned with chemicals, preserved with additives, and irradiated. To compound this, many foods have been selectively bred and genetically modified with more thought of profit than of digestibility. In so doing these things we have produced such poor-quality food, so far from its original genetic origins, that it is not surprising that the body rebels!

An example of this is any of the modern varieties of wheat, which perhaps more than any other food has been selectively bred and modified. Many people notice intolerance to bread made with cheap flour, yet they find they can eat old variety flours (e.g., spelt, kamut) with no problems.

This is only part of the picture. As we have stressed throughout this book, it is the state of the body that is all-important in how a child reacts to an illness. Allergies are exactly the same. If the child is healthy and the body is in balance, the likelihood of having a bad reaction to foods, no matter how poor in quality, is greatly reduced.

Realizing this opens the way for a totally new approach of how to treat allergies: to change the balance of the body so that it can tolerate a wider variety of foods. This makes sense in the short term in that it allows the child to visit friends who are not so ecologically minded. It also makes sense in the long term because it will improve the child's overall health.

Food: Trigger or Cause?

As in asthma, children diagnosed with food allergies are encouraged to go to great lengths to discover what the offending articles are and to eliminate them all from their diet. For some people this appears to be the only solution. However, allergy to food is now so common it begs the question whether other factors are involved.

Our observation in the children's clinic is that all children and babies with allergies have a significant imbalance in their digestive system. The food itself is the trigger that initiates the allergic reaction. It is

---

*A neighboring farmer reported that 20 years ago he fertilized his crops from the manure of his animals. As a result of European Community policy, he can no longer afford to keep animals, so he has to use chemical fertilizer. He has noticed that his plants are less resistant to disease and pests, so he now must use pesticides *and* fertilizer.

the final step in a long chain of events. What is more, we have found that by correcting this imbalance to improve the digestive system, often with very simple advice and herbs, these children can often rid themselves of the allergy completely and eat more or less anything. At the very least herbs can cure violent reactions to a particular food. This is an enormous relief to many parents. Therefore, to find a cure for a food allergy, you must look beyond the specific food. In most cases the food in itself it is not the sole cause of the allergy.*

Poisons

It is perhaps also worth pointing out that although most governments would have us believe that the food sold in stores contains very little pesticides and other noxious chemicals, this is not always the case. Some more delicate children may never be able to tolerate the levels of poisons in certain cheap foods, and these may need to be kept out of the diet. Their digestive system may never become strong enough to cope with more than minimal amounts. This is simply the makeup of some children. An early example of this in our practice was provided by a 6-year-old girl who developed eczema every time she ate nonorganic meat.

Allergy or Intolerance?

We start by an explanation of terms. In particular we wish to make a distinction between food allergy and food intolerance.

FOOD ALLERGY
We consider allergy to food when dramatic, terrible symptoms occur after ingestion of the tiniest amount of food. A common example of this is

---

*Having said this it should be pointed out that some people simply cannot digest certain foods, and to stay healthy, they should eliminate the offending foods from their diet. For example, many people from Africa do not have the enzymes to digest cow's milk, nor do many Asian people. This is genetic and cannot be changed. For most the allergy is not severe, but for some it is and cannot be changed.

allergy to peanuts. Many people with peanut allergy (adults included) have an asthma attack or, even worse, go into anaphylactic shock if they have as little as 10 mg of peanuts or peanut oil—almost less than one can taste.

FOOD INTOLERANCE
We consider food intolerance to be different from allergy. An intolerance to a food means the child cannot digest the food well. Instead of feeling more energetic after a meal, the child may feel tired or out of balance in some way. An excellent example of this is lactose intolerance. Many children have difficulty in digesting lactose, and this difficulty gives rise to the common symptom of catarrh. Instead of the milk giving them more energy, in the long term it weakens them by creating so much catarrh in the system that they have a permanent runny nose, chronic cough, or even asthma.

◼ Case History

Food intolerance can lead to food allergy. One patient of ours had been intolerant or mildly allergic to gluten throughout her life but was unaware of it. In her case the reaction manifested as tiredness; she had reached the age of 30 without ever feeling well, and she had always felt tired. At 30 she had her first baby, and unfortunately the birth was difficult and she lost a lot of blood. She recovered slowly and then started to get diarrhea. Nothing seemed to help the diarrhea, and she grew thinner and thinner. It was her good fortune to find someone who suggested avoiding gluten, and from that day on she started to get better. A year later her digestion had improved so much that she could eat a slice of bread every few days without experiencing any severe symptoms.

This is an example we like to give because it illustrates not only how intolerance can lead to allergy but also how allergy can be cured and revert to mere intolerance.

ADDICTION TO THE ALLERGEN
A strange feature of allergies is that people crave the very food that is worst for them. You may find this

in children who are addicted to milk. They may crave milk with a passion they show for nothing else.

One possible explanation is that when the child drinks the milk, there is a sudden rush of allergens into the bloodstream. This in turn produces a sudden reaction of the immune system, and with it a rush of adrenaline. Soon after, the adrenaline rush subsides and the debilitating effects of allergens in the bloodstream start to take over. To overcome this the child asks for more milk, to get another rush of adrenaline. This leads to a craving for the unsuitable food.

This presents serious problems in changing a child's diet and eliminating the offending food. If the child is old enough to forage, he or she may sneak into the refrigerator to see if any of the forbidden food is available. Similarly, when changing the type of milk given to bottle-fed infants, the baby will make the most plaintive wailing noises, which would melt the hardest of hearts. In addition, these children will stop taking any other foods, and although it is only for a few days, most mothers start to worry about the child wasting away (even though the child may be bursting with health). Worse still, toddlers may wake in the night gasping for the old type of milk.

When this happens, it is a real problem for parents. They have to adhere to a strict regimen for a *minimum* of 5 days. After about 5 days, the child starts to accept the new food. When giving advice to parents, it may be helpful to advise them to continue for 7 days so that they are mentally prepared for a difficult time.

> Allow at least 5 days for the child to overcome a food addiction, even if he or she refuses other food during this time.

■ INTERNAL CAUSES OF FOOD ALLERGY AND INTOLERANCE

Constitutional

Some children simply inherit a familial problem in digesting certain foods. For example, some families cannot eat strawberries without breaking out in a rash. On a wider scale, many Chinese people break out in a rash if they eat too much lamb. If the allergy or intolerance is to only a few foods, it is probably best left alone.

Weak Digestion

If the digestion is weak, the main symptoms and signs are general lack of energy and poor appetite, as described in Part 1 (see Chapter 2), but in some children, it appears as a food intolerance or allergy.

Stagnant Food (Younger Than 3 Years Old)

In some children it is the stagnant food pattern that leads to allergy. The stagnant food pattern may develop simply as a result of overeating or eating a diet that is too rich. This pattern irritates the intestines and opens the way for a food allergy because the food is poorly absorbed.

Accumulation of Mucus in the System

The mucous lining of the intestines is an active transporting agent. If this becomes too thick, the transport of molecules from the partly digested food to the portal circulation will be disrupted, allowing allergens to reach the bloodstream. This is often accompanied by disturbance in other mucous membranes, resulting in excess mucus everywhere—in the nose, the chest, the stools, and so forth.

Antibiotics

There is little doubt that the overconsumption of antibiotics is a contributory factor to food allergy. As a clinician, one can observe the gradual rise in mucus in a child who takes course after course of antibiotic. In the laboratory it has been shown that antibiotics exacerbate the leaky gut syndrome by killing beneficial bacteria as well as the harmful ones.

Immunizations

Immunizations are often given as injections, and a drug or poison* is introduced into the blood-stream. In some children this leads to excessive mucus, with corresponding food intolerance. In others it leads to a permanently overactive immune system, which can cause much stronger symptoms of allergy and sometimes anaphylactic shock.

Echo Pattern

The echo pattern, which arises from a severe illness, produces virtually the same effects as an immunization. The immune system never quite finished its work in eliminating an illness and is still somewhat overactive.

Leaky Gut Syndrome

In the causes previously discussed, we have emphasized the energetic pattern. Another perspective is the leaky gut syndrome discussed in Chapter 2. We have put this cause last, for when it comes to prescribing herbs, we find it more helpful to identify the pattern. The cause is important, but even more important is the way that the cause affects the body.

▨ COMMON ALLERGENS AND THEIR SIGNS

We now discuss the commonly observed symptoms and signs of intolerance or allergy to various foods. These are not the only ways in which they can present, but they are among the most common. (See also Table 15-1 for more details.)

- Ear infections
- Lethargy

---

*Many chemicals are used to preserve immunizations before they are administered. These include formaldehyde and mercury-containing compounds. These are all destined to be injected into the blood, in addition to the immunization itself.

- Vomiting
- Diarrhea
- Constipation
- Eczema

If a child presents with one of these conditions, consider a food allergy.

▨ STEPS IN THE CURE OF FOOD ALLERGY AND INTOLERANCE

Finding the Allergen

The first step is to determine which food or foods are causing the reactions. Sometimes this is obvious from the symptoms, as described in Table 15-1. Sometimes it is obvious from the addiction the child has to a particular food. In other cases it is more difficult to be certain, and there are different ways of proceeding. The first is to have the child go on an exclusion diet. This requires that the child exclude all foods from his or her diet except those foods that very few people are known to be allergic to. A common initial diet is lamb and pears (for Caucasians; some Oriental people break out in a rash after eating lamb). A new food is then added each week, and the reaction noted. This is obviously difficult for a mother to enforce on an unruly child, particularly if the child normally eats meals at school.

Another way to determine specific allergies is to perform allergen-specific blood tests. If such testing is available, it may add a little to the cost of treatment, but if it quickly pinpoints the main allergens, it can save a lot of time and trouble for the stressed parent. The primary disadvantage of blood tests is that they are not entirely reliable; the scientific nature of the test gives it a credibility value that it should not have.

Yet another way is the skin prick test, where allergens are introduced into the skin and the histamine reaction noted. In our experience this has been one of the less reliable tests. This may be because testing the skin is not the best way to find a problem in the digestive system.

Alternative allergy tests, which are just as reliable, are kinesiology, radionics, and dowsing.

Table 15-1	**Common Allergens and Their Signs**
FOOD	**COMMON SYMPTOMS AND SIGNS**
Cow's milk	• Mucus may accumulate, especially in the lungs, causing chronic cough. • Eczema develops. • Premature growth of breasts occurs in girls from the hormones given to the cows that find their way into the milk.* • A minority of children develop violent behavior if they take too much cow's milk.
Sugar	• Hyperactivity occurs soon after the child eats sugar, followed by the "sugar blues," where the child is whiny and out of sorts. • In other children, overconsumption of sugar leads to a watery nasal discharge. • If sugar is a major food source, one commonly sees mouth ulcers initially, followed by spots and boils. • If this continues for any length of time, the child may become undernourished because the food contains only carbohydrates, without enough vitamins and minerals or proteins. Commonly this undernourishment appears as excessive deposits of fat accompanied by lethargy
Gluten (in wheat and other grains)	• When gluten is poorly digested in babies and toddlers, the most common symptom is eczema; the most severe symptom is diarrhea. • In older children it is more common to see greenish discharges (from the nose especially, the eyes to a lesser extent, and occasionally the vagina). Again, in severe cases the child may have diarrhea. • In teenagers and older children, the main symptom may be depression, with accompanying abdominal aches from time to time. At this age and older there is a dull color to the complexion and there may be premature streaks of gray hair.
Peanuts	• At the stage of food intolerance, peanuts give rise to a yellow-tinged mucus. This may result in nasal catarrh or in severe cases may lead to asthma. The child may also have mucus discharge (i.e., "sleep") in the corner of the eyes. • In some children the external symptoms are greater, and atopic eczema may be present. Some children even develop contact dermatitis to peanuts. • At the allergic stage, peanuts can lead to anaphylactic shock.
Eggs	• Eggs are very rich and can easily give rise to the stagnant food pattern. After this stage the main symptom is the tendency to produce pus. • At the allergic stage, eggs can lead to anaphylactic shock. • Other signs of egg intolerance include purulent conjunctivitis and the appearance of boils and spots on the skin, especially those containing pus.
Seafood (crabs, lobsters, shrimps, prawns)	• When these foods are well digested, they are considered slightly cooling (hence the pleasure of a prawn cocktail on a hot day). When the digestive system is not functioning well, they can give rise to red wheals on the skin. In some cases they can affect the nervous system and give rise to insomnia with great unhappiness. • In severe cases, prolonged use of these foods can make the childhood diseases much worse. This advice is particularly important for nursing mothers because it is rare for toddlers and older children to enjoy these foods.
Food additives	• Children's reactions to food additives such as artificial flavorings and colorings is variable. Among the most common is hyperactivity, but some children react in the opposite direction, becoming completely lethargic and depressed.

*We have seen 2-year-old baby girls developing breasts. The condition was cured simply by removing milk from the diet.

Once the offending foods have been identified, they should be eliminated from the diet. Doing so will considerably speed the cure.

Finding the Contributory Foods

When children are allergic to one food, the root cause of the allergy is often to be found in another food not initially suspected. For example, we treated a child who was allergic to the chlorine in tap water. At first he simply felt tired every time he drank tap water. Gradually, his condition worsened, and by the age of 4 years, he had a severe asthma attack each time he drank a mouthful of chlorinated water. The allergy to chlorine was very marked and very clear, but we found the root cause of the allergy to be cow's milk. Once he stopped drinking cow's milk, his symptoms improved rapidly.

Another example is a 2-year-old boy we treated who was allergic to coffee. Every time he came into contact with the smallest amount of coffee, such as in a coffee-flavored cake, he had a severe nosebleed for hours. In his case the root cause was found to be the combination of cow's milk and muesli made from raw oats with nuts and raisins. Once he was put on a diet of cooked food, the allergy to coffee disappeared.

Improving the Digestive System by Treating the Pattern

The next step is to improve the digestive system so that the offending foods can be better digested. Herbs can be enormously helpful in doing this. The first step is to identify the main pattern affecting the child because this is helpful in determining the most suitable herbs to use. This often involves herbs that work on the liver, the blood, and the lymph system. Sometimes the allergen suggests which herbs will be of most use, but more often than not the best approach is to see how the child reacts to the allergen. Thus, when it comes to prescribing herbs, more attention should be paid to exactly how the individual child is affected than the particular offending allergen.

■ COMMON PATTERNS OF FOOD ALLERGY AND INTOLERANCE

We now turn to the common ways in which food allergy and intolerance manifest in children. Under each pattern we have included a paragraph on the "causes," and among these some foods are mentioned. Sometimes these foods are the primary factor causing the allergy or intolerance, but sometimes they are contributory factors. Whichever they are, they should be eliminated from the diet.

The following patterns are commonly associated with food allergy. It is a long list, but even this does not cover every eventuality.

- Fluid imbalance
- Mucus
- Echo pattern (thick mucus)
- Heat
- Cold
- Stagnant food pattern
- Weak digestion

■ SYMPTOMS AND SIGNS*
Fluid Imbalance

One of the most common patterns in Britain, fluid imbalance is characterized by the accumulation of fluids in the body. Often, there is an imbalance in the sugar levels, which contributes to a fluid imbalance.

- Pale face
- Nasal discharge (nose runs like a tap)
- Persistent watery cough if the respiratory system is weak
- A bit overweight and subjectively feels heavy when carried
- Lumbering walk
- Somewhat flabby arms and legs

---

*Facial color reveals a lot about a child's energy. See p. 54 for a discussion of facial colors and variations among racial groups.

CAUSES
- Damp climate
- Too much sugar and sweet foods
- Not enough exercise
- Aftereffects of an illness
- Many courses of antibiotics

COMMON ALLERGENS
- Milk
- Bread
- Commercial fruit juices
- Sugar
- Molds

Mucus

The mucus pattern is similar to the previous pattern and can be a further development of it. Instead of the retained fluids being watery, they become somewhat thick.

- Gray face
- Nasal discharge like glue
- Persistent, productive cough if respiratory system is weak
- Mouth breathing
- A bit overweight and feels heavy when carried
- Lumbering walk
- Somewhat flabby arms and legs

CAUSES
- Damp climate
- Too much cow's milk and produce from cow's milk
- Too many peanuts and peanut butter
- Too much sugar and sweet foods
- Too many bananas
- Too much ice-cold food
- Not enough exercise
- Aftereffects of an illness
- Aftereffects of immunizations
- Many courses of antibiotics

COMMON ALLERGENS
- Milk products
- Bread
- Eggs
- Peanuts
- Gluten

Note that when the nasal discharge is green, the cause may be gluten allergy.

Echo Pattern (Thick Mucus)

Echo pattern is a variation on the previous pattern. For a further description, see Chapter 5. The mucus is not nearly as obvious as in the previous pattern, for it is very thick. Some of these children do not show any obvious signs of mucus at all. Typically, one may see the following:

- Occasional stuffed-up nose
- Occasional cough that is dry or harsh and usually unproductive
- Slightly glazed look in the eyes
- Characteristic rough patch on the cheek
- Rough skin (like sandpaper) in places
- Swollen glands

CAUSES
- Any long illness, especially if treated with antibiotics
- Immunizations
- Cow's milk
- Gluten allergy

COMMON ALLERGENS
- Milk
- Pollen
- Molds
- Bread

Heat

In some cases something happens to upset the child's Heat balance inside, resulting in subacute inflammation in most of the body.

- Red face
- Impetuous behavior
- Hyperactivity (in some children only)

- Sleep problems (may be difficult to get to sleep or wakes in the middle of the night because of bad dreams)
- Withdrawn (not always seen; when present, may even be withdrawn to the point of being autistic)
- Anaphylactic shock (in severe cases)

CAUSES
- Immunization (in almost all cases); occasionally the aftereffects of a high fever

CONTRIBUTORY FACTORS
- Cow's milk
- Gluten allergy
- Colorings and flavorings in food
- Overconsumption of sugar

COMMON ALLERGENS
- Animal hair
- Shellfish
- Chlorine in drinking water
- Peanuts

Cold

The Cold pattern may have started during infancy or toddlerhood and lead to colic. If the colic was left untreated, the child continues with intense Cold energy in the digestive system, which disrupts the normal digestive process.

Typical symptoms are as follows:

- White face
- Occasional abdominal pains, even cramps
- Worsening of abdominal pains by the allergen and by Cold-energy foods and cold water
- Cold hands or feet (a lot of the time)
- History of colic when a baby
- Very ticklish

CAUSES
- Many courses of antibiotics
- Polio immunization
- A diet of ice cold food and drinks

- A diet containing Cold-energy foods such as bananas, cucumbers, and tomatoes

COMMON ALLERGENS
- Fruits
- Fruit juices
- Cow's milk
- Tomatoes
- Wheat

Stagnant Food Pattern (Younger Than 3 Years Old)

The stagnant food pattern is described in more detail in Part 1 (see Chapter 2). In this pattern, the food accumulates in the abdomen, remaining there only partially digested. When this happens, it is easy for food allergies to develop because the partially digested food often irritates the intestines.

Typical symptoms are as follows:

- Red cheeks
- Green around the mouth
- Nasal discharge
- Swollen abdomen (looks like a drum)
- Foul-smelling stools
- Constipation alternating with diarrhea

CAUSES
- Usually caused by one of the three factors of overeating, irregular eating, or unsuitable food (In our experience, it is most often caused by giving a young child food that is too rough, such as muesli or brown rice.)
- Sometimes caused by cow's milk
- Sometimes caused by gluten intolerance

COMMON ALLERGENS
- A wide range of foods

Weak Digestion

Weak digestion is described in more detail in Chapter 2. In this pattern the child does not have quite enough energy to cope. This means that there is not quite enough energy for the digestion, which is the source of energy. The child may prefer unsuitable foods, either because they are easy to assimilate (e.g., sugar and fruit juice) or because they are highly flavored (e.g., burgers and chips).

Typical symptoms are as follows:

- Thin
- Pale face
- Lacking in vital warmth (e.g., may want to wear wooly clothes and stay indoors)
- Poor appetite
- Frequent snacks
- Lack of energy *or* hyperactive when tired

CAUSES
- A long illness
- Too many immunizations in a row
- Irregular feeding patterns when young
- Not enough sleep

COMMON ALLERGENS
- Sugar
- Flavorings and colorings
- Hormones and chemicals in nonorganic food

Note that allergy tests will show allergies to many unrelated foods.

▪ TREATMENT AND RESULTS

Dosages*

Dosages are given for 3-year-olds (Table 15-2). The tinctures are given three times a day in about 25 to 50 ml of warm water. The medicine may be sweetened as desired.

The dosages we suggest are *suggestions only.* Each child may need something different.

Caution

When treating children who have violent allergic reactions, bear in mind that it is possible that they

---

*For more detailed information about dosages, see Chapter 8.

■ Table 15-2	
AGE	MULTIPLY 3-YEAR-OLD DOSE BY
6-12 months	$\times \frac{1}{3}$
1-2 years	$\times \frac{1}{2}$
2-4 years	$\times 1$
4-7 years	$\times 1\frac{1}{2}$
7-14 years	$\times 2$
14+ years	$\times 3$

will have such a reaction to the herbs they are given. It is very unlikely—it has never happened to us—but it is possible. It is therefore prudent to start by giving only one drop of the medicine to see what the reaction will be. Then the quantity can gradually be increased to the recommended dosage. A Chinese proverb best sums up this caution: "Better too little medicine than too much."

Comment

These prescriptions are meant only as a guide. Our experience has been that even within these categories there are enormous variations. For example, one child allergic to wheat had the thick mucus pattern but also had lower abdominal pains every time he ate wheat. Another with the same basic pattern had a feeling of heaviness in the stomach that was accompanied by nausea. Although the same basic prescription was used for each, it was modified to take account for their different symptoms.

When it comes to writing a prescription for a child, there are two main steps:

1. Decide which is the most important underlying pattern and use herbs accordingly.
2. Choose specific herbs to treat specific symptoms. For example, if the child has a cough, add herbs for cough (as detailed in the relevant chapter).

Fluid Imbalance

Bayberry *Myrica cerifera*	3 drops tincture
Agrimony *Agrimonia eupatoria*	3 drops tincture

Cleavers *Galium aparine*	2 drops tincture
Aniseed *Pimpinella anisum*	3 drops tincture
Ginger *Zingiber officinalis*	2 drops tincture

VARIATIONS

See Variations section later in this chapter.

Explanation. Bayberry is an astringent that dries up excess fluid, especially fluid in the stomach. Agrimony is an astringent that dries up fluid in the rest of the digestive system, and it is particularly indicated in children who have diarrhea. Cleavers is a diuretic to help pass the excess water out through the kidneys. It is also an alterative. Aniseed is a general digestive tonic. Ginger warms and tones the digestive system, and it also harmonizes the other herbs.

Results. The first results may be that the child urinates frequently and becomes thirstier. After that the child's energy should pick up. Continuing progress is somewhat variable. Some children get better quickly, and others take a long time—some take months. It may ultimately take a bad cold or cough to finally rid the child of the imbalance (see Chapter 4 for an explanation).

Mucus

Golden seal *Hydrastis canadensis*	4 drops tincture
Elderflower *Sambucus nigra*	2 drops tincture
Angelica *Angelica archangelica*	2 drops tincture
Burdock *Arctium lappa*	2 drops tincture

A possible addition is the following:

| Elecampane *Inula helenium* | 2 drops tincture |

VARIATIONS

See Variations section later in this chapter.

Explanation. Golden seal clears mucus from the entire body, and elderflower clears it from the upper respiratory tract. Angelica is a tonic for the digestive system. Burdock is a tonic and an alterative that stimulates the liver. Elecampane has a very similar function to that of burdock, with more effect on the lungs and less on the skin.

Results. Initially, there may be more signs of mucus, but over the next few weeks this should clear gradually. After some months, the allergies should be much reduced.

Echo Pattern (Thick Mucus)

Poke root *Phytolacca decandra*	2 drops tincture
Blue flag *Iris versicolor*	2 drops tincture
Elecampane *Inula helenium*	2 drops tincture
Golden seal *Hydrastis canadensis*	2 drops tincture
Ginger *Zingiber officinalis*	2 drops tincture

VARIATIONS

See Variations section later in this chapter.

Explanation. Poke root and blue flag soften phlegm and clear the entire system. Elecampane and golden seal prevent the phlegm that was released from overwhelming the system. Ginger is used to warm and circulate, and it also harmonizes the other herbs.

Results. Changes are slow to come when treating the echo pattern. The small signs that the herbs are actually working are listed in Chapter 17. After 3 to 6 months, the allergies should be considerably reduced.

Heat

Meadowsweet *Filipendula ulmaria*	4 drops tincture
Marshmallow *Althea officinalis*	4 drops tincture
Elecampane *Inula helenium*	2 drops tincture
Golden seal *Hydrastis canadensis*	2 drops tincture

If the child is also hyperactive, add the following:

Pasque flower *Anemone pulsatilla*	1 drops tincture
Passion flower *Passiflora incarnata*	2 drops tincture
Valerian *Valeriana officinalis*	2 drops tincture

VARIATIONS

See Variations section later in this chapter.

Explanation. Meadowsweet and marshmallow are both very cooling herbs and cool the stomach and intestines. This may release much of the phlegm, so golden seal and elecampane are added. Pasque flower brings the heat to the surface. Although a small dose, it is a strong herb. Passion flower and valerian help calm the child.

Results. Changes are usually noted within a week or so. At first they will be small changes, but then gradually the child starts to calm down. Full cure may not be achieved until the heat is expelled through a fever.

Cold

Prickly ash *Zanthoxylum americanum*	4 drops tincture
Aniseed *Pimpinella anisum*	3 drops tincture
Ginger *Zingiber officinalis*	3 drops tincture
Burdock *Arctium lappa*	3 drops tincture
Wild yam *Dioscorea villosa*	3 drops tincture

VARIATIONS
See Variations section later in this chapter.

Explanation. Prickly ash is the main herb, and it warms and tones the digestive system. It also increases the circulation of warmth throughout the body. Aniseed is a warming tonic for the digestive system. Ginger is used especially for the stomach and is harmonizing. Burdock is included as an alterative. Wild yam is optional. It is an antispasmodic and is included for any colic or griping pains that the child might have.

Results. Some small changes should be noticed in the first week in young children and after 2 to 3 weeks in older children. The face should become pinker, and other small signs will be noticed. After a few months, the child should be much better and it will be safe to try the allergen in small quantities.

Stagnant Food Pattern

Black root *Leptandra virginica*	4 drops tincture
Yellow dock *Rumex crispus*	2 drops tincture
Burdock *Arctium lappa*	2 drops tincture
Marshmallow root *Althea officinalis*	2 drops tincture

VARIATIONS
See Variations section later in this chapter.

Explanation. The main herb is black root, which is specific for the stagnant food pattern. Yellow dock and burdock both stimulate movement of the digestive system. Marshmallow is included as a demulcent to soothe any irritation of the digestive lining.

Results. As with all stagnant food patterns, spectacular evacuations may occur during the first 2 days. If this is excessive, the medicine should be stopped and then introduced at a smaller dosage when the bowels have normalized. A few days after that, the medicine may be increased back to the normal dosage. Once the stagnant food pattern has been cleared, the way is open for the allergy to go, although it may take several weeks before it is safe to try suspect foods. As always with the stagnant food pattern, the child must eat suitable food, eat regularly, and not eat too much.

Weak Digestion

Fennel *Foeniculum vulgare*	4 drops tincture
Burdock *Arctium lappa*	2 drops tincture
Ginger *Zingiber officinalis*	2 drops tincture
Licorice *Glycyrrhiza glabra*	2 drops tincture

VARIATIONS
See Variations section later in this chapter.

Explanation. Fennel is a digestive tonic. Burdock regulates the digestive system. Ginger is tonic and is warming, and licorice is a tonic and harmonizing.

Results. Results are often slow to come with the Weak digestion pattern. After a month, one may see an improved appetite, but it is unusual for it to be large for at least 6 months. It may be necessary to continue taking some type of tonic or supplement for several years to build up the child's strength to an optimal level.

Variations

Add in herbs for the following symptoms. In addition, consult the relevant chapter in this text (where there is one).

Cough (see Chapter 18)

Angelica *Angelica archangelica*	2 drops tincture
Hyssop *Hyssopus officinalis*	2 drops tincture
or	
White horehound *Marrubium vulgare*	2 drops tincture

Excessive mucus (including nasal catarrh)

Hyssop *Hyssopus officinalis*	2 drops tincture
Elderflower *Sambucus nigra*	2 drops tincture

Skin rash (see Chapter 26)

Marigold *Calendula officinalis*	2 drops tincture
Nettles *Urtica dioica*	2 drops tincture

Constipation (see Chapter 10)

Yellow dock *Rumex crispus*	2 drops tincture
or	
Butternut *Juglans cinerea*	2 drops tincture
or	
Cascara *Rhamnus purshiana*	2 drops tincture

Eye irritation

Eyebright *Euphrasia officinalis*	2 drops tincture

Obvious inflammation

Marshmallow *Althea officinalis*	2 drops tincture

GIVING ADVICE TO PARENTS

In this discussion we have made a distinction between allergy and food intolerance. This is an unnecessary distinction for most patients, and it may be simpler to use the single term *allergy*.

■ ESSENTIAL OILS

Essential oils are not the principal treatment but can be useful adjuncts, especially to relieve some specific symptoms such as excessive mucus or blocked sinus. Normally, we use them in massage oils, 2 drops of each oil to 30 ml (1 oz) of oil.

The following oils will be found useful:

Chamomile *Chamomilla matricaria*	Strengthens the digestive system and relieves colic
Lavender *Lavandula officinale*	Calms
Melissa *Melissa officinalis*	Strengthens the digestive system and is calming

■ APPENDIX: *CANDIDA*

Candida albicans is a yeast. Many people become infected by this yeast, and it causes them much misery. The yeast lives especially in the gut, but it is also present in other mucous membranes, particularly the mouth and the vagina. If it is present in the gut for a long time, it starts to grow into the lining of the gut and is then very difficult to dislodge. It is a problem that affects adults, but children also can suffer from it. Typical symptoms include the following:

- Low energy
- Tiredness
- Feelings of heaviness
- Itching

We have included this condition under food allergy because *Candida* thrives on certain foods and may be the agent that gives rise to food allergies. The foods that favor the growth of *Candida* are those that favor the growth of all yeast, in particular, foods containing sugar (even fruit sugars) and foods that give rise to fluid imbalances. It is also encouraged by the overuse of antibiotics.

The normal pattern that is seen when a child has a yeast infection is the fluid imbalance pattern, and it should be treated accordingly. It is especially important to avoid sugar in the diet and, for some people, gluten. The cure can sometimes be hastened by the use of orthodox antifungals, such as metronidazole (Flagyl), but the condition will recur if the underlying imbalance has not been corrected.

16

Fevers

Fevers are part of childhood. It is rare for a child to reach age 3 years without ever having some type of fever. The fever may be only mild, not requiring any treatment, but some type of fever is to be expected. For a child to continue in good health, these fevers should not be suppressed but rather should be led to a satisfactory conclusion. Sometimes this means just allowing them to run their course; sometimes this means treating the child with herbs. Only in rare cases should suppressants such as paracetamol be used. The reasons for this are discussed in Chapter 4. Most can be treated at home, without the need for specialist intervention, provided that the parents are prepared to do so. It does make life difficult for parents because they must simultaneously fill the roles of doctor, nurse, and parent. The task of a practitioner is also complicated. The practitioner should do the following:

First, teach the parents how to treat mild fevers themselves.
Second, teach parents the danger signs of when fevers are beginning to get out of control.
Third, treat fevers that are becoming dangerous.

Teaching Parents to Treat Mild Fevers

Most parents will never see many of the illnesses covered in this book, but they are bound to see their child with a fever sooner or later. They have to look after their child through such minor ailments, and it is a responsibility that most parents gladly take on. However, many parents find themselves in a quandary, for most of the advice they receive is to take over-the-counter orthodox medicines—most of which are known to cause side effects. Many parents are only too glad to learn of other treatments that do not carry the same risks of harming their child's body.

It is for this reason that we have extended the scope of this chapter to include other therapies beyond herbal remedies and herbal derivatives. We have included some massage strokes and some homeopathic remedies in addition to herbs and essential oils. For practitioners who are not yet familiar with these treatments, we encourage them to learn more, and this chapter (with Chapter 9), which introduces both homeopathy and massage, provides a starting point. It also improves the ability of practitioners to communicate with their patients who are already using these therapies.

When Are Fevers Dangerous?

Whether a fever is becoming dangerous is a matter of judgment. As a practitioner, one develops experience from seeing many children survive fevers, and with this experience comes a sixth sense. Parents, especially first-time parents, do not have this experience and need to be given rules. This is somewhat unsatisfactory, for there are so many different children that rules that apply to one family do not apply to another. The situation is further complicated by the enormous increase in litigation, which means that if anything goes wrong, the person who gave advice is likely to be sued. Consequently, there is a feeling that it is better to give very safe rules. There is obviously a compelling reason to do this,

Table 16-1	Danger Signs for Fevers in Weak and Strong Children	
CONDITION	**RULES FOR WEAK CHILDREN**	**RULES FOR STRONG CHILDREN**
When the fevers persist for a long time	More than 2 days	More than 4 days at 40° C (104° F)
When the fevers go very high	More than 39° C (102.2° F)	More than 40.5° C (104.9° F)
When the temperature rises very rapidly	To 39° C (102.2° F) in 4 hours	To 40° C (104° F) in 2 hours

but we believe that it is beneficial to encourage self-reliance, so we provide two sets of rules: one set for Weak children, who are prone to sickness, and another set for reasonably Strong, healthy children.

In general, fevers are rarely dangerous. There are, of course, certain conditions when you can expect them to become dangerous, and these are listed in Table 16-1.

The last condition in the table, that of rapidly rising fevers, requires further explanation. If the temperature rises slowly, children can withstand a surprisingly high temperature (even as high as 42° C) without sustaining any damage. If the temperature rises rapidly (within a few hours), then quite low fevers, even those below 40° C (104° F), can cause convulsions.

There are other signs that the fever really is going out of control. These include the following:

- The child is vague and confused or loses consciousness.
- One side of the body seems hot, but the other seems cold.
- The child starts to twitch.
- Fever is a common prelude to something serious, such as an asthma attack or epileptic fit.

What Are the Dangers?

If a fever goes too high for too long, the child becomes weakened. In the past, when a child may have a fever for weeks at a time, this could mean that the child simply gave up fighting. This is rare today, but a prolonged fever does open the way for complications. The most common complication is the development of febrile convulsions, which can lead to brain damage. This may progress into delir-

ium, coma, and eventually death. In other situations there is the risk for meningitis.

Danger Signs

A fever in a child who develops a purpuric rash must be taken seriously, as this may be a sign of meningitis. Other signs commonly seen with meningitis include the following:

- Headache
- Stiff neck
- Lethargy
- Vomiting
- Convulsions

Are Febrile Convulsions Dangerous?

Surprisingly, febrile convulsions in themselves are not usually dangerous. They certainly seem dangerous, and there is a strong feeling of panic that communicates itself to the parent and practitioner alike when a child has convulsions, but if the convulsions are only occasional and of short duration, then they usually leave no lasting mark. It is only when the convulsions last for more than 5 minutes or come very frequently that there is a greatly increased chance of developing brain damage.

■ TREATMENT OF FEVERS

Refer to Chapter 4 for a more in-depth discussion of the principles of treating fevers.

The Basics

We start our discussion with the basics of treating fevers. This is based on what fevers used to be like in the past and what many fevers are like now. It is based on the assumption that the child is reasonably healthy before the fever and succumbs to a viral or bacterial attack. In these strong children, the following patterns are seen:

- Mild
    Whining
    Sleepy
- Strong
    Shivery
    Boiling

▪ SYMPTOMS AND SIGNS

Mild

Appearance | The main feature with a mild fever is that the child is not overwhelmed by the infection. The face may be white, or it may be red, but this largely depends on what the color of the child was before.

Behavior | The child may be clingy and insecure but is usually prepared to go off and do something. An older child will feel a bit shivery if in a draught, but younger ones do not seem to notice.

Temperature | The forehead is hot, but the body usually is not especially hot. You may be a little unsure of whether the child has a fever without taking the temperature.

There are two subdivisions of this pattern: restless and sleepy. Some children become more and more restless and clingy, whereas others, although clingy while awake, may spend many more hours than usual sleeping.

Strong and Shivery

In children who have strong fevers and are shivery, there is no doubt that the child is ill. If this is the first time a mother has seen it, she may be very worried and think that something is seriously wrong. The child has been overwhelmed by terrible feelings of cold and cannot get warm.

Appearance | The child is very pale and is often frightened. The pupils are typically contracted.

Behavior | There is no question of the child engaging in any activity. All he or she wants to do is to curl up in mother's arms. The child feels very cold inside and shivers uncontrollably from time to time. Usually, the child does not sweat and, when resting at night, likes to curl up in a ball.

Temperature | The temperature is usually quite high (40° C [104° F]).

Confusing sign | The child often feels hot to the touch, so you or the parent may think that it is a Hot condition, but it is really a Cold condition. The child may feel cold inside because so much heat is being lost through the hot skin.

Strong and Boiling

Once again, there is no doubt that the child is ill. The main difference is that the child is not overwhelmed by feelings of cold but rather is overwhelmed by feelings of heat. The child is boiling up and simply cannot get cool. This gives rise to the following:

Appearance | The face is very red, and there may be some mild perspiration. The pupils are usually dilated.

Behavior | The child is difficult to be with and very restless, constantly tossing and turning. He or she wants to be close to mother when not being held, but when being held, he or she wants to be put down. No position is comfortable. When resting and at night, the child lies on back and throws off the covers.

Temperature | The temperature is usually quite high (40° C [104° F], maybe even higher).

▣ TREATMENT*

The dosages we give are for children aged 3 years (Table 16-2). The dosages we list are *suggestions only*. Each child may need something different.

Mild

AIM OF TREATMENT

The main purpose here is to prevent a mild fever from becoming a strong one. At this stage there is no real need for herbal remedies. All that is needed is frequent drinks of honey[†] and lemon juice.

If you can catch the fever in the early stages, then you may try the following:

Echinacea	3 drops tincture taken in
Echinacea angustifolia	warm water every 3 hours

ADVICE

Perhaps the most important part of treatment is advice. Children with mild fevers should be kept at home, kept quiet and warm,[‡] and kept out of the cold and the wind. This will enable the child to get through the fever and become stronger. As may be expected, this advice is often unwelcome, especially if both parents work. They may believe that their child is nearly well enough to go to school and may send the child back sooner than is prudent.

Table 16-2	
AGE	**MULTIPLY 3-YEAR-OLD DOSE BY**
6-12 months	$\times \frac{1}{3}$
1-2 years	$\times \frac{1}{2}$
2-4 years	$\times 1$
4-7 years	$\times 1\frac{1}{2}$
7-14 years	$\times 2$
14+ years	$\times 3$

---

*For more detailed information about dosages, see Chapter 8.

†Note: The honey should be pasteurized for children younger than 1 year. See note on p. 67.

‡Take care not to wrap the child in *too* many warm layers.

▣ Case History

Patrick was 7 years old and had recently joined the school football team. It was something that he had been longing for ever since he was small. At the time in question it was the beginning of autumn, and an epidemic fever was going around. Patrick was not especially Weak, but like many others he caught the fever. It was in these very early stages that he was brought to me for a routine checkup. I strongly advised them to keep him at home and, above all, not to expose him to wind. Unfortunately, the lure of the football pitch was too strong, and after school the next day, he went out for training. This involved prolonged standing in cold winds, wearing just football clothes. The consequence was that his fever shot up that night, and he had to spend the next 3 days in bed. It was 2 weeks before he was fully back to normal.

Strong and Cold

Treatment consists of two parts. First is the obvious one: warming up the child. As long as the child is shivering and feeling desperately cold, there is no chance of getting better. The second part of treatment is to promote sweating.

TREATMENT

The herb of choice is an herbal simple:

Yarrow *Achillea millefolium*	See following text for dosage

This is best given as a sweetened infusion, but tincture taken in hot water works almost as well. It should be taken as hot as possible every 1 or 2 hours and will gradually warm the child. The main difficulty with this herb is its very unpleasant taste.

If the fresh herb is not available or the child will take only a tincture, then give 1 ml of tincture in each dose and give in warm, sweetened water, as described.

DOSAGES

Add 3 tsp of fresh herb to 500 ml (20 oz) of boiling water and allow to stand until lukewarm. Sweeten and give a cupful (100 ml/4 oz) every 2 hours until the child starts to feel warm and perspiration has started.

Continue to give this medicine every 4 to 6 hours (except when the child is asleep), until the fever has decreased. Then give three times a day for 3 days.

EFFECT

Over the next few hours (maybe as long as 12 hours), the child should gradually feel warmer and warmer and then start to sweat. When the sweating occurs, the child is starting to get better and the fever has "broken." The infusion should be taken every 2 hours or so until the fever is well past. This dosage is necessary because yarrow is also a tonic, and it will sufficiently maintain the child's energy to keep on fighting the fever.

An alternative to yarrow follows:

Catmint *Nepeta cataria*	20 drops tincture
Ginger *Zingiber officinalis*	20 drops tincture

EXPLANATION

Catmint on its own helps get rid of fevers, but it does not warm the child, so ginger is added. Alternatives to ginger include the following:

Cayenne *Capsicum minimum*	10 drops tincture
or	
Prickly ash *Zanthoxylum americanum*	20 drops tincture

Strong and Hot

In the Cold pattern the first step in treatment is to warm the child, so with the Warm pattern, the first step is to cool the child. In orthodox medicine this may be done by the crude method of simply putting cold water bottles under the child's arms or immersing the child in tepid water, but we consider these inferior methods. They are indeed effective in lowering the temperature when it is going dangerously high, but they impede the sweating process and therefore increase the time taken to get over the fever. A superior method is to use cooling herbs and to promote perspiration.

The second part is to transform the sweat into a beneficial sweat.* Different herbs are used because the child is sweating already. Some of these herbs have been demonstrated to have antiviral or antibacterial effects.

TREATMENT

There are two well-established prescriptions. The first is the herbal simple:

Catmint *Nepeta cataria*	See following text for dosage

The second is the following compound:

Elderflower *Sambucus nigra*	See following text for dosage
Peppermint *Mentha piperata*	See following text for dosage

DOSAGES

The best way to give these herbs is as an infusion. Make a tea from 1 tsp of each herb in a cup of water and sweeten well. Give half the mixture while it is still warm every 2 hours (for 3-year-olds; for other ages, see Table 16-2), and then make up some more.

A good second best, which avoids the necessity of keeping dried herbs, is to take a syrup. These are commercially available in many places. Once again, give the mixture in warm water every 2 hours, following the instructions on the bottle.

Tinctures may also be used and are certainly effective. Dose $\frac{1}{4}$ tsp each dose for 3-year-olds. In view of the relatively large quantities needed, it is usually a good idea to evaporate off some of the alcohol. See Chapter 8 for details of this procedure.

RESULTS

What one is hoping for is for the mild nature of the sweat to become profuse. Often, the sweat seems a bit oily or greasy before the herbs are given; when the herbs take effect, the child becomes drenched. This sweat is the best way for the child to cool down. Sometimes this happens very quickly,

---

*This is what is meant by a *diaphoretic,* as opposed to a *sudorific.*

within minutes of giving the herbs. Sometimes it takes a few hours to work. If nothing has happened within 6 hours, other remedies (e.g., homeopathy, massage) should be added.

ADVICE ON NURSING

The child should be kept in bed and kept warm enough for the sweating to continue. In the Strong and Cold condition, this may mean wrapping the child up well. In the Strong and Hot condition the child should still be kept lightly covered (which may go contrary to one's instincts). The child is so restless and hot that the urge is to take the warm clothes off and cool the child, but what is needed is for the child to keep sweating. (Obviously, the child should not be allowed to get too hot.)

In both conditions, make sure the child is not in a draught. Also, the child should drink plenty of liquids to replenish what is being lost through sweating. The best drink is honey* and lemon, but any sweet drink is good. This should be given at room temperature or warmer, never ice cold.

RECUPERATION

The child should be kept at home after the fever for as long as the fever has lasted. For example, if the fever lasted 3 days, then the child should be kept at home for an additional 3 days after the fever has subsided. Once again, this is often unwelcome advice, but this course of action results in the best long-term health of the child. Parents who follow this advice find that they take fewer days off work because their child does not succumb to the next infection so severely.

■ FURTHER DEVELOPMENTS

So far we have discussed the very basic principles of treatment. When treating very young children, it is common for fevers to develop in a slightly different way than adults. In particular, the following three patterns may develop:

---

*Note: The honey should be pasteurized for children younger than 1 year. See note on p. 67.

- Panic reaction
- Cough
- Stagnant food pattern

PANIC REACTION

A fever is an unfamiliar sensation for children and can be very frightening. In some children the fear is so fierce that they lose all control and panic. The panic is so strong it is almost tangible. Commonly, this panic overwhelms the mother as well and can even affect practitioners who are seeing it for the first time. When this happens, the panic itself becomes part of the disease, for it is responsible for generating more and more heat from the energy the child puts into screaming. Without specifically treating the violent emotion, it is difficult to reduce the fever.

COUGH

Sometimes a spring fever affects an entire family, with the adults and older children merely experiencing a temperature. In younger children the temperature may be accompanied by a cough. If the cough is only mild, it may not need treatment, but when it is severe, it disturbs the sleep and consumes so much energy that herbs must be included to treat the cough.

STAGNANT FOOD PATTERN

In babies and toddlers the onset of a fever may precipitate the stagnant food pattern, just as happens when the teeth come in. The child becomes very irritable and angry; the abdomen bloats; and in addition to the fever produced by the infection, extra heat is produced by fermenting food. It is difficult to get the fever to go down if it is being continuously fueled in this way.

Panic Reaction

SYMPTOMS AND SIGNS

The child is hysterical with fear, weeping and burying his or her head in the mother's bosom. Usually, the mother is very distressed too, making it difficult for a practitioner not to be drawn into this state of hysteria.

TREATMENT

A number of herbs can be used to calm panic; among these, one stands out: passion flower *Passiflora incarnata*. Even better than conventional tinctures, though, is the Dr. Bach Rescue Remedy, which often has an effect within minutes.

ADMINISTRATION

Passion flower *Passiflora incarnata*	Add 1 or 3 drops of tincture to each dose of herbs. If the child is in too great a panic to take a normal dose, dilute the tincture 1:10 and squirt some in the child's mouth.
Rescue Remedy	Put 1 or 2 drops on the tongue of both the child and the mother. You can also put 1 or 2 drops in a glass of water and leave it for the parents to give to the child. When the level of panic is great, take sips every 5 minutes.

ADVICE

When panic of this kind arises, the mother's panic affects the child and the child's panic affects the mother, so both need to be treated. It can be helpful to separate the mother and child for half an hour or so. This can make it easier for each to control their panic. It can be helpful for the mother to take Rescue Remedy too. This will calm her panic, although more slowly than the child's.

RESULTS

Once the panic has been overcome, the fever usually subsides quickly, often within a few hours. If it does not, then at least it is relatively straightforward and easy to see what to do next.

Cough

SYMPTOMS AND SIGNS

Besides the main symptom of fever, the child has a cough.

TREATMENT

If the cough is mild, add the following:

Hyssop *Hyssopus officinalis*	2 drops tincture

If the cough is more severe, consult Chapter 19.

If the child needs sleep to get over both the fever and cough, add the following:

Wild cherry *Prunus serotina*	2 drops tincture or ½ tsp syrup

RESULTS

The fever usually goes down quickly, but the cough can linger on, in which case it should be treated like a chronic cough.

Stagnant Food Pattern

SYMPTOMS AND SIGNS

The child has the typical look of the stagnant food pattern: red cheeks, swollen abdomen, and so on (see Chapter 2). More often than not, the child is constipated because he or she has not had much to eat for a day or two, but even so the abdomen is enlarged. The child's mood is usually very difficult, being unsatisfied with everything.

TREATMENT

There are two herbs that stand out:

German chamomile *Chamomilla matricaria*	Taken as a tea
Black root *Leptandra virginica*	3 drops tincture

Of these chamomile is the place to start, because in addition to helping the digestive system, it is also a diaphoretic. It is best to give it as a tea, although tincture can be used. Black root has a stronger effect on the digestive system and is also a diaphoretic. It is more commonly given as tincture.

An alternative is as follows:

Elecampane *Inula helenium*	3 drops tincture

Elecampane will treat both cough and the stagnant food pattern at the same time.

RESULTS

Results are somewhat variable, depending on how severe the digestive disturbance is. If the child is not sweating, then sweating should start within an hour or so. Also, digestion should start to move, and the child should start to feel more comfortable. If nothing happens, keep repeating the dose every hour.

ADVICE

The child should not be given any solid food until either the fever has gone down or the abdomen is no longer swollen and the child has no abdominal pains. The child should be encouraged to drink a lot.

■ OTHER VARIATIONS

The Fever Goes On and On

Occasionally, a fever will go on and on despite correct treatment. There are two reasons for this:

- The child is not responding to the herbs.
- The fever is not merely straightforward influenza.

The Child Is Not Responding to the Herbs

This is the situation one dreads. All the books say that this herb or that is excellent for fevers, and yet despite persuading the child to take large quantities, no improvement is seen.

This is surprisingly common and may happen regardless of the therapy being used. Do not feel discouraged. What you have done with the herbs will certainly help. Even though nothing appears to be happening, unnoticed changes will be taking place. This will open the way for other therapies to work. The same is true no matter what therapy is used first. If you start with homeopathy, although you may notice no improvement initially, this will increase the herbs' ability to work. It is for this reason that we include the treatment of fevers by other therapies.

The Fever Is Not Merely Straightforward Influenza

This is also common, and once again there are various possibilities. The first, which should be considered immediately, is that the fever is a secondary effect of something more serious, such as appendicitis. It is obviously beyond the scope of this book to cover all of the possibilities.

The second, which is by far the most common, is that the fever is the body's way of rebalancing and of burning off excess Hot or Cold energy in the system. In particular, the fever may be related to the expulsion of an echo pattern. See Chapter 5 for a more detailed discussion.

In these circumstances it is appropriate simply to continue giving the herbs and wait for as long as it takes. This can be difficult as a parent, with no one to ask a second opinion. If the fever does persist, parents should be encouraged to try to find someone who can provide some sensible advice.

> If, as a parent, you are in the slightest doubt, you should call for help immediately.

Exhaustion during Fevers

One of the common causes for fevers is exhaustion. Some children simply do not have the energy to fight off an infection. When this happens, the fever is likely to be rather low. The child is miserable and whiny. Exhaustion can also occur during a fever. The fever wears out the child, and the temperature goes down without the benefit of any real relief. In both of these cases, the treatment is to give a tonic (e.g., yarrow, which may already be one of the herbs the child is taking), which is likely to increase the temperature again. This is not to be feared. The increased temperature is a sign that the body is fighting the illness.

> **Note:** The increase in temperature may also be caused by the disease taking a deeper hold, rather than the child getting better. When the child is fighting the disease, there is a sense of increased

vitality and determination to overcome the illness; on the other hand, when the disease is getting worse, there is a sense of further diminished vitality and despair. If the slightest doubt exists about what is happening, it is time to seek a second opinion quickly. If the doubt is significant, consider going to the emergency room.

Growth Spurts

It is common for a fever to develop in a child at a time of rapid growth. Sometimes, after a child has been in bed with fever, he or she seems to be at least 2 cm ($^3/_4$ inch) taller when finally getting up. Developmental changes may also be noticed at the same time.

Fevers with Teething

Teething time is dreaded by many mothers, for there is a period of a week or more when each tooth comes through and the child is miserable. In some children the condition is even more severe, and a fever develops; a minority even develop febrile convulsions when a tooth comes through.

The fevers that occur at this time can be treated in the same way as fevers mentioned previously. Especially look out for the stagnant food pattern, which often accompanies teething. In addition, to reduce the severity of symptoms during teething, care should be taken regarding the diet to reduce any possibility of the stagnant food pattern developing. That is, steps should be taken to avoid overeating, irregular feedings, and unsuitable foods (see Chapter 2).

Some simple home remedies may also help:

- Chamomile tea
- Homeopathic Chamomilla teething granules
- Essential oils rubbed into the gums, particularly clove or chamomile (2 drops of oil in an eggcup of ice-cold water)

■ PROTECTING AGAINST FEVERS

The instinct of many parents is to try to protect their child against fevers, especially if there has been a bad experience in the past. We would greatly encourage parents to try to get the child through a fever without resorting to Western medical drugs such as paracetamol* (Tylenol, Calpol). Many over-the-counter drugs are harmful, even for a healthy child, and they have the major disadvantage of suppressing a fever, rather than leading it out. In contrast, the effect on a child who has used his or her own immune system to overcome a fever can be truly remarkable. A previously weak or frail child can be transformed into a child with more energy who is less susceptible to disease.

Fevers, as we have said, are a perfectly natural part of childhood. It is as if the fever helps burn out the toxins that keep a Weak child ill.

Having said that, there are times when it is appropriate to suppress a fever, such as the following:

- There is a history of life-threatening asthma that is precipitated by fevers.
- The child has a history of severe febrile convulsions.

It is obviously better to suppress the fever than to run the risk of permanent damage. The long-term way to approach both of these conditions is to treat the child when a fever is not present to strengthen overall health. Then when the next fever comes along, the child will be that much stronger and the fever can be allowed to run its course. We have seen many children overcome a history of disease by means of a final high fever.

■ Case History

This story describes how a 10-year-old child managed to correct the underlying imbalance by means of a fever. This child had some degree of attention deficit disorder and paralysis of the arm (caused by an infection of streptococcus B, which she acquired at birth). This
Continued

---

*Paracetamol can cause death from liver failure or kidney failure. Aspirin is contraindicated for children because of the small but significant risk of allergic reaction and Reye's syndrome.

■ Case History—*cont'd*

illness had affected her by making her very dreamy and causing very poor concentration. She was not stupid. In fact, she learned things very easily, and on the few occasions when she did concentrate, she had no difficulty in doing her homework. Unfortunately, most of the time she was desperately slow. The mother had to sit with her for an hour and a half while they painfully ground through 10 very simple questions in mathematics—questions that would take as little as 5 minutes on a good day.

It is always difficult to clear out the echo effects of an infection that a child has had early in life, and hers was no exception. What we were able to do for her was to help the paralysis that the infection had left behind, but we could do little to improve her concentration.

Then one Christmas, when we were away visiting our family, the child got a very high fever. Fortunately, the mother sat with the child and waited for the fever to subside, but even she became a bit alarmed as it persisted. The girl had a temperature of 40° C (104° F) for 5 days, and nothing would bring it down. After this, the child was naturally rather tired for a week or two, but most wonderfully, her concentration was enormously improved. When it came to doing her homework, she sat down, did it in 5 or 10 minutes, and then got on with life. The fever was a turning point in her academic life, and after that it became clear that she was really intelligent and could go to any of the best schools. She would not need special schooling.

This is an example of an echo pattern coming out. As it came out, the underlying imbalance was finally cured. It took nearly 2 years of treatment for the child to reach the point where the body was strong enough to correct the imbalance that had been there since she was a baby.

Febrile Convulsions

With the use of the herbs presented earlier, it is unlikely that a child will get febrile convulsions. If convulsions do develop, we recommend that parents call for help immediately.

The treatment of febrile convulsions is outside the scope of this book for many reasons, not the least of which is because it is rare for a practitioner to be called to the bedside of a convulsing child, and it is even rarer for him or her to have brought the right medicines to be useful. Likewise, we do not advise that parents treat this condition by themselves. The difficulty in making clear decisions when your own child is suffering terribly is beyond the scope of most of us. Much more common is for parents to bring their children to a practitioner after the crisis has past and to ask if anything can be done to prevent them from happening again. In these circumstances there are three factors to look out for:

- Constitutional weakness
- Heat in the system
- Mucus in the system

The details of what to look out for and the corresponding treatments are described in Chapter 23.

■ OTHER THERAPIES

Essential Oils

There are two types of oil that can be used:

- Oils that are warming and induce sweating
- Oils that are cooling

OILS THAT ARE WARMING AND INDUCE SWEATING
These are suitable for treating Cold conditions. They should be used if the fever is less than 40° C (104° F) and when your child is cold, shivering, and not sweating.

Chamomile	See following text for
Chamomilla matricaria	dosage
Lavender *Lavandula officinalis*	See following text for
	dosage
Ti-tree *Melaleuca alternifolia*	See following text for
	dosage

These herbs may be used in a room diffuser, or if the child is well enough, they may be given in a bath, using 2 drops of each oil. (This dose is for 3-year-olds; adjust according to age.)

Alternatively, create a mixture of these oils in a base oil, 3 drops of each in 30 ml of oil, and use it in one of the massages described later in this chapter.

OILS THAT ARE COOLING

These oils are used when the fever is rising rapidly to 39.5° C (103° F) or above, and when the child is hot, red faced, and restless.

Eucalyptus *Eucalyptus globulus*	3 drops tincture
Lavender *Lavandula officinalis*	3 drops tincture
Peppermint *Mentha piperata*	3 drops tincture

Place the herbs in a bowl of cool, not cold, water and use to sponge your child's forehead and body. Use 3 drops of each oil per 30 ml.

See Chapter 8 for a further discussion of the uses and dangers of using essential oils.

Massage Techniques for Fevers

See Chapter 9 for further details and advice about how to prepare yourself to perform a massage.

The massage techniques can be done on their own or combined with another therapy. It is convenient to include some essential oils in the massage oil. The only disadvantage is that most essential oils completely ruin the effects of homeopathic remedies. You have to choose either homeopathy or aromatherapy (essential oils).

SPINAL STROKE

1. Lie the child face down.
2. With your thumb and index finger, massage gently down the spine from the base of the head to the tip of the "tail" just above the buttocks.
3. Take 2 to 3 seconds for each stroke, and do it 100 times.

Indications. Fevers, headaches, and red or sore eyes.

Comment. The connection between these symptoms is that they are all related to congestion and excess energy in the head. The effect of the massage is to draw the excess away from the head and get it circulating. If you can keep this thought in your head while doing the massage, it will help the results.

ELBOW TO LITTLE FINGER

1. Hold the child's hand in your left hand (if you are right-handed) and gently stroke down the forearm from the inside of the elbow to the little finger, using your index and middle fingers.
2. Take about 1 second to do each stroke, and repeat 30 to 50 times on each side.

Indications. Fevers, hot head, and panics; especially effective in children younger than 3 years.

Comment. Once again, the action is to stroke away from the head to relieve congestion in the head. The outside of the arm is chosen, for this corresponds to the channel associated with the heart. This is why this massage has the special indication of panic, which affects especially the heart.

UP FOREHEAD

1. Hold the child's head, with both hands, so that he or she is facing you.
2. Stroke upward, with alternate thumbs, from the bridge of the nose to the hairline.
3. Repeat 50 times.

Indications. Fevers and headaches.

Comment. This is very soothing when a child has a feverish headache.

ACROSS FOREHEAD

1. Hold the child's head, with both hands, so that he or she is facing you.
2. Using your thumbs, gently stroke across the forehead, from the center out. The stroke takes about half a second.
3. Repeat 50 times.

Indications. Fevers and headaches.

Comment. This is also very soothing when a child has a feverish headache.

BACK OF HEAD

1. With both thumbs or a thumb and index finger, massage the points in the hollows just below and

to the sides of the lower rear lump on the skull. The points are just outside the ridges of muscle that hold up the neck; they are often tender.
2. Vibrate for 1 to 2 minutes or rotate 50 times.

Indications. Headaches, eyestrain, and fevers.

Comment. This is harder to do than the other massages, but if you do it correctly, it can provide great relief when the headache is at the back of the head.

MIDDLE OF FOOT
1. Find the point on the sole of the foot, on the midline, one third of the way from toes to heel.
2. Grasp the child's foot with your left hand (if you are right-handed) and massage the point with your thumb for 1 to 2 minutes.
3. Repeat on the other foot.

Indications. Fevers, hot head, red or sore eyes, vomiting, and diarrhea.

Comment. The effect of this massage is similar to that of the spinal stroke massage in bringing energy away from the head and down. It is for this reason that all forms of foot massage (e.g., reflexology) are beneficial in children with fevers. As with the spinal stroke massage, it is helpful to think of this while you are doing the massage.

Homeopathy

See Chapter 9 for a discussion of doses and cautions for homeopathic remedies.

> **Note:** Essential oils nullify the action of homeopathic remedies, so do not use them at the same time. Choose one or the other.

Choose 6X potency if available. Give the remedy every 30 minutes at first, for up to six doses. If it works, the first change will be improvement of mood. Some symptoms may worsen, especially sweating, as with herbal remedies.

There are a few main remedies that appear again and again in the treatment of fevers. These are as follows:

- Aconite
- Belladonna
- Chamomilla
- Gelsemium
- Merc. sol.
- Sulfur

The approximate indications for these follow:

Remedy	Indications
Aconite	Sudden fevers, fear, shivering, white faced, cold. In our classification, it corresponds approximately to the Strong Cold condition. It is also suitable when panic is beginning.
Belladonna	Longer fevers, great heat, red faced, dry skin or minimal sweating, dilated pupils. In our classification it corresponds approximately to the Strong Hot condition.
Chamomilla	One cheek red, irritable and angry, swollen abdomen, maybe teething, foul-smelling stools. In our classification it corresponds approximately to development of the stagnant food pattern.
Gelsemium	Low-grade fever, lots of watery or mucus discharge; dusky red complexion. In our classification it corresponds approximately to the Heat with damp condition, which is described in more detail in the section on coughs. The child feels heavy and lethargic and looks dazed. There are also signs of mucus.
Merc. Sol.	Greasy perspiration that does not seem to bring any relief; yellow mucus discharges.
Sulfur	Stagnant food pattern. May be alternated with other remedies when stagnant food pattern has developed. Child's mood will help differentiate between Sulfur and Chamomilla. Give Sulfur if the child is more grumpy and irritable and Chamomilla if the child is more strongly angry.

RESULTS

The first thing one notices when giving homeopathic remedies is the mood of the child. Almost as soon as the remedy has been given, something changes. The child may be more docile, less frightened, or less clingy; sometimes the child becomes more angry and vociferous. When this happens, you know you have the right remedy. Wait for 15 to 30 minutes before giving the remedy again, and then continue to give the remedy until physical changes take place, namely that the child starts to perspire freely. When this happens, you know the child is well on the way to health. At this stage do not repeat the same remedy—after all, the symptom picture has changed.

When the remedy has finished doing its work, all changes will stop. If the child still has a fever, you will have to search for another fever remedy that fits the new picture.

When the fever has finally subsided, it may be appropriate to give a tonic. A discussion of remedies is beyond the scope of this book but can easily be found in books on homeopathy.

17

Chronic Cough

Chronic cough, together with asthma, accounts for nearly half of all the patients we see in the clinic. Orthodox medicine has little to offer for a chronic cough, apart from decongestants. In contrast, herbs are very effective in eradicating the problem once and for all.

This chapter divides chronic cough into three easily recognizable types, each with its own subdivision. Each of these types requires a slightly different prescription, and the results from the medicine vary significantly. Our experience has been that it is worthwhile making these distinctions. It is not always necessary, and some broad-spectrum prescriptions will work on many different types of chronic cough; indeed, we give one such prescription later in this chapter. However, as a practitioner, if you are able to make the distinction clearly, you will find that the cure is much more rapid and that you can give much clearer advice to parents. If you are a parent, you will be much clearer about what is going on in your own child.

What Is Chronic Cough?

What we mean by *chronic cough* covers a range of conditions:

- A cough that lingers for weeks, without getting any better
- A cough that gets better, but keeps coming back, either weeks or months after it had seemed to clear up or at a particular time of the year (e.g., autumn).

Danger Signs

The signs to watch out for are those of the following:

- Acute infection, such as fever and malaise, superimposed on the chronic cough (detailed in Chapter 19)
- Difficulty in breathing or wheezing, which may be early signs of asthma

■ CAUSES

Chronic cough has many causes, and each of these may give rise to a slightly different pattern. The different factors are discussed according to each different pattern, but there are some overall common causes of chronic cough.

- Incomplete recovery from a previous cough
- Immunizations
- Cow's milk intolerance

Incomplete Recovery from a Previous Cough

It is common for a child to get a cough that then becomes severe enough for the doctor to prescribe antibiotics, which clear it up. Although the antibiotics eliminate the bacterial infection, they leave behind mucus in the lungs, which is an ideal breeding ground for bacteria. It is then just a matter of time before new bacteria come along, and the child once again has a cough. One cough follows another in a downward spiral.

Immunizations

Another common cause is reaction to immunization (see Chapter 5). With immunization, the child is exposed to a mild version of a very severe illness, and in some cases the reaction to the introduced disease is not complete and the illness is never completely expelled. For example, when an immunization is given for whooping cough, a mild form of whooping cough is injected. After such an immunization, symptoms similar to a mild form of whooping cough may develop. Likewise, it is common for a child to get mucus in the lungs 3 to 4 weeks after a polio immunization, and this mucus can remain for a long time. This mucus can be the starting point for the downward spiral of repeated coughs treated with antibiotics, as described earlier.

Cow's Milk Intolerance

We cannot emphasize enough the role of cow's milk in causing chronic cough. It does not cause all chronic coughs, but it is involved in more than half of them. This is in part because of the poor quality of cow's milk available to most people, a matter that has been touched on before (see Chapter 3). It is also partly related to intolerance to cow's milk and products made from cow's milk, including cheese and, to a lesser extent, yogurt.

▪ PATTERNS

There are three easily recognizable patterns of chronic cough:

- Lots of mucus
- Weak energy
- Echo pattern (thick mucus)

Lots of Mucus

The main characteristic of children with lots of mucus is just that—the seemingly endless quantities of mucus that they generate. Their cough sounds wet and gurgly, and they may even cough some of it right out (although more commonly they swallow it). In addition, they often have a runny nose.

You suspect that if only you could somehow empty their lungs, perhaps by turning them upside down, they would feel much better. These children are fairly strong. They have to have strength to expectorate the mucus. If they were weaker, they would hardly be able to cough at all.

Weak Energy

Weak children do not have enough energy. Their lungs may be full of mucus, and if you listen with a stethoscope you will hear this. Often, they do not cough much—at least when they are in the clinic. When they do cough, it is not a very forceful cough and they often stop coughing even though you can hear that the trachea is still far from clear.

Echo Pattern (Thick Mucus)

An echo pattern is perhaps the most common complaint in the clinic, for children with this pattern may have a cough for many years. This pattern is also the one seen at the later stages of treating the first two patterns. Once most of the mucus has been eliminated and the energy has been returned to normal, one often finds the underlying echo pattern.

Children with an echo pattern are easily distinguishable from those with the previous patterns, for there is *not* a lot of mucus and they are *not* exhausted. These children have quite a lot of energy, but when they cough, very little comes up. The cough often is harsh. There may be a constant tickling in their throat that is difficult to alleviate, so they may cough and cough until finally a very small plug of thick mucus comes up (although with younger children you may not know, for once again they tend to swallow the mucus).

Further Subdivisions

The three types are further subdivided. Making these distinctions is worthwhile when you begin to prepare a prescription, as will become clear (Table 17-1).

Table 17-1 Checklist for Chronic Cough

PATTERN	MUCUS	MUCUS WITH STAGNANT FOOD	WEAK	WEAK WITH OVERSTIMULATION	ECHO PATTERN: HOT	ECHO PATTERN: COLD
Behavior	☐ Heavy, solid	☐ Restless, irritable, grumpy	☐ Underactive, tired	☐ Overactive	☐	☐
Cough	☐ "Fruity," productive	☐ "Fruity," productive	☐ Weak	☐ Weak	☐ Dry, harsh	☐ Dry, harsh
Mucus	☐ White and a bit thick	☐ Usually green and like glue	☐ Watery, but the child has no strength to cough it up	☐ Watery, but the child has no strength to cough it up	☐ Very thick or even nonexistent	☐ Very thick or even nonexistent
Nasal discharge	☐ White, like glue	☐ Green like glue	☐ Watery or none	☐ Watery or none	☐ None, some crusts in nose	☐ None, yellow crusts
Lymph glands	☐ Large and soft	☐ Large and soft	☐ May or may not be swollen	☐ May or may not be swollen	☐ Hard	☐ Hard
Stools	☐ Normal or a bit loose	☐ Sour or foul smelling, diarrhea alternating with constipation	☐ Normal or loose or constipated	☐ Normal or loose or constipated	☐ Normal	☐ Normal
Appetite	☐ Normal to a little reduced	☐ Good	☐ Poor	☐ Poor	☐ Variable	☐ Variable
Energy	☐ Adequate	☐ Tired but on the go	☐ Poor	☐ Endless	☐ Normal, with sudden drops	☐ Normal, with sudden drops
Face color	☐ Gray	☐ White with red cheeks	☐ Pale	☐ Pale	☐ Tends to red; patch on cheek	☐ Tends to pale; patch on cheek
Color of lips	☐ Pale, dull	☐ Red	☐ Pale or blue	☐ Pale or blue	☐ Red	☐ White or blue
Abdomen	☐ Normal, flabby	☐ Swollen	☐ Flat	☐ Flat	☐ Normal	☐ Normal

- Lots of mucus
    - In the lungs only
    - With a digestive disturbance (stagnant food pattern)
- Weak energy
    - Simple
    - Overstimulated
- Echo pattern (thick mucus)
    - Cold
    - Hot

LOTS OF MUCUS: IN THE LUNGS ONLY

Children with an accumulation of mucus in the lungs often look gray or even white. They run around and have a lot of energy, and their digestion is usually reasonable. In particular, you notice the absence of two factors that are seen in the next pattern, namely that the abdomen is not swollen and the stools are generally well formed and regular.

LOTS OF MUCUS: WITH A DIGESTIVE DISTURBANCE (UP TO THE AGE OF 3 YEARS)

It is one of the great observations of the Chinese that if the digestive system is not functioning well, it is easy for mucus to build up in the whole body. (This is discussed further in Chapter 2). In this case the digestive disturbance is the stagnant food pattern. The characteristic signs are a red face; an irritable, swollen abdomen; and irregular stools (often diarrhea alternating with constipation and stools that smell sour or foul).

WEAK ENERGY: SIMPLE OR OVERSTIMULATED

We mention the simple and overstimulated patterns as being distinct, but the same remedy suits both types. As we mentioned in Chapter 2, these two patterns have almost the same symptoms. If you simply made a list of the symptoms, you would find it difficult to distinguish between the two. The distinction is in the behavior. Children with the simple type behave just as you would expect exhausted children to behave. They are limp and droopy and are often whining. In contrast, children of the overstimulated type seem to have an abundance of energy (as is discussed more fully in Chapter 2). The key sign to distinguish this pattern is that there is a mismatch between energy level and the amount of food consumed. Upon reflection, you will notice that they could not possibly be getting all that energy from the tiny amount of food that they eat.

ECHO PATTERN (THICK MUCUS): HOT OR COLD

In the early stages of treatment, it is not always that important to make a distinction between the Hot and Cold types. The behavior and symptoms are often the same. They can be distinguished by small things, such as the color of the face, the color of the lips, or the color of the tongue. Children with the Hot type have at least some red somewhere, whereas those with the Cold type have none at all. The main difference is evident when the herbs start to take effect. As the herbs gradually begin working, children with the Hot type will become increasingly agitated, almost to the point of hyperactivity. Once this happens, it is easy to recognize and to correct. This is discussed later in the section on the results of treatment.

Other Variations

These patterns are the key for guiding which prescription to use. There are also some other variations that may require slight changes, the details of which are given later in this chapter.

NIGHTTIME COUGH

A cough may occur at night if there is an excess of mucus and this starts to settle in the lungs.

WINTER COUGHS

In England it is very common for chronic coughs to develop in the winter. Many parents begin to get concerned at about at the end of October, when the days are becoming shorter and the weather is turning cold.

The underlying pattern is usually internal Cold combined with some weakness. As the weather turns cold and dark, the Cold inside the body comes to the surface and the child gets a cough. The cough recurs in the winter because with each cough, the child's energy is reduced somewhat by the sheer effort of throwing off the cough. The body does not then have enough time to recover its energy before the next cough comes along.

▪ SYMPTOMS AND SIGNS OF THE PATTERNS*

Mucus

- Croaky, rattly cough
- Thick nasal discharge
- Gray face
- Swollen glands (not in all cases)
- Variable appetite (may eat a lot but is choosy about food)

CAUSES

- Incomplete cure of a previous cough
- Aftereffects of a polio immunization
- Excess intake of dairy products (e.g., cow's milk, cow's cheese)
- Excess intake of sugar, peanuts, oranges, or bananas
- Wheat intolerance

With Stagnant Food Pattern (Up to 3 Years Old)

- Croaky, rattly cough
- Thick nasal discharge
- Red cheeks
- Swollen abdomen
- Either regular stools that are green and sour or foul smelling or constipation

EXPLANATION

Many of the symptoms and signs are the same as those of the straightforward mucus pattern. What is different is that much of the mucus is being generated by the faulty digestive system. How this happen is discussed in detail in Chapter 2.

CAUSES

Causes for this pattern can include both those listed previously for the straightforward pattern and those of the stagnant food pattern. The causes for this pattern are discussed at length in Chapter 2. They are as follows:

- Overfeeding
- Irregular feeding
- Unsuitable food

Here we give a brief review of these causes.

Overeating. All parents are happy to see their child eat a lot. There is a deep-seated instinct that relates a large appetite to a state of health—we even call it a *healthy appetite.* Consequently, many mothers encourage their children to continue eating even after they are full. The pattern is more common after children have been weaned, but it can even occur in breast-fed children if the mother has a copious supply of milk or if the milk is too rich.

Irregular Feeding. The digestive system works best if food is eaten at regular times, and the stomach works best if it is allowed time to empty before being refilled. The exact pattern of feeding is not important. Different families and different countries have widely varying feeding patterns. The important thing is that the pattern be regular and that there be no snacks between meals. An easy trap to fall into with small children is to give them something to eat when they are unhappy or tired. This may start off as a one-time treat, but it can easily develop into a habit of snacking all the time and not eating proper meals. This opens the way for the stagnant food pattern.

Unsuitable Food. This means different things at different ages. In babies who are bottle fed, this means that they cannot easily digest the milk that they are receiving. For example, many children have cow's milk intolerance; others cannot easily digest soya milk. In toddlers younger than 3 years unsuitable food can be food that they simply cannot digest, but more often it means that the food is too rich for them (it may be too fatty or too high in protein). It

---

*Facial color reveals a lot about a child's energy. See p. 54 for a discussion of facial colors and variations among racial groups.

may also mean that the range of foods they are eating is too great. Toddlers should eat very simple foods.

Weakness

- Weak and wet cough
- Watery nasal discharge
- Pale face
- Poor appetite or choosy about food
- Lack of stamina
- Frequent nighttime awakenings
- Small for age (or growing rapidly*)
- Dark lines or rings under eyes
- Dribbling from the mouth

EXPLANATION

The cough is weak because the child does not have enough energy to produce a really good cough, even though the mucus is watery. The pale face, poor appetite, and lack of stamina are the result of the child not having much energy. The sleeping pattern is characteristic of having Weak energy (see Chapter 25). The child may be small for age because not enough food is being consumed for growth. The dark lines or rings round the eyes are a sign of deep exhaustion. Dribbling from the mouth is a sign that the digestive system is not working because there is too much water in the system.

CAUSES

- Long labor
- Exhaustion of the mother
- Long illness
- Excessive immunizations
- Unstructured nursing and feeding

All of these are exhausting or weaken the energy.

Overstimulated

- Weak and wet cough
- Watery nasal discharge

- Pale face
- Small for age
- Poor appetite or choosy about food
- Many nighttime awakenings
- Dark lines or rings under eyes
- Dribbling from the mouth

The child's behavior, is quite different:

- Restless
- Alternating shy and bold
- Coy
- May show signs of extreme distress or fear toward practitioners
- Willful
- Likes to be the center of attention

EXPLANATION

The symptoms and signs are the same as those for the previous pattern, but the behavior is characteristic of being overstimulated.

CAUSES

The root causes are the same as those that give rise to the Weak pattern discussed previously.

Echo Pattern (Thick Mucus): Cold

This pattern is characterized by mucus that is very hard and "congealed." In the straightforward mucus pattern, the mucus had become rather thick. In this pattern it has further thickened, becoming viscous to the point of being hard. Consequently, there are often no external signs of mucus: There is no nasal discharge nor does the cough sound gurgly. The mucus is simply too thick to flow.

SYMPTOMS

- Hard, hacking cough that is worse when tired
- Swollen glands in the neck and under the jaw
- Tendency to rough skin
- Depigmented patch on face (see Plate 1-4)
- Difficulty in concentrating
- Occasional drops in energy for no reason
- Abdominal aches from time to time

---

*In some cases the child is undersized because the digestive system is not strong enough to absorb enough food. In other cases digestion appears to be weak because so much energy has to go into rapid growth.

CAUSES

- Repeated infection
- Infections treated with antibiotics
- Immunization, especially the pertussis and polio immunizations

In addition, this pattern is often seen at the last stage of treating any chronic cough, whatever the original pattern. These causes have been discussed in detail in Chapter 5.

Echo Pattern (Thick Mucus): Hot

SYMPTOMS

Symptoms are the same as those for the cold echo pattern, but with small differentiating signs.

- Pale face with red lips, red cheeks, or red tongue
- Behavior that is alternately polite and wild
- Dream-disturbed sleep

CAUSES

The causes of this pattern are very similar to those of the cold echo pattern:

- Repeated infection
- Infections treated with antibiotics
- Immunization, especially measles and *Haemophilus influenzae* type B immunizations
- Constitutional Hot energy
- A diet of greasy food or of junk food

Again, this pattern is often seen at the last stage of treating any chronic cough, whatever the original pattern.

▪ TREATMENT

Dosages*

The doses we suggest are *suggestions only.* Each child may need something different. Dosages are given for 3-year-olds (Table 17-2). The tinctures

---

*For more detailed information about dosages, see Chapter 8.

Table 17-2	
AGE	MULTIPLY 3-YEAR-OLD DOSE BY
6-12 months	$\times \frac{1}{3}$
1-2 years	$\times \frac{1}{2}$
2-4 years	$\times 1$
4-7 years	$\times 1\frac{1}{2}$
7-14 years	$\times 2$
14+ years	$\times 3$

are given in about 25 to 50 ml of warm water three times a day. The medicine may be sweetened.

Lots of Mucus

When preparing a prescription for a child with a lot of mucus, you may need to exercise caution. If the lungs are very full of mucus, you must avoid giving any herbs such as golden seal *Hydrastis canadensis* or Oregon grape *Berberis aquifolium,* which may aggravate this condition. If there is any doubt, start by giving a simple, such as hyssop *Hysoppus officinale.* It is wise to stick to this until you are confident that there is no danger if the symptoms could temporarily be aggravated. When this danger is past, the following prescriptions will provide a useful starting point.

MUCUS IN THE LUNGS ONLY

Thyme *Thymus vulgaris*	4 drops tincture
Elecampane *Inula helenium*	4 drops tincture
Angelica *Angelica archangelica*	2 drops tincture
White horehound *Marrubium vulgare*	2 drops tincture
Golden seal *Hydrastis canadensis*	2 drops tincture

Explanation. Thyme and elecampane are both stimulating expectorants that help clear mucus from the lungs. Thyme is also an astringent and helps dry out excess dampness, and angelica is added as a digestive tonic. Angelica is also a warming expectorant. White horehound assists the aforementioned herbs, being both a stimulating expectorant and a digestive tonic. Golden seal does not have a special action on the lungs, but it is a wonder herb for clearing mucus from the entire system. It is also slightly stimulating to the digestive system, which is what these children often need.

VARIATIONS. If the mucus is very watery and the child is a bit miserable and whiny, add the following:

Cleavers *Galium aparine*   2 drops tincture

Cleavers has the effect of eliminating the dampness by promoting the flow of urine.

Results. There should be a gradual improvement. You may be lucky and notice some changes in the first few days, but more often it takes a week or two before any significant change is seen. As the herbs take effect, the amount of mucus is reduced. After 1 or 2 months of treatment, the child may be left with the hard mucus (echo) pattern, in which case the prescription will need to be changed. During this long time, there may be many setbacks. See the following for a further discussion.

MUCUS WITH A DIGESTIVE DISTURBANCE

Elecampane *Inula helenium*	3 drops tincture
Thyme *Thymus vulgaris*	3 drops tincture
White horehound	3 drops tincture
Marrubium vulgare	
Black root *Leptandra virginica*	2 drops tincture
Oregon grape *Berberis aquifolium*	2 drops tincture

Explanation. Elecampane, thyme, and white horehound are stimulating expectorants that help eliminate mucus from the lungs, and they are also gentle digestive tonics. Black root is specific for the stagnant food pattern, and Oregon grape helps clear mucus from the digestive system. It is also a digestive tonic.

VARIATIONS. If the child is constipated, add the following:

Butternut *Juglans cinerea*	2 drops tincture
Cascara *Rhamnus purshiana*	2 drops tincture

Results. In the "pure pattern," when you see a "textbook" case of the stagnant food pattern, the results are very good but somewhat unpredictable. In some children there is a gradual evacuation of the stagnant food, but in others sudden and violent diarrhea ensues as the accumulated food is cleared out. Whatever happens, most of the digestive component should be cleared out within 2 weeks. If the pattern remains after this time, the cause of the problem may not have been corrected. The parents may not have understood your advice about diet, they may have been unable to put it into practice, or there may be some other component of the diet that has not been considered.

During the time that the stools are moving with exceptional vigor, it is common for the cough to get considerably worse as the mucus is expelled from the entire body. It is also common for the child to have some sleepless nights at this time. Parents should be well advised to prepare for this. Practitioners must warn their patients; otherwise, parents may lose trust in them, thinking that the practitioner made their child worse.

Once digestion has been regulated, the cough is usually greatly reduced. In most cases it disappears altogether. In a minority of cases there is still some cough, in which case you need to look for one of the other patterns.

Advice. The most important advice to give to parents of these children is to ensure that their child eats regular meals, suitable food, and not too much food. One of our colleagues summed this up as "a diet of bread and water, with not too much bread." This is of course a rather extreme and pessimistic point of view, but the importance of very simple food and not too much cannot be overemphasized.

Weak Energy

White horehound	4 drops tincture
Marrubium vulgare	
Mullein *Verbascum thapsus*	4 drops tincture
Fennel *Foeniculum vulgare*	2 drops tincture
Licorice *Glycyrrhiza glabra*	2 drops tincture

Explanation. White horehound is an all-purpose herb for the lung and is both a tonic and an expectorant. It contains bitter principles, which make a bit unpleasant to take but are of great help to the digestive system. Mullein is another wonder herb for the lung, and it complements white horehound. Fennel helps the digestive system, and licorice, besides helping the digestive system and the lungs, is an all-purpose tonic.

This prescription is useful for both types, the main difference being that overactive children will find it much easier to wriggle out of taking the herbs.

Results. When children are persuaded to take these herbs, you will see a gradual improvement. After about 2 or 3 weeks, their color should improve, as should their energy. At this stage the cough may still be present; it may even start to get worse as they start to expectorate more. You may then need to change the prescription to include herbs such as elecampane *Inula helenium*, which will help clear the lungs. It may be very difficult to get children to take the herbs; after all, their appetite is poor at the best of times. In these cases you may have to resort to using herbs that have a more pleasant taste, and this may take some time in experimentation. The other alternatives are to put the herbs in bath water (as is discussed in Chapter 8) or to use essential oils, applied externally or used in massage oil (see later discussion).

The herbs should be continued until the appetite improves (usually a few months); otherwise, there is a real danger that the condition will return. In the later stages you may need to reduce the quantity of herbs that work on the lungs and increase the quantity of herbs that strengthen the digestive system. Thus in the later stages, a prescription such as follows may be useful:

White horehound *Marrubium vulgare*	3 drops tincture
Elecampane *Inula helenium*	3 drops tincture
Aniseed *Pimpinella anisum*	4 drops tincture

You may even be able to persuade the child to take the following:

Gentian *Gentiana lutea*	3 drops tincture
or	
Wormwood *Artemisia absinthium*	3 drops tincture

Both of these are powerful digestive tonics, but they are bitter.

During this long time, there may be many setbacks. This is discussed more later in this chapter.

Echo Pattern (Thick Mucus)

The aim of treatment is to soften the thick mucus or, to put it another way, to clear out the lymphatic system. A suitable prescription is as follows:

Poke root *Phytolacca decandra*	2 drops tincture
Blue flag *Iris versicolor*	2 drops tincture
Queen's delight *Stillingia sylvatica*	2 drops tincture
Hyssop *Hysoppus officinale*	2 drops tincture
Elecampane *Inula helenium*	2 drops tincture
Golden seal *Hydrastis canadensis*	2 drops tincture

The first three, poke root, blue flag, and queen's delight, soften the mucus, and given on their own, these herbs result in the lungs being filled with the mucus and may even upset the digestive system. The child may get a really bad cough and possibly diarrhea. Therefore you need to add herbs for the lungs and to resolve mucus. Both hyssop and elecampane clear mucus from the lungs. Elecampane and golden seal (or Oregon grape *Berberis aquifolium*, which is a possible alternative to golden seal) resolve mucus.

VARIATIONS: HOT OR COLD

If the child is noticeably a Cold type, with white face, and so forth (as outlined in Chapter 1), add the following:

Ginger *Zingiber officinalis*	4 drops tincture

If the child is noticeably a Hot type, then replace hyssop with Mullein *Verbascum thapsus*. It may also be necessary to add lobelia *Lobelia inflata* to calm the child.

OTHER VARIATIONS

If the cough is very harsh and dry, you may not need to use either elecampane or golden seal. You may prefer to add the following instead (a general relaxant):

Lobelia *Lobelia inflata*	4 drops tincture

To relieve an irritating cough, add the following:

Gum weed *Grindelia camporum*	4 drops tincture

If the child has loose stools, this is probably because there is mucus in the stools. If this is a reaction to the herbs, it is a beneficial evacuation, but if the stools were loose beforehand or if the child has loose stool for a long time, it may be appropriate to replace golden seal with the following:

Agrimony *Agrimonia eupatoria*	2 drops tincture

Agrimony is a tonic for the digestive system and helps reduce mucus and loose stools.

Results. The results here are somewhat unpredictable, for it is sometimes difficult to get the proportions of herbs right the first time. In particular, if you give too much of the herbs for softening mucus and clearing the lymphatic system, you run the risk of drowning the child in mucus and leaving the child exhausted. On the other hand, if you do not give enough, relatively little effect will be achieved. A good place to start is with the standard dosage, but it may need to be varied for each individual child. In addition, some children may need rather smaller doses at the beginning of treatment and larger ones toward the end.

The length of treatment is very variable and depends on the thickness of the mucus, the child's energy, and the child's situation in life.

THICKNESS OF THE MUCUS

The thickness of the underlying mucus can be determined by how hard the lymph nodes in the neck are. Another indicator is the stringiness of the child's saliva. If it is very stringy, then all of the body fluids are thick and affected by mucus. Another indicator is the skin. If it is rough and dry, there is very thick mucus in the system.

CHILD'S ENERGY

If the child is bubbling over with energy, then there is a lot to spare for healing the body. If, on the other hand, the child is still somewhat weak or has a weak constitution (with rather thin bones and is perhaps a little small for age), then there is much less energy available to make changes in the body and the cure will take much longer.

SITUATION IN LIFE

Some children are very happy in their life; others are less so. The reasons for unhappiness are many and varied. The child may have a difficult family situation, sibling rivalry, stressed parents without enough time, or difficulties at school. Whatever the reason, if the child is unhappy, his or her condition is harder to cure because there is less enthusiasm for life.

Taking all these factors into account, the length of time for a cure can be predicted with some accuracy. The shortest time that a cure is likely to take is approximately 6 weeks. At the other extreme, it can take 1 year or more of treatment before the child is well. A cure may not even be possible until the next major transition in life.

■ SIGNS AND INDICATORS ON THE WAY IN CURING AN ECHO PATTERN

Giving herbs for many months in a row demands energy and commitment on the part of the parents. If you are practitioner, you will need to be able to reassure the parents and give them some idea of how things are progressing. If you are a parent, you will need to have something to look for to know that the herbs are working. There are some obvious indicators that parents can observe for but that are easily overlooked, such as energy level, spirit, skin, behavior, and resistance to disease.

Energy Level

The child's energy gradually increases. The child needs less sleep, gets up earlier in the morning, and goes to bed later at night. The child does not get as exhausted as before. The inexplicable drops in energy are less and less frequent.

Spirit

The child is more enthusiastic and complains less. The eyes also have more of a twinkle.

Skin

The skin tone should change. At first, it may get a little worse, but then the rough quality should give way to smooth and supple skin.

Behavior

Often, the child becomes very difficult and obstinate after about a month of taking the herbs. If this happens, it is a very good sign and indicates that the herbs are working (see Chapter 5).

Resistance to Disease

As time goes on, the repeated coughs that the child used to get are fewer and farther between. The child manages to get over the acute attacks more quickly, and toward the end of treatment, the child may not get a cough when other members of the family do.

Other Signs

Signs that a practitioner may notice but that the parents may not include changes in face color and the lymph nodes.

FACE COLOR*

Often, these children look gray or yellow when they are first seen in the clinic. This gray color

---

*Facial color reveals a lot about a child's energy. See p. 54 for a discussion of facial colors and variations among racial groups.

gradually disappears. At first, there is improvement in color in parts of the face, especially the cheeks. As treatment continues, the overall face color improves: If there were bags or dark patches under the eyes, these gradually go; the green/yellow color around the mouth goes; and the pale color in the forehead gradually goes. The pathologic colors are replaced by a glowing color over the entire face.

LYMPH NODES

The lymph nodes change only very slowly. As treatment progresses, the nodes should become smaller (although initially they may become larger). Above all, they should become softer as the hard mucus softens. The hardness of the nodes is an indication of the hardness of the remaining mucus. Sometimes (especially in children who have a weak constitution) it is impossible to clear the swollen nodes completely. In these cases the best you can do is to improve their health, energy, and resistance to disease.

ROLE OF INFECTIONS

During the course of treatment, it is common for a child to catch an infectious cough. (After all, a course of herbs may last 6 months. It would be surprising if a child did not get a cough during this time.) In the early stages of treatment, before the effect of treatments has really built up, these infections are not at all beneficial and may set the treatment back. This is especially the case if the cough is treated with antibiotics. However, in the later stages, an attack of cough from outside can be beneficial, especially if the child gets over the attack unaided or with natural therapies. What seems to happen is that the external pathogen has the effect of mobilizing the immune system. The immune system then recognizes the echo pattern as alien and expels it. The result is that after such an attack, the child may be left with a bad cough as a result of all the phlegm being loosened at once, but the deep, hard phlegm has been softened and is no longer there. The way is then open for a complete cure.

An All-Purpose Prescription

A good all-purpose prescription that is helpful in the early stages of all chronic cough follows:

Coltsfoot *Tussilago farfara*	2 drops tincture
Hyssop *Hyssopus officinale*	2 drops tincture
Elecampane *Inula helenium*	2 drops tincture
Golden seal *Hydrastis canadensis*	2 drops tincture

ADVICE

For all cases of chronic cough, the child has to avoid mucus-producing food. There should be a near-total ban on cow's milk and related products. Peanuts, peanut butter, oranges, and bananas should also be avoided. Regular meals with no snacks between should be encouraged.

Stagnant Food Pattern. Children with the stagnant food pattern should eat less food, regular food, and suitable food (see Chapter 3 for details).

Weak Energy. You may find that Weak children are addicted to milk, cheese, and yogurt. The mother may be desperate to find something that the child will take, and if you remove these foods, the mother may be concerned that the child will simply stop feeding and fade away. In fact, this does not happen. It may take up to 5 days, but after this the child starts to take an interest in other foods.

TIMES TO TREAT

During an Acute Cough. When a child is brought for treatment for a chronic cough, there is a good chance that the child will also have an acute cough. It actually may be the recurrence of the acute cough that has finally driven the parents to seek alternative help. In these cases one must address both the acute cough and the chronic cough at the same time. The difficulty posed here is that when herbs are given for the chronic condition, they may aggravate it. This is the last thing that the child needs during an acute attack, especially at nighttime. One possible solution to this is to give two medicines: one to be taken before 4 PM and one to be taken at bedtime. A good example is to give herbs for the chronic condition during the daytime and to administer the other prescription, which contains essential oils, topically on the chest in the evening. These oils may be used at any time and will reduce the effect of any aggravation. Alternatively, the evening prescription may contain antitussives or even cough suppressants such as wild cherry *Prunus serotina*.

Nighttime Coughs. The most common cause for nighttime coughs is mucus accumulation in the lungs. One way of overcoming this that may work for older children is to prop them up in bed with pillows so that the mucus stays in the bottom of the lungs and does not interfere with breathing.

There are some variations that can be made with herbs. The first is to use antitussives, as just described, to stop the symptom of cough. Another is to give herbs that work on the digestive system before noon and to give herbs that work more on the lungs in the afternoon. The morning prescription would contain golden seal *Hydrastis canadensis*, which would then be omitted from the afternoon prescription. The reason for this is that golden seal clears mucus out of the entire body, but in doing so, it may temporarily increase the amount of mucus in the lungs.

Another way is to put some drops of essential oils, such as eucalyptus *Eucalyptus globulus,* on a pad of cloth and keep it on the child's chest during the night. This will help keep the bronchi open.

Winter Coughs. The best time to treat winter coughs is before winter starts. Start giving herbs at least 3 months before the expected time of the cough, if possible. You can of course treat at any time, but toward the end of summer, the child's energy should be at a maximum because of the summer break. If you treat at this time, there is the possibility of ridding the body of the main imbalance that would cause a cough.

Echo Patterns. Treat echo patterns as soon as they appear. When treating an echo pattern, one sometimes makes great strides at first, having impressive results, but comes to a plateau after some months of the child taking the herbs. The obvious first step is to have a careful look at the prescription and see if it can be changed. In particular, it may be time to concentrate more on improving energy by working on the digestive system.

If that fails, the best thing to do is to wait until the next major transition in the child's life. If the child is 4 years old, this transition is likely to be that of going to school. If the child is 5 years old and already going to school, it may mean waiting until the 7-year transition. If the child is 10 years old, it almost certainly means waiting until the 14-year transition. This means that the best thing to do is to ask the child to come back at about 12 years of age to resume treatment.

▪ ESSENTIAL OILS FOR COUGH

The following prescriptions will be of help. (See Chapter 8 for details of prescribing essential oils.)

Acute Cough with Much Mucus

Thyme oil *Thymus vulgaris*	3 drops tincture
Hyssop oil *Hyssopus officinalis*	3 drops tincture
Eucalyptus oil *Eucalyptus globulus*	3 drops tincture

Add these to 30 ml (1 oz) of carrier oil, such as olive or almond oil.

Tickling, Irritating Coughs

Sandalwood oil *Santalum album*	2 drops tincture
Thyme oil *Thymus vulgaris*	2 drops tincture
Marjoram oil *Origanum majorana*	2 drops tincture
Lavender oil *Lavandula officinalis*	2 drops tincture

Add these to 30 ml (1 oz) of carrier oil, such as olive or almond oil. When the cough is dry and painful, add the following:

Benzoin oil *Styrax benzoin*	2 drops tincture

These oils are very helpful as a chest rub.

18

Asthma

The incidence of asthma in children has increased to epidemic proportions. Asthma in one form or another has always existed, but the sheer scale of the problem is quite new. We believe that this is a refelection of changes in the nature of the disease.

From our point of view, asthma is a very deep disease. It is not a disease like a cold or a cough, which simply involves a mild infection. It is more than just the symptoms of breathlessness and wheezing. It is something that has affected the very core of a person's being. This means that for treatment to be effective, deep changes need to take place, and these inevitably take time.

A New Approach

In this chapter we offer a new approach. In orthodox medicine, all that can be offered is symptomatic relief. Orthodox medicine focuses on "managing" asthma rather than curing it. As such, the best that can be offered is to identify an external "cause," such as allergy to dust mites or pollen, and to keep asthmatic children away from such "causes."

We believe this to be a faulty approach. Looking for an external cause of asthma is looking in the wrong place. The cause is to be found inside. It is clearly true that dust mites provoke an asthma attack in some children, as can pollen in others, but this must be considered as the trigger factor, the final act in a long chain of events.

Our approach is to address some of the components of this long chain, to eliminate the factors that predispose a particular child to an attack, and

to strengthen the lungs. We have found this approach to be very effective. The only proviso is that the treatment should be started at a young age. The longer a condition is left untreated, the harder it becomes to cure.

Treating between Attacks

A review of the traditional treatments for asthma prescribed in herbal practice, ranging from the seventeenth century to present day, reveals that nearly all of the herbs suggested are those that relieve an acute asthma attack. In very few books is anything prescribed to build up the child's constitution between attacks. We believe that initiating treatment between attacks is of the greatest importance and that an understanding of how to do this opens the way to truly curing asthma. This is especially true when treating children, in whom there is great potential for growth and change. By pointing the child in the right direction with herbs, you give that child the possibility of growing up to be a healthy adult rather than an asthmatic adult.

Different Treatments for Children

The treatments we describe for building up the constitution between attacks are treatments specifically for children. Again, we present something rarely mentioned elsewhere, namely the importance of the digestive system in producing energy. This is a factor for adults too, but for children it is of overriding importance. Adults have reserves of energy that they can mobilize to overcome short-term problems. Children do not have these reserves and depend on a continuous supply of energy. If the digestive system is not functioning well, the energy supply is disrupted and it is easy for the child to become ill.

In this chapter we first explain what we believe must happen for a child to develop asthma. We then discuss the factors in life that encourage this. Once this is understood, the treatment becomes self-explanatory.

◼ WHY ASTHMA HAPPENS: AN ALTERNATIVE VIEW

We mentioned earlier that we consider asthma to be a deep disease and that profound changes must take place for it to appear. We now cover some of the factors that we believe have to change for the disease to take hold.

Underlying Factors

LUNG WEAKNESS

For asthma to develop in a child, something must have happened to weaken the lungs. Asthma does develop in a child with strong lungs. Illnesses may occur, but they appear in other parts of the body. Weakness in the lungs may be hereditary, but the lungs can also be weakened by an external event, such as whooping cough.

This child in Figure 18-1 has hereditary lung weakness, as evidenced by his flat and narrow chest. It is made worse by his posture (droopy shoulders).

ENERGY WEAKNESS

Energy weakness affects children more frequently than adults. For asthma to take hold, something must be interfering with the overall production of energy. If the energy is reasonably good, it is rare for the child to develop asthma, and any lung illness usually stays at the level of chronic cough. This means that not only is the lung weakened but also, in children, the digestive system is weakened.

MUCUS ACCUMULATION

Our experience has been that mucus is always present when a child has asthma. In certain types of

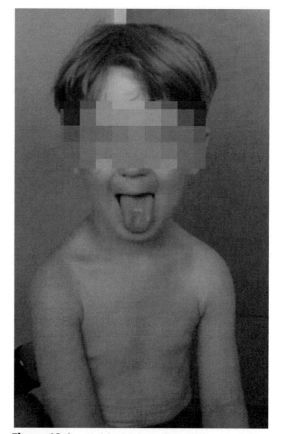

Figure 18-1   Child with hereditary lung weakness.

asthma—those associated with frequent coughing—it is very obvious. In other conditions with very few signs of mucus it is less obvious. In these cases we consider the mucus to come in the category of an echo pattern, whereby the mucus has become so thick that it cannot be coughed up. There are no obvious signs of mucus because it does not move. Its presence becomes clear only during the course of treatment.

IRRITATION OF THE LUNGS

A further factor is irritation of the lining of the lungs. This is very obvious in cases of allergic asthma, in which the lining is so irritated that it needs only the tiniest trigger to cause a major reaction. In all forms of asthma, however, there is some degree of irritation there all the time.

EMOTIONAL TENSION

When children feel free and safe, they are able to relax. When children feel restrained, tension arises and often finds its way to the muscles. Two situations are common. First, some children are very polite and dare not say what they are thinking. The effort of holding back feelings causes physical tension. The other situation is when children are not given clear boundaries. The uncertainty that this creates can also lead to tension.

FEAR

Fear is a major component of asthma. It is one of the things that allows an attack to proceed so quickly. The panic that one feels when suffocating can in itself cause the pectoral muscles to seize up and turn mild wheezing into a life-threatening attack.

Body Imbalances Predisposing Children to Asthma

- Lung weakness
- Energy weakness
- Mucus accumulation
- Irritation of the lungs
- Emotional tension
- Fear

The Trigger

So far we have covered the factors that predispose children to asthma. To precipitate an asthma attack, one more thing—one extra stress—is required to finally tip the balance and cause these children to struggle for air.

Many different factors have been found to be triggers: air pollution, pollen, molds, house mites, and perfumes to name a few. The importance of these is discussed later in this chapter.

Many people believe that the trigger, such as allergy to cat's hair or dust mites, is the single factor causing asthma in children. So much emphasis is put on the external factor that some of our patients have been persuaded to spend large sums of money on expensive equipment to eradicate dust

from their homes. Others have been persuaded to get rid of the family pet. Although these measures are preferable to seeing a child suffering repeated life-threatening attacks, we believe that the actions are founded on a misunderstanding of the true causes of asthma.

Contributing Factors

There is no single cause for asthma. It arises from the sum of many different causes. Each of these factors contributes a small part to the deep changes that need to take place. Some are hereditary and cannot be changed, but many arise directly from the life that the child leads. The next paragraphs outline a few of these factors and show how they contribute to one of the body imbalances predisposing to asthma.

CONTRIBUTORY CAUSES

- Heredity
- Whooping cough
- Frequent lung infections
- Antibiotic and inhaler use
- Immunizations
- Diet
- Lack of exercise
- Poor posture
- Irregular eating patterns
- Lack of sleep
- Excessive television watching
- Suppression of skin diseases
- Sadness
- Air pollution

Heredity. Lung conditions often run in families. Even when there has been no asthma in a family, if you look back a generation or two, you may find family members who suffered from the scourge of their times: tuberculosis of the lungs.

Whooping Cough. If a child has whooping cough very badly, the prolonged coughing (month after month) can weaken the lungs. This is uncommon now, but it used to be common in the past, when living conditions were worse.

Frequent Lung Infections. Frequent lung infections are perhaps the most common route for getting asthma. This may start as young as 3 months of age, with a child getting an infection that he or she never quite gets over. Then one infection leads to another. This is a particularly fast route if the infections are treated with antibiotics, for, as we described in Chapter 4, treating with antibiotics can stop a disease in the middle, without allowing it to go to completion. The child is then likely to develop another illness soon after. If this too is treated with antibiotics, then one illness can rapidly follow another and the child soon becomes asthmatic.

Antibiotic and Inhaler Use. Some children can take antibiotics with no ill effects, but many react badly. The most common reaction is for the child to feel tired and have upset digestion; in addition, mucus commonly appears. The tiredness and the excess mucus both contribute to asthma. Some inhaled medicines, particularly the steroids, tend to damage the lining of the lungs. Therefore, although they may temporarily relieve the symptoms of asthma, they may aggravate the condition in the long run.

Immunizations. Immunizations are often the trigger for starting the cycle of lung infections. As we describe in Chapter 23, it is common for immunizations to give rise to excess mucus in the respiratory tract. This is an ideal breeding ground for bacteria and opens the way for an infection.

Immunizations can also predispose children to asthma by causing a general irritation in the lungs. The mechanism for this is the same as that which gives rise to the echo pattern, described in Chapter 5.

Diet. The factors in diet that are likely to contribute to asthma are the foods and feeding patterns that encourage the formation of excess mucus in the entire system. The most common of these is cow's milk, followed by peanuts and sugar and, for some children, wheat. This is discussed more fully in Chapters 3 and 15.

Lack of Exercise. Another change that has taken place in the last generation is that children get very little exercise. Most no longer walk to school; many no longer even walk to the bus stop but rather are taken everywhere by car. This means that their lungs never get filled with air properly, from one end of the day to the other. The lung is like any other part of the body; if it is not used, it never grows strong.

Poor Posture. Fifty years ago posture was considered very important. One hundred years ago it was considered so important that children might even be strapped to boards for some hours each day to straighten their backs. There has been a natural reaction against these cruel practices, but the reaction has gone to the opposite extreme and posture is now completely ignored—a problem compounded by the design of school desks. A straight back is important for good functioning of the internal organs. In particular, if the upper back is bent over, the lungs will not function well. For example, it is difficult to take a deep breath with a bent back (Figure 18-2).

Irregular Eating Patterns. This is especially a problem for children, in whom proper digestion is so important for health. The digestive system works better if meals are eaten on a fairly regular basis. It is now common for children to eat by themselves, with food taken directly from the freezer and warmed in the microwave, a practice that may lead to the child eating irregular and sporadic meals.

Lack of Sleep. In many families children are allowed to choose their own bedtime. Some believe that if children are tired, they will go to sleep. This is true for many children, but others never seem to feel tired and will find ways of keeping themselves awake. These children can often be recognized by the dark rings under their eyes. If a child does not get enough sleep, the entire system is generally weakened, opening the way for illness.

Excessive Television Watching. Television watching encourages many of the previous factors at the

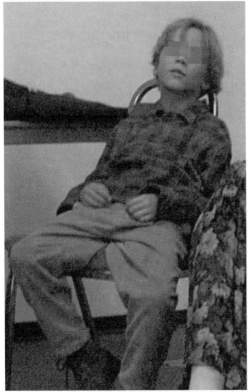

Figure 18-2 An asthmatic child with a combination of low energy and poor posture.

same time. Slouched in front of the screen, the couch potato gets no exercise, has poor posture, and builds up great tension from watching images of violence and death hour after hour. The effects may be compounded by a diet consisting of instant food from the fridge, taken at irregular times to suit intervals in the programs rather than the needs of the body.

Suppression of Skin Diseases. The skin and lungs are very closely related, as has been discussed Chapter 2. It has long been noticed by homeopathic and naturopathic practitioners that suppression of skin diseases such as eczema can encourage lung diseases such as chronic cough—and by extension asthma. In orthodox medicine a common treatment of eczema is suppression with drugs such as hydrocortisone. This can aggravate any tendency to asthma.

Sadness. Generally we do not emphasize the role of emotions in children's problems, but asthma is an exception. The emotion of sadness affects the lungs more than any other organ. This can be seen by the way people get bowed over by grief and by the way people sigh when they are sad. For some children this may be a significant factor, for example, after the death of a grandparent or possibly after the parents divorce. It may take 6 months or 1 year before the suppressed grief affects the functioning of the lungs.

Air Pollution. Air pollution, especially from smoke and chemicals, is a factor in asthma. Pollution obviously damages the lungs. In addition, increases in the levels of pollution tend to provide the trigger for an attack.

SOME COMMON TRIGGERS
As we have said, external factors are less important as causes for the underlying condition of asthma, but once asthma has taken a hold, they are very real factors in precipitating an attack. Some common triggers include the following:

- Increase in levels of pollution
- Allergy to a food
- Allergy to animals, pollen, mold, smoke, or other inhaled substances
- Allergy to dust mites
- Emotional stress
- Cough or cold
- Change in weather
- Change in air temperature (e.g., going from inside to outside)

If a certain substance is known to be a trigger, it makes sense to avoid it. As treatment progresses and the lungs become stronger, the effect of the trigger is reduced.

▪ MANAGEMENT OF AN ATTACK

By the time parents consider herbal treatment for their children's asthma, the children are probably already taking orthodox drugs. Almost certainly they will have secured a steady supply of bron-chodilating inhalers. As far as the parent and child are concerned, they are indispensable. Indeed, for some, they truly are indispensable. However, there will come a time during the course of treatment when they wish to be rid of their inhalers. At this time, it may be possible for the child to replace the orthodox medicines used for acute attacks with herbal medicines.

In this section we outline some treatments that may be effective for treating an acute attack. These can be tried before resorting to orthodox medicine. However, we would like to emphasize that *asthma is a dangerous disease.* We have both known people (not our patients, we are glad to say) who died from throwing away their ortho-dox medicines without having anything suffi-ciently strong to replace them. If a child relies on orthodox drugs during an attack, they should not be abandoned until it is *certain* that the alterna-tives will work.

> If a child relies on orthodox drugs during an attack, they should not be abandoned until it is *certain* that the alternatives will work.

Before it is attempted to treat an acute attack with natural remedies and herbs, some efforts should have been made, between attacks, to strengthen the child. Orthodox drugs may be nec-essary during this time, but their use should gradu-ally be reduced. When noticeable changes for the better are seen in the child, it is time to try an herbal remedy for treatment of an acute attack.

When the first signs of attack appear, try one or more of the cures described here. If it works, then that is excellent and it can be used next time. If it does not work or if it only partially works, one should not hesitate to use the orthodox drugs that have worked in the past.

There are many things that can help avert an asthma attack. The following are a few suggestions:

- Herbs taken by mouth
- Essential oils rubbed into the chest or back

- Special massage techniques
- Shower steam
- Butyeko method
- Blowing up a balloon

Herbs Taken by Mouth

The following prescription can be very helpful in relieving an attack. Do not wait until the attack is fully under way because the herbs do take some minutes to work. The herbs should be given as soon as there are signs that an attack may be forth-coming.

Ephedra *Ephedra sinensis*	4 drops tincture
Lobelia *Lobelia inflata*	2 drops tincture
Hyssop *Hyssopus officinalis*	2 drops tincture
Coltsfoot *Tussilago farfara*	2 drops tincture
Licorice *Glycyrrhiza glabra*	2 drops tincture

The dosages given are for 3 year-olds. Vary the dosage according to Table 18-1. The tincture should be preprepared and may be taken with a small amount of water. If the child is going on an outing or will be somewhere where it will be difficult to take a drink, the tinctures should be diluted to a strength that the child can take directly from the bottle. The herbs may be taken every half-hour for five doses.

Explanation. The Chinese have used ephedra for acute attacks of asthma since antiquity. Since the 1930s it has been used in the West. It stimu-lates the lungs into action, thus drawing on the reserves of the body. It has the disadvantage also seen with albuterol in that it can make the child

Table 18-1	
AGE	**MULTIPLY 3-YEAR-OLD DOSE BY**
6-12 months	$\times \frac{1}{3}$
1-2 years	$\times \frac{1}{2}$
2-4 years	$\times 1$
4-7 years	$\times 1\frac{1}{2}$
7-14 years	$\times 2$
14+ years	$\times 3$

hyperactive. In contrast, lobelia is a powerful relaxant and works especially on spasmodic conditions of the lungs, so it helps counteract the stimulating effect of ephedra. Hyssop and coltsfoot are herbs that improve lung function and promote expectoration. Licorice is a general tonic and harmonizer and is also a mild expectorant. There are of course many other herbs that can be of use, but the preceding prescription provides a starting point.

VARIATIONS
If exercise provokes a catarrhal cough, add the following:

Horehound *Marrubium vulgare*	2 drops of tincture

Horehound has the specific effect of clearing out mucous plugs from the bronchi.

If the attack comes with a viral infection, add the following:

Echinacea *Echinacea angustifolia*	2 drops of tincture

In addition, see Chapter 19.

For an attack accompanied by an acute cough, add the following:

Wild cherry bark *Prunus serotina*	3 drops of tincture

For an attack with feverish bronchitis, add the following:

Marshmallow *Althea officinalis*	4 drops of tincture
Bloodroot *Sanguinaria canadensis*	2 drops of tincture

Marshmallow is soothing to the lungs and reduces inflammation. Bloodroot will help relax a harsh barking cough.

If the child is very weak, add the following:

Gingko *Gingko biloba*	4 drops of tincture

Gingko is a great tonic for the lungs and is particularly indicated for children who are gasping for breath.

If the child is very anxious, add the following:

Passion flower *Passiflora incarnata*	2 drops tincture
Valerian *Valeriana officinalis*	2 drops tincture

If the chest is very tight and goes into spasm, add the following:

Gum weed *Grindelia camporum*	3 drops tincture

ALTERNATIVES
If it is any difficult to obtain some of the herbs mentioned here, the following herbs may be useful.

- Sundew *Drosera rotundifolia* is specific for harsh, tight coughs of nervous origin.
- Pill-bearing spurge *Euphorbia pilulifera*, also known as *Queensland asthma-weed*, is a tonic for the lungs and can also reduce inflammation. It is therefore useful in asthma brought on by infection.
- Gum weed *Grindelia camporum* is a relaxant. This is particularly useful when the chest is very tight and there is no mucus. If a lot of mucus is present, this herb should be used with caution because it may loosen the mucus, thereby temporarily increasing the amount of mucus present.

Essential Oils Rubbed into the Chest or Back

Essential oils are particularly useful in the treatment of asthma. They have the immediate effect of relaxing the child. They also have a very powerful effect in opening the airways. The following oils are often useful:

Cypress *Cupressus sempervirens*	
Marjoram *Origanum marjorana*	See following text
Frankincense *Boswellia carteri*	for dosage
Lavender *Lavandula officinalis*	

Put 2 to 3 drops of each oil in a 25-ml (1-oz) bottle of almond oil or olive oil. Put $\frac{1}{2}$ to 1 tsp of the oil on the child's chest and gently rub it in. The treatment can be repeated every hour or so. If the oils are preprepared, the massage can be done straight away.

VARIATION

If exercise provokes a catarrhal cough, add the following:

Eucalyptus *Eucalyptus globulus*	Add 2 to 3 drops of essential oil to the mixture

If an attack is precipitated by a viral infection, add the following:

Ti-tree *Melaleuca alternifolia* or eucalyptus *Eucalyptus globulus*	Add 2 to 3 drops of essential oil to the mixture

Special Massage Techniques

In the following paragraphs we describe some special massage techniques developed in China specifically for overcoming asthma attacks. These massages are very effective. The only disadvantage is that the young children may resist the massage, particularly if they have a tendency toward hyperactivity, in which case the very act of making them do something may provoke a contrary reaction.

Practitioners should teach parents to keep calm and take control, firmly but gently reassuring the child. Parents should help the child relax in any way they know how and in such a manner that vital energy is not dissipated through crying. Asthma attacks commonly occur at night, when one's concentration may be lacking, so it is recommended that parents practice these massages during the day. See Chapter 9 for further details and advice about how to prepare to do a massage.

CHEST

1. Sit the child on your knee, facing you, and hold him or her firmly under the arms.
2. Use your thumbs to massage the chest between the nipples, gently stroking away from the midline toward each nipple.
3. Massage for 3 to 4 minutes.

Indications. Coughs and asthma.

SHOULDER

1. Find the points midway between the backbone and the outer edge of each shoulder.
2. Press down firmly with your index fingers and rotate vigorously. This may be uncomfortable for the child, but it can often relieve the attack.

Indications. Wheezing and struggling for breath.

TIANTU (WINDPIPE)

1. Sit the child upright (if massaging a baby, hold the baby almost vertical and support the head).
2. From behind, massage the hollow at the base of the front of the neck and the top of the chest with your index finger.
3. Vibrate gently 200 times.

Indications. Coughs, wheezing, and asthma.

SHOULDER BLADE

1. Sit the child on your knee, facing away from you, and hold him or her firmly under the arms.
2. With your thumbs, massage the back between the shoulder blades.
3. Stroke firmly, from near the top of the back to between the bases of the shoulder blades.
4. Repeat 50 to 100 times.

When you do this massage, you will notice that the child wants to sit up immediately.

Indications. Coughs, asthma, wheezing, and general weakness.

RESULTS

Time goes very slowly during an acute attack, so keep an eye on the clock. At the beginning of a massage, changes may not be noticed for the first 5 minutes. The massage should be continued for at least 15 minutes. If it is helping, the massage should be continued until the attack is over.

Shower Steam

If a child often has a dry cough and dry lungs, it can be very helpful to moisten the lungs by putting the child in a steamy environment. The easiest way to do this at home is to turn the shower on to very hot so that a lot of steam is produced.

Butyeko Method

The Butyeko method is suitable for children 5 years and older, although we have seen it used with success by a 3-year-old. It is a method developed by the Russian physician Butyeko, who noted that carbon dioxide is needed in the lungs for the absorption of oxygen. When a child (or adult) has an asthma attack, they often hyperventilate, resulting in the poor absorption of oxygen because there is too *much* oxygen in the lungs—not too little; carbon dioxide, on the other hand, is in too short of supply. Butyeko's method involves ways of increasing the amount of carbon dioxide in the lungs through simple methods such as breathing into a paper bag. The method also involves learning to control one's breathing, learning to relax, and learning ways to overcome the panic associated with an attack. Many people have been helped by this method.

Blowing Up a Balloon

Blowing up a balloon 10 times a day every day has been shown to be as effective as bronchodilators for treatment in the long term.*

▪ PATTERNS BETWEEN ATTACKS

The principle of treatment at the time of attack is essentially the same for all the patterns. All of the body's reserves must be mobilized to enable the child to breathe. Between attacks a different approach is called for. The prescription should be based on the child's constitution. What is more, the herbs that children require are often different from those that adults require because of the importance of digestion for children.

Sometimes merely adjusting the digestive system is enough to free up the energy to overcome a long-standing history of asthma. The reason for this is that a good digestion is essential for a good supply of energy. Without that supply of energy, the lungs cannot work well. This is reflected in the patterns that we describe:

- Mucus
- Weak lungs and digestion
- Echo pattern (thick mucus)
- Emotional (older than 7 years)

▪ SYMPTOMS AND SIGNS*

Mucus

The dominant factor in some children's asthma is the mucus that blocks the windpipe and prevents them from breathing. The children are not weaklings, but you get the impression that they are overwhelmed by the quantities of mucus present. There is more than they can possibly cough up. Often, the asthma is made worse by exercise because it shakes up even more mucus into the system.

- Productive cough
- Nasal discharge
- Bubbles from the nose
- Bubble blowing (like chewing gum) with the saliva (not seen in all children)
- Gray face

VARIATION: MUCUS PLUS STAGNANT FOOD PATTERN†

Here you get the same feeling as with the previous pattern. The main difference is that the mucus is coming from stagnant food pattern.

---

*Quoted in Gascoigne S: *Manual of conventional medicine for the alternative practitioner*, Dorking, England, 1993, Jigme Press.

---

*Facial color reveals a lot about a child's energy. See p. 54 for a discussion of facial colors and variations among racial groups.
†For children younger than 3 years.

The symptoms include those for mucus plus the following:

- Swollen abdomen
- Whitish face (instead of gray) with bright red cheeks
- Irregular stools (green, smelly)

Explanation. The cough, nasal discharge, and bubbles from the mouth are all related to the mucus. The face appears gray when the circulation is impaired by mucus. The symptoms for stagnant food pattern are explained in detail in Chapter 2.

Weak Lungs and Digestion

You get a different feeling here. You may think that if the child had only a bit more energy, he or she would start to get better. Often, these children have mucus in their lungs, but they simply lack the energy needed to produce a decent cough.

- White or gray face
- Weak, small, possibly undersized
- Nasal discharge
- Small voice
- Shortness of breath
- Poor appetite or choosy about food
- Frequent infections
- Frequent illnesses and difficulty in recovering

VARIATION: WEAK LUNGS AND DIGESTION WITH NERVOUS ENERGY

This is the pattern described in Chapter 2. There is an additional cause for this pattern: the use of bronchodilators. Bronchodilators are powerful stimulants, and some children become hyperactive for some hours after taking them.

The symptoms are the same as those listed for weak lungs and digestion, with the following exceptions:

- The child apparently has a lot of energy.
- The child likes to be the center of attention.
- The child is always pushing the boundaries.
- The parents are often exhausted.

VARIATION: DEEP EXHAUSTION*

If asthma has been present for a long time and the child does not get enough sleep, he or she may become deeply exhausted. In this case you will see the following additional symptoms:

- Face white like a ghost
- Black circles around the eyes
- On palpation, weak back and concave lumbar region

Explanation. The reason for most of these symptoms is described in Chapter 2. The dark circles around the eyes and a weak back are characteristic signs of deep exhaustion. The extremely pale or white face is a sign of great lung weakness.

Echo Pattern (Thick Mucus)

The echo pattern with thick mucus is perhaps the most common pattern of asthma. The child is not especially weak and tired and is not especially full of mucus. Some children do not appear to have any mucus at all. As explained earlier, the mucus has become congealed. This pattern often appears in the second stage of treatment, after most of the mucus has been cleared from the lungs and when the child's energy has been strengthened.

- Gray face
- Slightly glazed eyes
- History of repeated attacks, usually treated with antibiotics
- History of immunizations
- Swollen lymph glands
- Worsening of asthma in cold, damp weather
- Allergies to molds and penicillin (can precipitate attacks)
- Occasional abdominal aches with no obvious cause

VARIATION: ECHO PATTERN WITH HEAT
- White forehead and red cheeks or lips
- Tendency to fevers

---

*For children older than 7 years.

- Worsening of asthma in hot weather
- Allergy to animals

Explanation. All of these symptoms are characteristic of an echo pattern, as explained in Chapter 5.

Allergic Asthma

Allergic asthma falls under the heading of the thick mucus pattern. One can make a distinction between a child who is allergic to something taken by mouth, such as peanut butter or artificial flavorings, and a child who is allergic to something touched or inhaled, such as animal fur. Such a distinction is somewhat arbitrary, for in our opinion the pattern is almost the same. It is the allergic reaction that is important, not the route by which the allergen enters the body. When it comes to treatment, both the lungs and the digestive system need to be treated.

When one is trying to make a diagnosis, the substance to which the child is allergic can sometimes provide useful information. In general, those allergic to pollens have a more inflammatory and Hot condition, whereas those allergic to molds and damp things tend to have a Colder and wetter disposition.

Extra Pattern for Children Older Than 7 Years: Emotional Tension

With any illness or disease, there is always an emotional component. Even with something as common as influenza or a cold, there is at the very least a change in the emotional state of a person. This is true of asthma as well. What distinguishes the emotional pattern from the other patterns is that any strong emotion can provide the trigger for an attack. For example, a child may get an attack when faced with a particularly unpleasant situation, such as having lessons with an overbearing teacher.

EMOTIONAL TENSION
- Attacks are brought on by or aggravated by external stress or high emotion.
- Often, there is stress between parents or in the family environment.

- The child may look frightened when he or she first sees you.
- Attacks coincide with changes in the weather or occur during stifling weather.
- Attacks precipitated by rapid changes in temperature, such as when going from a hot room to the cold outdoors.
- The face is usually pale with a greenish tinge.
- The child may be especially green around the mouth.
- The lips may be red.
- Often, there are dark pools around the eyes.

Explanation. Many of the signs are simply those of emotional tension. There are one or two interesting ones. Attacks brought on by changes in the weather and from going out into the cold occur because the body has lost its ability to adapt. The tension is a sort of "holding on," and this interferes with adaptability on the physical level and the emotional level. A green appearance around the mouth is often seen in this pattern; the red lips are caused by an underlying echo pattern.

■ TREATMENT

Dosages*

The dosages we give are for children aged 3 years (Table 18-2). The dosages we suggest are *suggestions only*. Each child may need something different.

Table 18-2	
AGE	**MULTIPLY 3-YEAR-OLD DOSE BY**
6-12 months	$\times \frac{1}{3}$
1-2 years	$\times \frac{1}{2}$
2-4 years	$\times 1$
4-7 years	$\times 1\frac{1}{2}$
7-14 years	$\times 2$
14+ years	$\times 3$

*For more detailed information about dosages, see Chapter 8.

Mucus

In both of the mucus patterns, it may be necessary to start with expectorants only. The reason for this is that if herbs such as golden seal *Hydrastis canadensis* are given to start with, they can often aggravate the situation. If the bronchi are already filled with mucus, this aggravation can lead to an asthma attack. For the first week or two, it is wise to give simples such as coltsfoot *Tussilago farfara* or horehound *Marrubium vulgare*. After this, one may proceed to herbs that have a deeper effect on clearing the mucus from the system.

For the first 2 weeks, try the following:

Coltsfoot *Tussilago farfara*	4 drops tincture
Thyme *Thymus vulgaris*	3 drops tincture

For the next 2 weeks, try the following:

Coltsfoot *Tussilago farfara*	4 drops tincture
Thyme *Thymus vulgaris*	3 drops tincture
Elecampane *Inula helenium*	2 drops tincture

A good all-purpose prescription to use after this follows:

Coltsfoot *Tussilago farfara*	4 drops tincture
Horehound *Marrubium vulgare*	4 drops tincture
Elecampane *Inula helenium*	2 drops tincture
Golden seal *Hydrastis canadensis*	2 drops tincture

If coltsfoot or horehound is unavailable, then hyssop *Hyssopus officinalis* may be substituted. If golden seal is unavailable, Oregon grape *Berberis aquifolium* may be substituted.

Note: An herb that can always be used for all cases of asthma is wild cherry bark Prunus serotina prepared as a syrup. This is normally used as a cough medicine, but it is very safe to use in the treatment of asthma and has the great advantage of having a pleasant taste. All of the tinctures listed may be added to the syrup.

Explanation. Coltsfoot and horehound are both expectorants and are tonics for the lungs. Horehound has the added advantage of relaxing the muscles of the chest to loosen up any mucus lodged there. If the effect of the medicine is to produce an abnormal amount of mucus, then horehound may be omitted. Elecampane clears mucus from the lungs and also works on the digestive system. It has a specific action in increasing the secretion of bile, and as such, it helps move digestion and clear excess mucus from the digestive system. Golden seal has little or no effect on the lungs themselves, but it is a tonic and mild stimulant to the digestive system, having the specific action of clearing mucus from the system.

VARIATION: MUCUS PLUS STAGNANT FOOD PATTERN*

Add the following:

Black root *Leptandra virginica*	3 drops tincture

Substitutes. If golden seal or black root is not available, you can start using the prescription without them, but find an appropriate substitute as soon as possible. For example, in some children the combination of yellow dock *Rumex crispus* with butternut *Juglans* cinerea will serve the purpose.

Dosages. These dosages are suggestions to start with. They may be reduced if the child has too strong of a reaction. Commonly, they can be doubled after a few weeks and in some cases doubled again after another few weeks.

Results. Some slight aggravation (e.g., the child coughing a little more) for the first week or two is common. During this time, it is unusual for any worse asthma attacks to develop.

After the first 2 weeks, if the aggravation is still there, reduce the amount of golden seal. On the other hand, if the aggravation has been reduced, it is time to increase the amount of herbs taken. This may be further increased after another 2 weeks.

---

*For children younger than 3 years.

Treatment is normally needed for several months. At the end of this time, if the child still has asthma, it is time to change the prescription. Often, a change to a prescription for the echo pattern (provided later in this chapter) is helpful, for by this time most of the mucus has been cleared from the lungs and the lungs are stronger. Herbs are then needed to treat the very thick tenacious mucus that remains.

If the stagnant food pattern is present, there may be spectacular evacuation of vile-smelling stools for the first week or so. If this is too dramatic, advise the mother to stop giving the child the herbs until it has settled down. The herbs may be resumed again in a smaller dose when digestion has settled down.

Weak Digestion and Lungs

The same all-purpose prescription may be used as a base, but the emphasis of treatment here is different. The main herbs are those that strengthen both the digestive system and the lungs. A suitable prescription to start with follows:

Coltsfoot *Tussilago farfara*	4 drops tincture
Angelica root *Angelica archangelica*	4 drops tincture
Licorice *Glycyrrhiza glabra*	3 drops tincture
Fennel *Foeniculum vulgare*	3 drops tincture
Golden seal *Hydrastis canadensis*	2 drops tincture

If the child shows signs of coldness, with a white face and cramping, then one may add the following:

Ginger *Zingiber officinalis*	3 drops tincture

If the child is mildly constipated, add the following:

Barberry *Berberis vulgaris*	3 drops tincture

If the constipation is more severe, add the following:

Buckthorn *Rhamnus cathartica*	2 drops tincture

If the child has diarrhea, add the following:

Agrimony *Agrimonia eupatoria*	2 to 3 drops tincture

Explanation. The herbs first in the list benefit the lungs most of all, and those later in the list benefit the digestive system more. Coltsfoot is a great tonic for the lungs. Angelica is more of a tonic for the digestive system, but it is also of great benefit to the lungs. Licorice is an overall tonic. Fennel is a gently soothing and warming tonic for the digestive system. Golden seal is a tonic-stimulant and has the special effect of clearing mucus from the system. Ginger is a warming tonic for the stomach. Barberry and buckthorn are laxatives, and agrimony is an astringent.

Results. Small changes are noticed at first, either in the mood or physical symptoms. For example, if the mood changes first, you will notice that the child has a more positive approach to life. If the symptoms change first, one commonly finds the child coughing up some mucus with a little more vigor than before. Gradually the lungs clear, the face starts to get some pink color, and the appetite starts to improve.

All this takes time—several months at the least—and at times one is not sure whether the herbs are working any longer. It can be helpful to increase the dosage of herbs gradually, week by week, carefully noting any reactions. The dosages may be increased up to five times our baseline recommendation.

Again, after 3 or 4 months, it may be time to change the prescription. At this stage, one may need the herbs for clearing mucus, or one may need the herbs for the echo pattern.

VARIATION: WEAK LUNGS AND DIGESTION WITH NERVOUS ENERGY

The basic prescription given earlier is suitable for this variation too. In principle the prescription should include an herb that helps calm these children down. One might expect passion flower *Passiflora incarnata*, lemon balm *Melissa officinalis*, or St. John's wort *Hypericum perfoliatum* to calm these children, but these herbs do not always seem to work or the children refuse to take them. One possibility that helps from time to time is to use massage with essential oils. Adding ginger to the massage oil and massaging both the abdomen and the soles of the feet can be a helpful addition.

Results. It is not unusual for these children to become very sad and burst into tears during the treatment because part of the reason for their slightly manic behavior is that they are trying to escape from some deep sadness. When they slow down, this sadness comes to the surface. If this should happen during the course of treatment or during the massage, it is an encouraging sign. The child will not like the experience, but if the sadness can be brought out, the benefits will be long lasting. There may be some temptation to try to talk about the sadness, but in our experience all that is necessary is for the child just to release it.

VARIATION: DEEP EXHAUSTION*
Add the following to the basic prescription:

Schizandra *Schizandra sinensis*	3 drops tincture
Siberian ginseng	3 drops tincture
Eleutherococcus quinquefolium	

Note: These dosages are standardized dosages for 3-year-olds and need to be increased according to the scale in Table 18-2 according to age.

Explanation. These two herbs are strong and deep tonics to the system and can be added to the prescription. Schizandra is not stimulating but rather is a tonic. Siberian ginseng *(Eleutherococcus)* is less stimulating than Chinese ginseng *(Panax).*

Results. The results vary widely. Part of the problem is that these children are deeply exhausted, but they are also slightly hyperactive as a result of the inhalers. If you give them tonics, the energy they receive will be spent in doing more and staying up

For children older than 7 years.

later, and there may not be much change to the health. For the herbs to be successful in restoring health, the child must reduce the amount of activity and increase the amount of rest.

Echo Pattern (Thick mucus)
TREATMENT
The extra herbs to be included are herbs for softening thick mucus. Traditionally, these are the same as herbs that cleanse the lymphatic system. We favor the following:

- Poke root *Phytolacca decandra*
- Blue flag *Iris versicolor*

Other herbs in the same category include the following:

- Queen's delight *Stillingia sylvatica*
- Cleavers *Galium aparine*
- Figwort *Scrophularia nodosa*

A typical prescription follows:

Coltsfoot *Tussilago farfara*	4 drops tinture
Elecampane *Inula helenium*	4 drops tinture
Poke root *Phytolacca decandra*	3 drops tinture
Blue flag *Iris versicolor*	3 drops tinture

Possibly with the addition of the following:

Golden seal *Hydrastis canadensis*	2 drops tinture

Again, the dosages listed here are for 3-year-olds.

Results. When poke root and iris are included, they have the effect of gradually and slowly softening the mucus. If these herbs are used on their own, it is common to get an increase in mucus in the system and the child starts coughing a lot. The addition of coltsfoot and elecampane helps keep the lungs clear. If there is an increase in coughing, even with the prescription we have given, the relative quantities of poke root and iris should be temporarily reduced.

For a few children, rather than loosening mucus, these herbs tire them out. A common symptom that one may see is a return of bedwetting. If this happens, the new herbs should be reduced or even eliminated altogether and one should return to the prescription for weak digestion and lungs, given earlier.

It takes a long time to clear this pattern. As we described in Chapter 5, it is common for the child to go through emotional changes. A docile child becomes more difficult and obstinate. A difficult and obstinate child may become quite impossible. Provided that the other symptoms and signs show that the child is in fact getting better, this bad behavior should be welcomed. The entire cycle of bad behavior to a more lovely and open child can take 2 to 4 months. The herbs should be taken during the whole of this time, gradually increased over these 2 to 4 months and possibly even after that.

If the child has any allergies, these should start to diminish after about 3 months of treatment. After about 6 months, the allergies may still be there, but they will be much less of a problem.

VARIATION: ECHO PATTERN WITH HEAT

Add the following to the prescription:

Pill-bearing spurge *Euphorbia pilulifera*	2 drops tincture
Black cohosh *Cimicifuga racemosa*	2 drops tincture
Lobelia *Lobelia inflata*	2 drops tincture

Explanation. When the thick phlegm is softened, the heat that was trapped is then released and can make the child very tense, angry, or wild. Pill-bearing spurge is a relaxant for the lungs that also helps take away heat. Black cohosh is a tonic for the nerves and is used in asthma as a relaxant. Lobelia is a general relaxant.

If these herbs are not available, an alternative prescription follows:

Passion flower *Passiflora incarnata*	2 drops tincture
Valerian *Valeriana officinalis*	2 drops tincture
Hyssop *Hyssopus officinalis*	2 drops tincture

Hyssop is a relaxant that has a special effect on the lungs. Passion flower is a general nerve tonic and relaxant, and its use is indicated for children who experience anxiety, fear, and panic. Valerian is a general relaxant.

Results. The results are similar to those seen with the echo pattern without heat. The main differences are that the child may have a series of fevers as the heat is released and that the child's behavior might become very bad.

Emotional Pattern

TREATMENT

There are two aspects to treating the emotional pattern. The first aspect is to relax the child. The child needs to be relaxed to breathe properly and to allow unwanted events to be shrugged off without the child getting too wound up. The second aspect is to strengthen the child. Strength is needed so that the child can stand up for himself or herself when the going gets difficult. The following prescription reflects these two components.

Lobelia *Lobelia inflata*	4 drops tincture
Lemon balm *Melissa officinalis*	4 drops tincture
Angelica root *Angelica archangelica*	2 drops tincture
Coltsfoot *Tussilago farfara*	2 drops tincture
Golden seal *Hydrastis canadensis*	2 drops tincture

Another herb that may be added as an alternative to the relaxing herbs is the following:

Passion flower *Passiflora incarnata*	2 drops tincture

This prescription is especially indicated when there is great tightness in the chest. This starting dosage is for 3-year-olds. Vary the proportions of the two parts according to whether the child needs more strengthening or more relaxing.

Explanation. Lobelia *Lobelia inflata*, lemon balm *Melissa officinalis*, and passion flower *Passiflora incarnata* are relaxing herbs. Angelica root *Angelica archangelica*, coltsfoot *Tussilago farfara*, and golden seal *Hydrastis canadensis* are strengthening herbs.

Results. Results for this pattern are sometimes disappointing for children younger than 5 years because these young children are emotional sponges, absorbing the emotions in their environment. The tension causing the symptoms is not their own tension but a reflection of tension in those around them. For example, if a child's parents are in the process of getting separated, it is likely that there will be a lot of tension in the house, and it is easy for a child to pick this tension up. Merely giving the child herbs is not going to relieve the underlying tension. However, it is worth giving the herbs, for by treating in this way, the child's health does not deteriorate. When circumstances later change, the cure is much more rapid.

In children older than 7 years, the position is more favorable, for these children are a little more independent. It is still more favorable if an outside stress can be identified and the child can be encouraged to overcome it in some way. For example, if the child has difficulty getting along with a teacher, it is often helpful for him or her to hear that you, as a practitioner (or parent), also had great difficulty with a teacher at one time in your life.

▪ ADVICE

Much of the advice has already been covered implicitly. This is to remove the major causes of asthma. Some of this, involving major changes in lifestyle, can be done only gradually. The easiest place to start is often dietary, and above all we advise the following:

- Avoid cow's milk and cow's milk products.
- Avoid peanuts and peanut butter.
- Reduce intake of bananas and oranges.

▪ HOW PATTERNS CHANGE

During the course of treatment, the pattern can change; in fact, it probably will. For example, as you treat the Weak child he or she becomes stronger and the pattern may evolve into the mucus pattern. As the mucus clears, there is still thick mucus left behind and you will need to treat the echo pattern. If you use too many dispersing herbs when treating the echo pattern, you will find that a lot of mucus is produced and you will need to change the prescription accordingly.

▪ ORTHODOX MEDICINES
The Value of Orthodox Medicines

The strong point of orthodox medicine is in dealing with life-threatening emergencies, which require fast-acting medicines. Nowhere is this more true than in the treatment of asthma. Inhaled bronchodilators have an almost immediate effect in opening the airways and allowing a child to breathe. There are herbal-based remedies that have an almost equally quick effect (e.g., an inhaler made from oil of mugwort *Artemisia vulgaris* or the smoke from cigarettes of coltsfoot *Tussilago farfara*), but they have disadvantages when compared with orthodox inhalers. A mugwort inhaler is difficult to obtain and has the disadvantage that for a few seconds it causes a suffocating feeling before being effective in opening the airways. As for coltsfoot, for most people, the sight of a 5-year-old smoking a cigarette is socially unacceptable, even though coltsfoot smoke is beneficial, whereas tobacco smoke obviously is not. For this reason, with some reluctance, we normally advise children to continue taking their inhalers when herbal treatment starts. In particular, unless you are positive that alternative medicines will be effective, a supply of the orthodox medicine should always be kept available in the event that a child has a life-threatening asthma attack.

However, the effectiveness or orthodox medicines in quickly relieving the symptoms of asthma is completely overshadowed by the absence of anything to cure the long-standing condition. The emphasis on speed means that diseases, which, by their nature, need a long time to cure, cannot be helped. It is here that herbal remedies come to the forefront. Herbs can treat constitutional problems and can correct functional imbalances in a way that orthodox medicine cannot. It is therefore our belief that herbal medicine is vastly superior for treating the underlying condition and in effecting a genuine, long-lasting cure.

The Effect of Orthodox Medicines

Most of the children who come for treatment are already taking a cocktail of medicines. At present, a common combination is an antiinflammatory based on sodium cromoglycate, a bronchodilator, and an inhaled corticosteroid. Each of these medicines has its use, but we believe that the long-term use of all these medicines together can harm the health. In addition, the steroids and bronchodilators are addictive, so in terms of treatment, one has to treat not only the asthma but also the drug dependency. Thus the patients usually have two diseases, not one. This is what makes asthma different from most chronic coughs, and it is one of the factors that makes it more difficult to cure. In the following section we give some advice on how to take the children off the drugs. At this point we confine ourselves to the effect of the drugs.

Sodium cromoglycate (Cromolyn) is an antiinflammatory, originally derived from the plant Kalmia. It is used to reduce the histamine reaction. The long-term effect of this is not really harmful. We have seen children taking this for years, with no ill effects.

Bronchodilators (albuterol, terbutaline sulfate) are powerful stimulants. For some children they work in much the same way as caffeine and make them hyperactive. We even had one patient who enjoyed the "buzz" that he got from taking his bronchodilator inhaler so much that he would take it whenever he wanted a "lift," not just when he could not breathe! The harmful effects of this are indirect in that they stimulate the child to excess activity. The excess activity and lack of sleep that the drug produces can gradually undermine overall health. For some children the drug does not overstimulate them, but even in these children we have noticed that the drug can weaken the vitality of lungs in the long term.

Corticosteroids are given in two ways. They are given in large doses by mouth for 3 or 4 days during an acute attack. On the whole this does not seem to be harmful, provided that the treatment is not repeated too often. The other way is through regular inhalation. It is our experience that this can really damage the lungs. The effect is much the same as the corticosteroids, which are used for external application in eczema. The effect is beneficial in the short term but in the long term actually weakens the lungs, making the asthma more and more difficult to cure.

■ DIFFICULTIES IN TREATING ASTHMA

Special Difficulties Facing Parents

There are special problems that arise for practitioners who are also parents treating their own children. These problems arise from the dual role of being both parent and practitioner. Some of the problems we have seen are discussed here.

HABITS

When you have a sick child in the family, especially one with a life-threatening disease, it is inevitable that the affected child will be treated somewhat differently than the other members of the family. How this manifests varies, but it is common for a more lenient approach to be taken in regard to the ill member compared with the siblings. Although no child wants be ill, a child may get used to these "perks" and may find it hard to give them up. We have certainly seen asthma attacks produced seemingly at will when a child is asked to do something he or she does not want to do. As a parent you may find tantrums and arguments as some habits are changed. This requires great strength of mind.

REBELLION

As explained in Chapter 5, a child's behavior can become difficult during the cure of an echo pattern. Here it is common for a child almost to rebel against the parents. To begin with, the parents find it refreshing to see their child have enough energy to rebel, but soon the rebellion is in real earnest and the parents wish that they had not started treatment. If the parent is the primary practitioner as well, it is difficult to be dispassionate about the unacceptable behavior of their child. This is not to say that it is impossible. Forewarned is forearmed, but if you can get some help, the chance of success is increased.

AGGRAVATION OF SYMPTOMS

Asthma takes time to cure, and on the road to recovery the changes that need to take place can involve aggravations of the symptoms. For example, a cough may get very bad as mucus is released. We have talked about how a child relies on his or her parents more than normal when ill. To be both practitioner and parent in such a chronic and long drawn-out disease can be very draining. Typical feelings are that the herbs are not actually working and may be making the child worse, even if it is only in the short term. Support from outside at this time is very helpful.

BAD BEHAVIOR

Another problem is that as mucus and toxins are cleared from the body, the child often starts to behave very badly. As the parent, you will bear the brunt of this, and it can be very exhausting! We have met many parents who have given up at this point. If only they had had the strength to continue for a few more weeks, the child could have been completely cured. Having help at this time can mean the difference between success and failure.

These difficulties also concern the practitioner. A parent who had an amiable docile child who has turned into an argumentative monster will ask the practitioner some very searching questions.

Caution

If a child's behavior becomes intolerable, it may be because the wrong herbs are being given. This can be determined on the basis of other symptoms and signs. If the right herbs are being given, you will notice all sorts of little improvements—in digestion, appetite, facial color, and brightness of the eyes. If the herbs are wrong, then all these little things will be worse.

SETBACKS

Perhaps the most common time for parents to give up treatment prematurely is when there is a setback. When parents seek treatment from an alternative practitioner, they pin great hopes on the success of treatment. They often expect the medicine to work in the same instant way that orthodox medicine does, and if there is a setback after 1 or 2 months, they can become disheartened. A common pattern is for the parents to seek alternative treatment at the end of autumn. They notice some immediate positive results, but then after a month or two, an epidemic goes around their child's school and the child becomes ill again. After 1 or 2 months, the herbs have not had time to complete their work. The depression that the parents feel in going through yet another round of hospital visits is often enough to make them lose heart.

When this happens, it is up to the practitioner to point out how things have changed. Comparison should be made with previous attacks and with other children at the same school. Normally, it is found that the attack is less severe or lasts a shorter time. There will be other little signs that the herbs are working. It has to be emphasized again and again that time is needed to cure such a deep disease.

Coming off Medication

As we mentioned earlier, the child who is taking a cocktail of medications has two diseases: asthma and drug addiction. There are very real problems in discontinuing drugs altogether—not least is the change in family dynamics. If there is one child who is sick in the family, there are often certain advantages to the child in staying sick. The sick child may get preferential treatment and may be able to avoid unpleasant chores. All this has to change if the child is completely cured. Each child presents different problems, and all we can do here is to give some guidelines of where to start.

Often, the parents are very keen to reduce drugs and will press for an early reduction. This we discourage. We believe that at least 2 months of treatment should pass before orthodox drugs are reduced. One should be sure that the herbs are doing what they are supposed to do, and there should be some definite signs that changes are taking place (e.g., better sleep, better appetite, and above all else, some signs that the lungs are working better, such as easier breathing). When you are sure of this, you may do the following:

Start by reducing the oral corticosteroids. These are damaging to the whole system. They should not be stopped suddenly, and this should be done only under medical supervision. If oral corticosteroids are reduced too suddenly, there is a danger of complete collapse. Fortunately, they are not commonly given now since the advent of inhaled steroids.

Next reduce the inhaled corticosteroids. These are the most damaging to the lungs. These should also be reduced slowly and under medical supervision.

Next reduce the bronchodilators. These too are harmful, but mainly by being a great stimulant to the system. It is not normally dangerous to stop them suddenly as it is with oral steroids, but nevertheless, you can notice a marked drop in energy.

Last reduce the antiinflammatory drugs.

All these drugs should be reduced *slowly*, step by step. Reduce the dosage by a small amount, maintain that dosage for a week or two (until the child has become accustomed to the lower level of drugs), and then reduce again.

The Placebo Effect of an Inhaler

The placebo effect of an inhaler has been estimated to occur 50% to 60% of the time*; that is,

*Weiss RF: *Herbal medicine*, Gothenburg, Sweden, and Beaconsfield, UK, 1988, Beaconsfield Publishers (English translation of *Lehrbuch der Phytotherapie*, 1985).

even if there is no active principle in an inhaler, the very act of inhaling something that is believed to be good can have a strong effect in overcoming an attack. This should be born in mind when treating a child. In particular, there is a right time to tell this to the child. If you tell the child too early in the course of treatment, you are taking away a useful prop. It is like taking away the crutch from someone with a broken leg. If you tell the child later on in the treatment, when he or she does not really need the support, it empowers the child to live a normal life without inhalers.

In practice there are some children who are comforted by having an inhaler available. I had one child who went 1 month without using his inhaler, but he carried it around with him. The day that he realized that he had left it at home, he had an asthma attack. When one is treating children such as this, it is helpful to give them an herbal remedy, such as the one listed earlier, to take in the unlikely event of having an attack. For example, one could give an herbal pill of Lobelia *Lobelia inflata*.

Healing Crisis

The great majority of asthmatic children have an echo pattern. There is some illness in the system that has never been completely cured. It is our experience that final cure for many children comes when this echo pattern makes its final appearance. A common way for this to happen used to be called a *healing crisis*. The child gets a very high fever, only this time there is something different about the fever. Despite using many different treatments, such as antibiotics, antivirals, herbs, massage, and other alternative medicines, the fever persists. This causes great alarm to the parents, who feel that all the work of the previous 6 months or year has come to nothing. What often happens is that far from being worse after the long (5 to 7 days), and high fever, the child is much better. Weak, obviously, but it often happens that this is a turning point and that the child never has a severe asthma attack again.

19

Acute Cough

The treatment of acute coughs is a big subject, and one that we can give only an introduction to here. The severity and danger of a cough varies from time to time and from child to child. At one end of the scale, a cough may be a relatively mild single event, where the child coughs through the night, and the main discomfort is that neither the child nor the family gets much sleep. At the other end of the scale, a cough may be the first step in a rapidly descending spiral in which the child will ultimately be hospitalized because of a life-threatening asthma attack. We cannot cover all eventualities, but we hope to give some general principles that will enable the reader to create suitable prescriptions in difficult cases.

In working our way through this subject, we start by considering simple coughs and their potential progression to bronchitis and pneumonia. We then continue by examining what happens when these illnesses are superimposed on chronic cough and asthma (the latter was discussed in the previous chapter).

Finally, we discuss at some length how a cough can actually be of benefit to a child. This is true when the cough is a symptom of expelling the accumulations of mucus and toxins. In such cases the child needs to be supported throughout the process rather than given a quick fix.

Why Do Children Get Coughs?

It used to be thought that all coughs were, like influenza, simply caused by changes in the weather. Today this aspect is almost completely ignored, and all attention is focused on a pathogen such as a virus or bacterium. As explained in Chapter 4, the state of the body is of equal importance as the infecting agent, and it is the interaction of the body, the weather, and the pathogen that gives rise to an infection. Thus the "internal" state of the child has a major influence on whether and when a child gets a cough. For example, children who have a Cold energy and who are habitually cold and pale are more likely to get a Cold type of cough, and they are likely to get it when the weather turns cold in autumn.

The lungs are particularly susceptible to changes in the weather, in a way that other internal organs are not. The reason is easy to see: The lungs are in direct contact with outside air. Any changes in the temperature or humidity have to be compensated for immediately by the lungs if they are to continue functioning effectively. It is for this reason that the main types of cough are related to the four permutations of these meteorologic factors, namely cold, hot, damp, and dry. Cold and damp are often combined, as are hot and dry. These changes can alter the balance in the lungs, resulting in a cough being able to take hold. We now provide descriptions and treatment approaches for these types of coughs.

Damp

Children affected by dampness have a productive cough with watery mucus. Older children cough the mucus up and expectorate; younger children normally swallow it. The connection between watery mucus, water collecting in the lungs, and a damp imbalance is obvious.

CAUSES

The external cause is damp weather. Obviously, this pattern is very common in England. Internally, the cause is usually dietary. Foods such as cow's milk, cow's cheese, and foods containing a lot of sugar all predispose children to dampness. Coughs of this kind may be caused by immunizations, especially the polio immunization, and also the side effects of antibiotics.

Cold

Children affected by the cold have a harsh cough. In extreme cases it is a barking cough. It is often worse at night and can wake the child, and even the whole family. The explanation for the harsh or barking nature is that the mucus in the lungs is "tight," that is, the opposite of watery. When mucus does come up, it is gelatinous. The connection between cold and rather thick mucus is traditionally thought to be related to the cold "freezing" the mucus.

CAUSES

The external cause is exposure to cold or a drop in the temperature. Internally, one finds that affected children have taken antibiotics or eat cold food such as ice creams and food straight from the refrigerator. Immunizations are a significant cause, especially the immunization for whooping cough.

Variation: Damp and Cold Combined

One often sees these two "energies"—of cold and damp—combined. This can give rise to a cough that reflects the worst characteristics of both. In practice, there is a whole spectrum of coughs between a damp cough and a cold one, with pure damp giving rise to a very watery cough; damp and cold together giving rise to a thick phlegmatic, but productive cough; and pure cold giving rise to the harsh and unproductive cough.

Hot

Children affected by hot weather have a nonproductive cough that is often painful from the very start. These children may even complain of a burning sensation in the throat. This is because the throat and windpipe are inflamed from the heat.

CAUSES

The external cause is a spell of hot weather or an overheated building. Internally, dietary factors, such as eating curries or red meat or simply overeating, are a cause. Many immunizations can give rise to a Hot type of cough, especially the measles, mumps, rubella vaccine.

Dry

Children affected by dryness have a nonproductive cough that begins as a tickling sensation and later becomes irritating rather than painful. The main characteristic is that the lungs have become too dry.

CAUSES

The external cause is very dry, dusty weather; exposure to dust; and central heating and air conditioning. The main internal cause is the echo pattern from an immunization or another illness.

Variation: Hot and Dry Combined

There is a whole spectrum of coughs between a hot cough and a dry one, with pure heat giving rise to painful hot cough with fever and pure dry giving rise to an irritating, tickling cough, without much pain.

Variation: Hot and Damp Combined

Children affected by hot and damp conditions have a productive cough and green or sometimes bad-smelling mucus. The external cause of hot, humid weather is rare in England. The internal causes are a combination of factors causing dampness (e.g., dairy products and greasy foods) and factors causing heat (e.g., spicy food, fried food, junk food, immunizations). These types of cough are summarized in Table 19-1.

Table 19-1 Type of Cough and the Related Imbalance

NATURE OF COUGH	CORRESPONDING IMBALANCE
Watery, productive	Damp
Tight	Cold
Hacking, barking, croupy	Very cold; echo pattern
Tickling	Dry
Spasmodic	Hot, dry

▪ OTHER SYMPTOMS AND SIGNS*

Damp (Wet Coughs)

- The face is pale and puffy.
- Watery nasal discharge is common.
- The eyes often water.
- The child may have a dull ache in the forehead.
- The child is rather miserable.
- The child feels tired.

Cold (Croupy Coughs)

- The face is white.
- The child feels chilly and may want to curl up.
- The child is miserable and sometimes seems rather frightened.
- The child may have a low-grade fever.
- The child may have a strong headache.
- At first the throat tickles or itches. Then after a lot of coughing, the throat and chest together may become painful when the child coughs.

Hot (Painful Coughs)

- The face is flushed.
- The throat is sore (even from the beginning the throat is sore and painful).
- The child tends to feel hot and does not want to wear a lot of clothes.

- The child may have a fever, which may start to rise.
- The child may have a mild headache at the top of the head.
- The child is clingy.
- The child is restless and fidgety.

Dry (Tickling, Raspy Coughs)

- The face may be a little flushed, but usually not much (sometimes it is gray).
- The skin may feel very dry.
- A tickling sensation is felt in the throat at first, but then the throat becomes sore.
- The child constantly asks for drinks but is never satisfied.
- Normally, there is no fever at first.

▪ TREATMENT

Dosages*

The doses we suggest are *suggestions only.* Each child may need something different. Dosages are given for 3-year-olds (Table 19-2). The tinctures are given in about 25 to 50 ml of warm water. The medicine may be sweetened as desired.

Frequency

The medicine may be given as frequently as needed for acute coughs. A minimum to be effective is three times a day, with a maximum of every hour (more frequently than this will not make

Table 19-2

AGE	MULTIPLY 3-YEAR-OLD DOSE BY
6-12 months	$\times \frac{1}{3}$
1-2 years	$\times \frac{1}{2}$
2-4 years	$\times 1$
4-7 years	$\times 1\frac{1}{2}$
7-14 years	$\times 2$
14+ years	$\times 3$

*Facial color reveals a lot about a child's energy. See p. 54 for a discussion of facial colors and variations among racial groups.

*For more detailed information about dosages, see Chapter 8.

the child better). If the child hates the medicine, you may find that only the minimum is sufficient. If the cough is very severe, the maximum dosage should be given until improvement is noted.

Cough Suppressants

The normal over-the-counter remedies for cough usually include a cough suppressant such as codeine or even chloroform.* On the whole we discourage the use of these because the ingredients are themselves harmful, and generally it is better to cough mucus out of the lungs than to leave it in the lungs. However, there are times when these are useful. One situation is when the child (or parents) have become desperately tired but cannot sleep because of the cough. In cases such as this, the damaging effect of the cough remedy has to be weighed against the damaging effect of loss of sleep.

Herbal Cough Suppressants

Herbal medicine has its own antitussives:

- Wild cherry *Prunus serotina*
- Wild lettuce *Lactuca virosa*

Wild cherry has long been used to ease and suppress coughs. It is not purely a cough suppressant; it also has some expectorant action in clearing the lungs.† In addition, it has a gentle tonic action on the digestive system, which speeds recovery. It may be used on its own or added to

---

*It is astonishing to us that such chemicals are allowed on sale, but safe ones such as comfrey are banned. Chloroform in quite small doses is known to cause various types of damage to the internal organs, including the liver, whereas comfrey has been shown to cause problems only in animals, and even then only when given in massive doses.

†Opinions are divided regarding the action of wild cherry. Some say it is purely a suppressant. This has not been our experience. It appears to us that it has some expectorant qualities as well.

any of the cough remedies listed later in this chapter, if the need arises to ease the symptoms of cough. It should not be used over an extended time (more than 1 month). Both wild cherry and wild lettuce are best given as a syrup $\frac{1}{2}$ tsp per dose for 3-year-olds.

Treating the Digestive System

Besides giving herbs to treat the lungs and to control the symptoms of coughing, all of our prescriptions contain tonics for the digestive system. This is for various reasons. The child usually has become a little weak before the cough developed—otherwise he or she would not have succumbed in the first place. More important, the digestive system is always affected when there is mucus in the system, and if the digestive system is working better, then excess mucus will be removed from the body more quickly.

Damp (Wet Coughs)

Elecampane *Inula helenium*	4 drops tincture
Thyme *Thymus vulgaris*	3 drops tincture
Angelica *Angelica archangelica*	2 drops tincture
White horehound	2 drops tincture
Marrubium vulgare	
Ginger *Zingiber officinalis*	2 drops tincture

VARIATION: SPASMODIC COUGH

Add the following herbs:

Lobelia *Lobelia inflata*	2 drops tincture
Pill-bearing spurge	2 drops tincture
Euphorbia pilulifera	

VARIATION: FEVER

Add the following herb:

Yarrow *Achillea millefolium*	2 drops tincture

Explanation. Elecampane and thyme are both stimulating expectorants that help eliminate mucus from the lungs. Thyme is also an astringent and helps dry out the excess damp. Angelica is added as a digestive tonic to help the body eliminate excess damp and is also a warming expectorant. White horehound assists the afore-mentioned herbs by being both a stimulating expectorant and a digestive tonic. Ginger is added to provide overall warmth and to circulate the energy of these herbs. It is also a mild expectorant. Lobelia and pill-bearing spurge are both antispasmodics and can be added if the child goes into paroxysms of coughs.

Many of the herbs listed here will help resolve a fever, but yarrow may be added if the fever is a significant part of the child's condition. It is of great benefit in treating all fevers with which the child feels cold and somewhat exhausted.

Results. A short time after these medicines are given initially there may be an increase in the amount of coughing as the lungs are stimulated to expel mucus. Soon after, however, the cough should improve. After an hour or two, the cough may start coming back again, so it is time to take more medicine.

If the child has a fever perspiration should start after taking a few doses, and the fever should then come down. At this stage it is very important to keep the child warm and away from draughts.

Cold (Croupy Coughs)

PRESCRIPTION 1
When the croup is more spasmodic, use the following prescription:

Gum weed *Grindelia camporum*	4 drops tincture
Hyssop *Hyssopus officinalis*	2 drops tincture
Thyme *Thymus vulgaris*	2 drops tincture
Ginger *Zingiber officinalis*	2 drops tincture

Explanation. In this prescription we use relaxing expectorants that help relax the bronchial muscles and facilitate the expulsion of mucus. Gum weed is specific for relaxing the muscles of the chest to ease the spasm associated with this type of cough. Hyssop and thyme are good expectorants to facilitate a productive cough. Thyme in particular is warming. Ginger is warming and improves the

general circulation of the body and the digestive system.

PRESCRIPTION 2
When the croup is more harsh and hard, use the following prescription:

Mullein *Verbascum thapsus*	4 drops tincture
Pill-bearing spurge *Euphorbia pilulifera*	2 drops tincture
Blood root *Sanguinaria canadensis*	2 drops tincture
Cayenne *Capsicum minimum*	2 drops tincture

Explanation. Mullein is both soothing and a tonic to the chest; in addition, it is an excellent all-purpose expectorant. Pill-bearing spurge is an antispasmodic, helps relieve the spasm associated with the cough, and facilitates loosening of and coughing up of the mucus. Blood root is a stimulating expectorant especially for croupy coughs. It has the effect of loosening very hard and tough mucus. Cayenne replaces ginger in this prescription. Although rather hot on the tongue, it is included to stimulate and warm the entire system.

Results. The first sign that the herbs are working may be a slight reduction in the severity of the cough. The key sign, which may take a day or two, is that the cough "breaks"; that is, it becomes less harsh and more productive. The child may still be troubled by the cough, for there will be a large amount of mucus to cough up, but the cough will not have the same barking, spasmodic quality. Once this change has taken place, the cough is on its way out. If you have free access to medicines, it may be worth changing to the prescription given under the previous pattern (damp), but the same prescription will still be helpful for this later stage.

Hot (Painful Coughs)

PRESCRIPTION 1: GENERAL

Coltsfoot *Tussilago farfara*	3 drops tincture
Mullein *Verbascum thapsus*	3 drops tincture

Marshmallow *Althea officinale*	3 drops tincture
Lobelia *Lobelia inflata*	2 drops tincture
Licorice *Glycyrrhiza glabra*	2 drops tincture
Peppermint *Mentha piperata*	2 drops tincture

PRESCRIPTION 2: BACTERIAL INVOLVEMENT

Gum weed *Grindelia camporum*	4 drops tincture
White horehound *Marrubium vulgare*	3 drops tincture
Marshmallow *Althea officinale*	3 drops tincture
Peppermint *Mentha piperata*	2 drops tincture
Golden seal *Hydrastis canadensis*	2 drops tincture
Echinacea *Echinacea angustifolia*	2 drops tincture

VARIATION: DIGESTIVE DISTURBANCE

If the child is constipated or has diarrhea, some of the herbs mentioned in Chapters 10 and 11 should be added.

Explanation. Coltsfoot, mullein, and marshmallow are all "demulcents" in that they reduce and soothe inflammation in the lungs. To some extent they are interchangeable, and if one is not available, it may be omitted. Lobelia is an antispasmodic and a relaxant; it also promotes perspiration. Licorice is a gentle expectorant, is a tonic, and helps harmonize the herbs. Mint promotes perspiration and helps reduce heat in the body.

Gum weed is the principal herb in the second prescription because it helps relieve spasms in the chest and promote expectoration. An alternative that has similar properties is pill-bearing spurge *Euphorbia pilulifera*. White horehound is useful for dry coughs because it loosens mucus.

Golden seal and echinacea are both antibacterials. Golden seal is especially good at soothing the mucous membranes and helps remove mucus via the intestines.

Results. The best way to reduce heat in the body is through perspiration, but the first effect of the medicines should be to soothe the cough. The feelings of heat should subside slightly, and the cough should become less spasmodic. Several doses may need to be taken before proper perspiration starts and the child starts to sweat the cough out.

Dry (Tickling, Raspy Coughs)

Coltsfoot *Tussilago farfara*	3 drops tincture
White horehound *Marrubium vulgare*	3 drops tincture
Mullein *Verbascum thapsus*	3 drops tincture
Marshmallow *Althea officinale*	2 drops tincture
Angelica *Angelica archangelica*	2 drops tincture
Licorice *Glycyrrhiza glabra*	2 drops tincture

Angelica may be replaced by aniseed *Pimpinella anisum.*

Explanation. Coltsfoot, white horehound, and mullein are included for their general effect on the lungs and their specific demulcent (soothing inflammation) properties. Marshmallow is a general demulcent. Angelica or aniseed is included as a tonic for the digestive system. Licorice is an expectorant and an all-purpose tonic, and it helps harmonize the other herbs.

VARIATION: DIGESTIVE DISTURBANCES

If the child has a significant digestive disturbance, this must be addressed. In younger children the stagnant food pattern is often the main cause of acute cough. This pattern may appear "out of the blue" or with teething. If diarrhea is present, the child will be losing a lot of the energy that is needed to fight the cough. If the child is constipated, toxins are building up in the body, which make matters worse. The details of treatment of these conditions are given in Chapters 10 and 11. As a simple suggestion, the herbs listed next will be of benefit.

For the child with diarrhea, add the following:

| Agrimony *Agrimonia eupatorium* | 3 drops tincture |

For the constipated child, add the following:

| Butternut *Juglans cinerea* | 3 drops tincture |

If the constipation does not respond to milder herbs, then add the following:

| Senna *Cassia angustifolia* | The easiest way to administer this is in pills, which are readily available at most pharmacies. |

VARIATION: BACTERIAL INFECTION

A number of herbs can be of benefit in children who also have a bacterial infection. Among these are the following:

Garlic *Allium sativum*   Capsules of garlic oil

Although the easiest way to administer garlic is in the form of capsules of garlic oil, be sure to look carefully at the label. Many capsules purporting to contain garlic contain many additional ingredients as well, which may be undesirable.

If the child also has a fever, the following may be added:

Echinacea *Echinacea angustifolia*   2-4 drops tincture

This is best given at the onset of a fever, as soon as some sort of infection is suspected. See also Chapter 16, which discusses rising temperatures.

▪ PROGRESSION TO BRONCHITIS

The progression of a simple cough to bronchitis was greatly feared in the past, for the next stage after bronchitis, which could follow with alarming rapidity, was pneumonia, which was often fatal. At the time of writing, when antibiotics are still effective, the progression to bronchitis does not carry the same risks for a relatively healthy person, but it is still a nasty experience.

From the traditional point of view this represented a transition to an excess of fire in the body. Although this explanation does not satisfy contemporary scientists, it is nevertheless a good description of what it feels like to patients. Patients unanimously describe a burning sensation in their chest and a general feeling of "boiling."

Typical symptoms are as follows:

- An irritating cough develops into a painful cough, causing the child to cry out every time he or she coughs. The pain is mainly behind the sternum.

- Older children will sit up to cough and may complain of a tight feeling in the chest.
- Fever is often present.
- At first there is little sputum, but then it becomes more and more copious and greenish yellow.

Treatment

Let us first of all say once again that bronchitis carries the risk of developing into pneumonia. The normal orthodox treatment is antibiotics, and it would be irresponsible of a parent to reject these if the situation appeared to be getting out of hand.* However, their usefulness in the majority of bronchitis cases is doubtful. It seems that antibiotics do not significantly shorten the course of bronchitis in relatively healthy children. If the child can get over the bronchitis without the need for antibiotics, in the end, the child's health will be much better. When a bacterial disease is treated with antibiotics, the disease is only half treated and usually leaves behind the echo pattern, as explained in Chapter 5.

PRESCRIPTION

Elecampane *Inula helenium*	4 drops tincture
Coltsfoot *Tussilago farfara*	4 drops tincture
Blood root *Sanguinaria canadensis*	4 drops tincture
Violet *Viola odorata*	4 drops tincture
Marshmallow *Althea officinalis*	4 drops tincture

In addition, add one of the following:

Wormwood *Artemisia absinthium*   4 drops tincture
or
Angelica *Angelica archangelica*   4 drops tincture

Explanation. Elecampane is an expectorant and an antibacterial. Coltsfoot is a demulcent and

---

*Note that the use of antibiotics may not shorten the course of the disease. "It is often said that acute bronchitis lasts around 7 days without the use of antibiotics, and one week with them" (From Gascoigne S: *Manual of conventional medicine for alternative practitioners*, Dorking, England, 1993, Jigme Press).

expectorant, so it reduces inflammation and helps clear the chest. Blood root is a powerful expectorant and antispasmodic. Violet, the new herb in this prescription, has the specific effect of cooling and soothing inflammation in the lungs. Marshmallow has a similar effect for the entire system. Wormwood or angelica is added as a tonic for the digestive system.

The herbs should be given frequently, possibly every 2 hours. Note that the dosage is doubled because of the urgency of the situation.

■ PROGRESSION TO PNEUMONIA

The word *pneumonia* covers a wide range of conditions. Pneumonia is usually a bacterial infection, but it may be viral. If a cough progresses to pneumonia it must be taken very seriously.

Pneumonia should be treated only with the help of a qualified practitioner. Herbs may be useful in combating the disease, but it must be said antibiotics are very effective and must be considered.*

The diagnosis of pneumonia is usually made through identification of the causative organism, but the simpler classification of lobar or bronchopneumonia with their accompanying symptoms is possibly of more use to the herbal practitioner. A detailed discussion of how to treat this condition is beyond the scope of this book, but it is important to recognize the danger signs. Pneumonia is especially serious in the young children, immunosuppressed patients, and elderly persons.

■ OTHER TREATMENTS
Applications to the Chest

Many of the herbs can be applied to the chest. The old-fashioned way was to make a strong tea and

---

Danger Signs Indicating Lobar Pneumonia

- High fever
- Coughing up blood-stained or reddish sputum
- Severe pain in the chest or under the armpit or scapula, which is worse on coughing
- Pleuritic pain
- Breathlessness
- Wheezing
- Loss of consciousness
- Sense that the child is fading away

---

soak a cloth in the tea. The cloth was loosely wrung out and applied to the chest while still warm. The application used to be changed every 20 minutes. In the preantibiotic era, this was a large part of a nurse's work in a hospital.

These methods are still as effective as they always used to be, although they have the disadvantage now that they are labor intensive and no one wants to do the work if there is an easier way. It is obviously much easier to give a pill than to do these repeated applications. As a very good second best, one can apply essential oils to the chest.

Essential Oils

Essential oils really come into their own in the treatment of acute coughs. They penetrate the skin quickly and have a very quick effect both in reducing the severity of a cough and in dissolving thick mucus. Being so volatile and diffusive, they can quickly reach very congested parts in a way that few other remedies can.

The oils may be mixed with a massage oil for rubbing onto the chest. An alternative way of using them is to place a few drops of each oil on a cloth or handkerchief and lay this on the chest for inhalation. They may also be used in steam inhalations. This method is easier for older children rather than younger ones.

---

*The symptoms of a child who has bacterial pneumonia but is not fighting it are very similar to those of a child with viral pneumonia. The difference is that the child who is not fighting the bacterial pneumonia may sink very fast. Because there is so little time, it may be better to give antibiotics.

PRESCRIPTION 1: ACUTE COUGH WITH MUCH MUCUS

Eucalyptus oil *Eucalyptus globulus*	3 drops
Thyme oil *Thymus vulgaris*	3 drops
Hyssop oil *Hyssopus officinalis*	3 drops

Add these to 30 ml (1 oz) of a carrier oil, such as olive or almond oil. Alternatively, put the oils on a handkerchief and inhale or inhale from a steam bath.

PRESCRIPTION 2: TICKLING, IRRITATING COUGHS

Sandalwood oil *Santalum album*	2 drops
Thyme oil *Thymus vulgaris*	2 drops
Lavender oil *Lavandula officinalis*	2 drops

Add these to 30 ml (1 oz) of a carrier oil, such as olive or almond oil.

Explanation. Eucalyptus is a wonder oil for clearing mucus and improving breathing. Thyme is good for coughs and is an antimicrobial. Hyssop is good for coughs and relieves spasms. Sandalwood is an antiseptic for the lungs. Lavender is a general relaxant.

■ WHAT ACTUALLY HAPPENS

More often than not, an acute cough needs treatment urgently when it is an acute episode of a chronic cough or, more seriously, when it is the prelude to an asthma attack.

An Acute Cough Superimposed on a Chronic Cough (Echo Pattern)

There is an old Chinese saying that "A time of crisis is a time of opportunity," and this saying applies here. This is especially true of the echo pattern of chronic cough.

HOW YOU SHOULD TREAT IT

When a child with an echo pattern has an acute flare-up, all of the mucus in the body is softened. Often, the occasional dry cough that came when the child was tired or upset suddenly becomes much more productive. In some senses this is marvelous because the external pathogen is doing what we have been trying to do with herbs such as poke root *Phytolacca decandra* and blue flag *Iris versicolor*. The problem arises when the release of mucus is too sudden and too much for the child to cope with. If that happens, the child will succumb to a bacterial illness and start to sink, necessitating the use of antibiotics. Knowing this, we can give guidelines on the principles of treatment.

1. At the first signs of infection, stop giving herbs to loosen phlegm (e.g., poke root *Phytolacca decandra* and blue flag *Iris versicolor*).
2. If the child is still early in the course of treatment and it is likely that he or she will succumb and have to take antibiotics, then at the first signs give herbs to strengthen the immune system and to strengthen the lungs, such as the following:

Echinacea *Echinacea angustifolia*	6 drops tincture
Coltsfoot *Tussilago farfara*	6 drops tincture
White horehound *Marrubium vulgare*	6 drops tincture
Aniseed *Pimpinella anisum*	6 drops tincture

In addition, add the following:

Garlic *Allium sativum*	$\frac{1}{2}$ to 1 capsule of oil

Notice the relatively larger doses required.

Explanation. Echinacea and garlic will help combat lung infection and boost the immune system. Coltsfoot and white horehound help strengthen the lungs and help expectorate any excess mucus. Aniseed is a general tonic for the lungs and the digestive system.

Frequency. This situation is relatively urgent, so the herbs should be given much more frequently (e.g., every 2 to 3 hours throughout the day). At this stage it may be helpful to put into action all the other therapies for overcoming cough, such as essential oils rubbed into the chest.

If the child is later on in the course of treatment and it is unlikely that the cough will become very severe, one can be more relaxed about the approach to treatment. There is not the same urgent need to take herbs to fight infection.

The herbs to take depend on what happens to the child during such an infection. There are two likely patterns: The child may have a large amount of mucus and revert to something similar to the mucus pattern of chronic cough, or the child may start to become weak and tired and revert to something similar to the Weak pattern of chronic cough. Slightly different herbs are given in the two cases.

LARGE AMOUNT OF MUCUS

Elderflower *Sambucus nigra*	4 drops tincture
Elecampane *Inula helenium*	4 drops tincture
Thyme *Thymus vulgaris*	3 drops tincture
Angelica *Angelica archangelica*	2 drops tincture
White horehound *Marrubium vulgare*	2 drops tincture
Golden seal *Hydrastis canadensis*	2 drops tincture

Explanation. This prescription is very similar to the prescription for the damp pattern, with golden seal replacing ginger and the addition of elderflower. Golden seal has that extra effect of resolving long-standing thick mucus, which is likely to be present in children with the echo pattern. Elderflower is specific for coughs that affect the upper respiratory tract.

Results. These herbs together should keep the airways clear of mucus. They may not eradicate the mucus up altogether, but the child should notice a definite improvement after taking the herbs. If the cough is severe during the night and causes the child to lose a lot of sleep, then the first thing to do is to put aromatic oils on the chest, as outlined earlier. If these do not work, it might be worth considering taking the occasional dose of a cough suppressant. We do not normally recommend taking these, certainly not for any length of time, but occasional use will enable a child to get a good night's sleep and the beneficial effects will outweigh the adverse effects. During the day one can return to the herbs that really are of benefit to the child (see Danger Signs box earlier in this chapter).

WEAKNESS

White Horehound *Marrubium vulgare*	3 drops tincture
Thyme *thymus vulgaris*	3 drops tincture
Coltsfoot *Tussilago farfara*	3 drops tincture
Mullein *Verbascum thapsus*	3 drops tincture
Aniseed *Pimpinella anisum*	2 drops tincture
Angelica *Angelica archangelica*	2 drops tincture
Ginger *Zingiber officinalis*	2 drops tincture

Explanation. White horehound and thyme are the main expectorants here to help rid the lungs of mucus. Coltsfoot and mullein are assistants and are also antitussives, which help prevent the cough from getting out of hand for a Weak child. Aniseed and angelica assists expectoration and tone the digestive system. Ginger is warming and tones the entire system.

Results. The purpose of these herbs is to maintain the child's energy so that the lungs can be kept clear (i.e., so that the mucus can be coughed up). The expectorant herbs should have the effect of clearing the mucus out of the lungs without producing too much coughing. It may happen that the cough may become more productive and appear to get worse. If this happens it is a matter of judgment what to do. The first thing is to increase the expectorant herbs. It will also be beneficial to rub essential oils into the chest, as described previously.

Note: Watch for the danger signs at all times.

■ AN ACUTE COUGH IN AN ASTHMATIC CHILD

The development of an acute cough in an asthmatic child is a situation that many parent fear. For many asthmatic children, this is the trigger that precipitates a serious asthma attack, possibly necessitating hospitalization for emergency treatment.

How You Should Treat It

The principle of treatment is somewhat different. Although the patterns for asthma and chronic cough are very similar, the priorities differ greatly. In chronic cough, one can use the infection as a wave of energy with which to rid the body of the echo pattern that has been lingering for so long. In asthma the condition is so much deeper that there is little chance of ridding the body in the same way. The first priority is to enable the child to fight the infection. This is especially a priority if succumbing to infection has become a habit.

There are various aspects to treatment:

1. Boost the immune system by using the following herbs:

Echinacea *Echinacea angustifolia*	2 drops tincture
Garlic *Allium sativa*	½ to 1 capsule of oil

2. Use a remedy for acute cough based on the pattern given earlier that the child is showing. Give the herbs every 2 to 3 hours in warm water. If necessary, use the prescription for acute asthma given in Chapter 18. When the immediate threat of an asthma attack has passed, proceed to step 2.
3. Treat the underlying pattern that has caused the asthma When much of the mucus has gone, you can then treat the underlying echo pattern.

RESULTS

The results of treating an infection in an asthmatic child are unpredictable. As explained in the previous chapter, the lungs have to be somewhat weak for a child to have asthma in the first place, and it is difficult to assess just how weak they are in each individual case. The success in fighting off infection depends very much on this. In some children, one is very successful; in others, the effect of taking herbs is helpful but may not avert an attack. Even in these children the treatment will not have been in vain, for it will be found that the severity and duration of the attack are less than expected. As treatments progress for the underlying condition, the next time an infection comes along, there will be a markedly improved response to the treatment for the infection.

If the child is able to get over the attack without taking suppressant medicines, you will notice a big improvement all around. The child's lungs will be cleared of much mucus.

USE OF ANTIBIOTICS IN ASTHMATIC CHILDREN

In some children the timely use of antibiotics may avert a life-threatening condition, such as when a Weak child has a severe bacterial infection. In this situation there is a real danger of the infection getting out of control.

However, in many cases antibiotics are given inappropriately. In addition, it must be remembered that antibiotics have their disadvantages in that they stop an illness half way through, thus giving rise to the echo pattern. In terms of treating asthma, this means that the child will overcome the asthma attack more quickly, but it almost ensures that another similar attack will come along within a few months.

If the infection is viral, antibiotics will have no beneficial effect. In fact, they may possibly make matters worse by upsetting the digestive system.

It is not always possible to tell whether a child has a bacterial infection without performing time-consuming tests, and time is often of the essence in asthmatic patients. This puts the parents in a difficult position—should they give their child antibiotics, knowing that it may do nothing to help in the long term, or should they struggle and struggle, hoping that the herbs will work? What we advise in these situations is that the parents obtain some antibiotics but give them only if the situation is getting out of hand.

▪ AN ACUTE COUGH THAT IS REALLY A TRANSITION

In Chapter 6 we discussed some of the great changes that happen during the life of a child. Growth is not continuous but rather goes in steps. Each of these steps on the way to adulthood involves changes at all levels—mental, emotional, energetic, and physical. These changes often lead to a cleansing of the body, with expulsion of toxins just before or soon after. As these toxins leave the system, they may give rise to the symptom of fevers or, more frequently, to coughs. This pattern is very common with children younger than 7 years. When a child gets a cough, it is easy to miss this pattern, for one never knows if this cough is a sign of infection or whether it is the cough making a significant change in the child's perception.

TYPICAL TRANSITIONS THAT MAY GIVE RISE TO A COUGH

- Potty training
- Growth spurts
- Walking
- Birth of a sibling
- Learning to like a younger sibling
- Learning social skills
- Learning numbers, colors, and grammar
- Going to school

How You Should Treat It

A cough that is a transition initially looks like any other cough. There is no way of knowing whether this one is a transition or not. It becomes clear only after a week or so, when the child has much less response to the medicines than you would expect. At this point it is helpful to examine all of the symptoms and signs closely and to ask (or think, if you are a parent) about the child and what is going on in his or her life—is the child going through an emotional or physical development?

The medicines will be based on what you find. The main difference now is that the condition should be treated as a *chronic cough*, not an acute one. This normally means choosing herbs that support the body and help rid the body of mucus and also omitting herbs that combat bacteria or viruses.

■ Case History

A child we know was born with a considerable amount of mucus in her system. Her stools always contained mucus, her stomach often made a splashing noise when she was bounced up and down, and she would occasionally vomit mucus. This was something that she was born with.

It was a long time before she acquired an infection. For the first 2 years she was hardly ever ill. Then she went to nursery school. It is hardly surprising that she succumbed to a cough within the first week. On the surface it appeared to be an acute cough, but the difference was that it took almost 6 weeks for her to get well again—and this was a healthy child. During this time she was treated with herbs, and a large amount of mucus was removed from her system. An enormous time of change in her life was accompanied by a transition on the physical level to a stronger child with less mucus. The use of herbs was not a waste of time, for they prevented the child from becoming worn out by the long illness and led her through to being a much healthier child.

■ SOME ALL-PURPOSE COUGH MIXTURES

If you find yourself confused by our discussion or if you have many members of the family who each have different patterns, you may wish to keep a bottle of an all-purpose cough mixture. The following prescriptions would be suitable:

Plantain syrup *Plantago lanceolata*	1 tsp

The fresh herb is chopped and steeped in hot honey.* Make sure that you get the long-leaved plantain, sometimes called *ribwort*. The broad-leaved plantain, *P. major,* can also be used but is less effective.

Alternatively, the following may be used:

Horehound *Marrubium vulgare*	1 part
Aniseed *Pimpinella anisum*	1 part

Give 1 tsp of syrup in hot water. The water should be as hot as child can comfortably drink it to help the warm the body.

---

*Note: The honey should be pasteurized for children younger than 1 year. See note on p. 67.

A simpler, nicer-tasting syrup, which will not act as quickly in expelling the cough but that will certainly soothe the symptoms and is easier for the child to take, follows:

Wild cherry *Prunus serotina*	1 part
Aniseed *Pimpinella anisum*	1 part

Give 1 tsp of syrup in hot water.
Alternatively, you may try the following:

Mullein *Verbascum thapsus*	4 drops tincture
Coltsfoot *Tussilago farfara*	4 drops tincture
White horehound	4 drops tincture
Marrubium vulgare	
Ginger *Zingiber officinale*	1-2 drops tincture
Licorice *Glycyrrhiza glabra*	2 drops tincture
Angelica *Angelica archangelica*	2 drops tincture

Mullein, coltsfoot, and white horehound are all lung tonics and expectorants. They have the virtue of being effective for many different types of cough. They are regulating in that they have the property of soothing inflammation and of warming the system when Cold is present. Licorice is included both for its role as an expectorant and as a general regulator and tonic for the entire system. Ginger helps spread warmth and circulate the energy of the herbs.

■ ADVICE FOR ALL TYPES OF ACUTE COUGH

- Keep the child at home. This is good advice for a cough that develops in a relatively healthy child. For a child with a chronic cough or asthma, this is essential. If the child is kept home, there is less chance of the child becoming exhausted by the acute attack.
- Make sure that the child has plenty of rest to conserve energy. Early nights are essential.
- Be stricter about keeping milk and other unsuitable foods out of the child's diet. As time passes in a chronic problem, it is easy to let things slip a little. Now is the time to tighten up—no milk, no ice-cold food, no junk food, and so on.

20

Measles

In Chapter 4 we outlined our view that childhood diseases are usually beneficial and that to try and prevent them is misguided. Whether you believe this to be true or not depends on your point of view. What is certain is that some children who have been immunized contract these diseases. Moreover, there are an increasing number of parents who do not immunize their children because they are fearful of the side effects. These children are open to diseases. The childhood diseases are rarely dangerous if they are nursed well, but knowledge of how to nurse them is no longer common. Therefore in this and the next two chapters we outline principles to be followed in nursing children through each of these diseases (measles, mumps, and whooping cough), and we give herbal treatments.

Of all the childhood illnesses, measles presents the greatest opportunity for benefitting the child. In developing countries it also presents the possibility of bringing the worst to the child, for at present, it is one of the major causes of infant mortality in these countries. However, this danger is considerably less in developed countries. All authorities agree that the mortality rate from measles had fallen to a very low level, long before the introduction of the vaccine. Since the vaccine was introduced, the mortality rate has continued to fall at exactly the same rate as before the vaccine was available, so it is far from proven that the vaccine has been instrumental in reducing deaths from measles in developed countries. What is clear is that the risks of measles, although significant, are now small.

Even though the risks associated with measles are small, the disease must be taken seriously. Good nursing is essential to ensure that the disease is beneficial to the child and ultimately leads to a better state of health. If you are a parent and feel unable to cope, seek the help of a qualified practitioner who has experience with the disease.

An Alternative View

The orthodox view of measles is simply that the child is attacked by a virus. The virus is then believed to generate poisons, which affect the body, especially the brain and spinal cord. The alternative view does not contradict this observation but casts it in a slightly different form. It is thought that the poisons are present at all times, and it is the action of the virus that stimulates the body to release the poisons.* The virus provides a trigger for the poisons that are waiting to come out in just the same way as we have seen with other infectious diseases (see Chapter 4). The main difference between measles and other fevers is in the severity and in the nature of the poison.

It might seem strange to think of a child being born with poisons in the body, yet this is how it seems to be. One possible explanation is that the poisons occur as a result of the rapid growth of the brain. During the first 3 years of life, the chemistry

*This concept is found in traditional Chinese medicine, as well as anthroposophical medicine, which originated in the West.

of the brain must be very different from that later on, when growth is minimal. During the growth phase it is easy for mild inflammations and waste products to accumulate if the body is not completely in balance.

Measles is therefore as much an internal disease as one caused by attack by a virus. A virus is needed for the disease to be initiated, but if the poisons were not present in the first place, measles would not develop. The health of the child will be much better once these poisons are cleared out of the system.

■ DESCRIPTION

First we give a description of the disease, as it used to be. Occasionally, children still get the disease in this manner, but more often they get a much milder version. The disease process is conveniently divided into four stages:

- First stage
- Rash stage
- Recovery stage
- Recuperation stage

First Stage

The virus can be passed by contact or through infected droplets released into the air from another child with measles. There is then an incubation period of 7 to 14 days before any signs of disease are noticed. The first signs are usually those of a cold, with watery eyes, sneezing, and nasal discharge. The child is usually irritable and miserable at this stage. Typically, the child's temperature rises over a day or two before the rash first appears.

Rash Stage

The rash initially appears behind the ears and then spreads in a day or two to cover the entire body. In mild cases the rash appears as a few red dots here and there, but in severe cases the red dots multiply and merge, resulting in whole areas of livid red with a few islands of yellowish green skin between. The child is usually very irritated and distressed. The child's eyes are swollen and often red, and the child becomes photophobic (i.e., dislikes bright lights). After a day or two of severe rash, the child may become listless and his or her consciousness dulled. The child usually has a cough with some yellow mucus, a red tongue with a yellow coating, and as the rash spreads, a fever of 40°C (104° F) or higher. The presence of white raised spots inside the mouth (known as *Koplik's spots**) confirms the diagnosis of measles.

Recovery Stage

The most voilent stage of the illness usually lasts between 3 and 6 days, after which the temperature starts to come down and the rash changes color from a livid red to a duller, slightly purple-red. As a parent there is a great feeling of relief to see the symptoms abate. Over the next few days to a week, the rash fades completely, usually leaving no trace. During this week the child is often confused and rather distant in behavior.

Recuperation

Once the recovery stage is over, the child is clearly well but is usually rather weak and easily tired. Over the next few weeks, the energy and strength gradually return, revealing a happier and more open child.

■ COMPLICATIONS

Complications are extremely rare, but they can occur in severe cases. They may arise because the poisons that are released come at too great a rate

---

*How to find Koplik's spots: Take the lip between the thumb and forefinger and pull it out and down. The spots are usually to be found there. Sometimes you may have to look on the inner surface of the cheek. Koplik's spots do not always appear in measles today. It is unclear whether measles itself has changed or whether illnesses have developed that look very similar to measles but that are in fact caused by another virus.

for the body to cope with. Some possible complications are discussed in the following sections.

Pneumonia

During a severe attack of measles, mucus is released and commonly gives rise to a cough. This mucus is an ideal breeding ground for bacteria, and the most common complication is pneumonia, where a secondary infection invades the bronchi. This tends to occur in children prone to lung weakness. The bronchi become inflamed, and severe pain is felt in the chest, often with shallow breathing or even wheezing. This is a serious condition, and help should be sought immediately.

Encephalitis

The child with encephalitis will be delirious or even in a coma as a result of inflammation of the brain, brought about by the toxins released by the virus.* Encephalitis is an emergency condition requiring immediate assistance.

Danger Signs of Encephalitis

- Severe headache with the inability to bend the head
- Sudden lethargy
- Convulsions
- Rash that is flat, dark red, and unchanged by pressure

Diarrhea

The poison that appears on the skin as a rash travels to the intestines. This inflames the lining of the intestines and disturbs their function, giving rise to diarrhea.

■ TREATMENT*

The dosages we give are for children aged 3 years. The dosages we suggest are *suggestions only.* Each child may need something different.

The most important aspect of treatment is to prevent the fever from rising. The details of this were outlined in Chapter 16, so at this stage we give a reminder of the key points.

First Stage

The symptoms during the first stage resemble those of a bad cold. The best medicine to give at this stage is the following:

Yarrow *Achillea millefolium*	See following text for dosage
Echinacea *Echinacea angustifolia*	See following text for dosage

Yarrow is best given as an infusion (well sweetened), but tincture taken in hot water works almost as well. The main difficulty with this herb is that it has an unpleasant taste and it is therefore difficult to get children to take it.

Dosage. Use 3 tsp of fresh herb. Add the herb to 500 ml (20 oz) of boiling water and allow to stand until lukewarm. Sweeten and give a cupful (100 ml/4 oz) every 2 hours until the child begins to feel warm and perspiration has started.

Keep giving the herb every 4 to 6 hours (except when the child is asleep) until the fever is down; then give three times a day. Echinacea may be added to the tea. Give 3 to 4 drops tincture in each cup. If you do not have the fresh herb or the child will take only a tincture, then give 1 ml of tincture in each dose and give in warm, sweetened water, as described earlier.

Explanation. Measles starts out by being somewhat cold and wet, and yarrow will help warm the

---

*A prevailing theory is that measles encephalitis results when the virus enters brain cells.

*For more detailed information about dosages, see Chapter 8.

child up and initiate perspiration. Yarrow also has the positive effect of bringing the rash to the surface, thereby speeding the transition to the second stage. Yarrow is also a tonic. At this stage, there should not be much need of a tonic, but as the disease progresses, it certainly will be needed. If there is one herb to choose, which can be safely given from beginning to end of measles, it is yarrow. Echinacea can also be given and can be effective. At present, it has the great advantage that it is very easy to obtain. Echinacea "rallies" the immune system and speeds the transition to the second stage. As a secondary property, it also has the effect of clearing poisons from the system. Echinacea may be given in the first two stages, but it is not as beneficial during the third and fourth stages.

Second Stage

During the second stage, the aims of treatment are as follows:

- To bring the fever down through perspiration
- To make sure the child is not constipated
- To make sure the child has enough to drink

Yarrow may still be given, but a better prescription would be the following:

Elderflower *Sambucus nigra*	Infusion
Peppermint *Mentha piperata*	Infusion

If the child is very restless, add the following:

Lime flowers *Tilea europea*	Infusion
Chamomile *Chamomilla matricaria*	Infusion

Dosage. The best way to give these herbs is as an infusion. Make a tea from 1 tsp of each herb in 1 cup of water and sweeten well. Give half the mixture while it is still warm every 2 hours (dosage for 3-year-olds; for other ages, see Table 20-1) and then prepare some more.

A good second best, which avoids the necessity of keeping dried herbs, is to give the herbs as a

Table 20-1

AGE	MULTIPLY 3-YEAR-OLD DOSE BY
6-12 months	$\times \frac{1}{3}$
1-2 years	$\times \frac{1}{2}$
2-4 years	$\times 1$
4-7 years	$\times 1\frac{1}{2}$
7-14 years	$\times 2$
14+ years	$\times 3$

syrup. Syrups are commercially available in many places. Once again, give the mixture in warm water every 2 hours, following the instructions on the bottle.

Tinctures may also be used and are certainly effective. Give $\frac{1}{4}$ tsp each dose for 3-year-olds. In view of the relatively large quantities needed, it is usually a good idea to evaporate off some of the alcohol. See Chapter 8 for details of this procedure.

Special herbs for measles include the following:

Burdock seeds *Arctium lappa*	$\frac{1}{4}$ tsp of seeds in infusion or tincture
Pasque flower *Anemone pulsatilla*	1 drop tincture
Marigold petals *Calendula officinalis*	1 tsp of petals piled high for the tea or 3 drops tincture
Echinacea *Echinacea angustifolia*	3 drops tincture

Again, burdock is best given as a tea. It is normally burdock root that is available. It may be possible to obtain burdock seeds at a pharmacy that sells Chinese herbs. Burdock root may be used as a second best. Pasque flower is better given as a tincture. It is a strong herb, so do not exceed the stated dosage. Marigold may be given on its own or together with other herbs, either as a tea or as a tincture. It helps reduce heat, clear poisons from the body, and reduce the rash. It is also bacteriostatic and will decrease the risk of a secondary infection. Echinacea may also be safely given throughout the second stage to decrease the risk of a secondary infection leading to pneumonia.

Explanation. Burdock is the herb most often used for skin complaints of all kinds, but burdock seeds have the special effect of resolving poisons. Pasque flower has the special effect of bringing the measles rash to the surface.

Results. If the child is younger than 5 years and is relatively healthy, measles usually resolves very quickly. Sometimes the healing process starts within a few hours of giving the herbs, so that within about 24 hours, the rash has almost disappeared. If the child's health has never been especially good, more time will be needed.

If the child is older than 7 years, the effects seem to be much slower. There seems to be a much bigger struggle, and the herbs do not have the same curative effect. This does not mean you should stop giving the herbs. The herbs are benefitting the child, even though there is not an obvious cure. The main benefit they are conferring is to stop the fever from getting too high, and they certainly shorten the course of the disease.

If the child is older than 7 years and is Weak as well, with a history of many other severe illnesses, there is real cause for concern. Seek the advice of a practitioner who has experience in treating such conditions.

Third Stage

Continue giving herbs that reduce the rash for several days after the rash has disappeared and gradually introduce tonic herbs. Once the fever has subsided, the febrifuge herbs elderflower, peppermint, and echinacea may be discontinued. Yarrow may be continued, for it is a great tonic. If a cough is present, this should be treated as an acute cough (see Chapter 19). If the appetite is poor, this should also be treated (see Chapter 14). Otherwise, ensure that the child receives nourishing food and is kept in bed (usually for a longer period than the child wants to stay in bed). Some people like to give vitamins at this stage, but it should not be necessary if the child is eating good organic food and has a good appetite.

Fourth Stage

Herbs are normally not be needed during the fourth stage of measles. If the third stage has been treated well, all that should be needed is rest and quiet. Occasionally, the child has a poor appetite or a residual cough, in which case the herbs given during the third stage should be continued until the symptoms disappear.

■ COMPLICATIONS

Pneumonia

The details of the treatment of lung complaints are provided in Chapter 19. If pneumonia develops, you must call for help. If the pneumonia becomes severe, do not hesitate to use antibiotics if they are prescribed, but also continue to give the herbs. Do not feel that you have failed. If you give both the herbs and the antibiotics, the child will get better much more quickly.

Encephalitis

Seek help immediately. The child will probably be admitted to hospital, but continue to give the herbs and treatments for fevers. In particular, perform the spinal stroke massage. Also make sure that the rash is coming out by giving the herbs listed earlier.

Diarrhea

Mild diarrhea is nothing to worry about, but if it becomes severe, seek help immediately. The place for the child is in the hospital, where it is easy to rehydrate.

■ SEQUELAE

If the attack has been very severe, the child may be left with an "echo" of measles. Some very common symptoms of this are described in the following sections.

Night Terrors

Instead of being more calm and peaceful after measles, the child is tearful and timid. Sleep is impaired, and the child wakes at night in fear. This is a combination of the "fright" pattern of insomnia and the "heat" pattern. See Chapter 25 for treatments.

Eczema

A mild form of eczema may be left behind, which is more severe when the child is tired. See Chapter 26 for treatments.

Impaired Vision

The poison that affects the system and gives rise to irregularities in the brain waves also affects the optic nerve. In severe cases the optic nerve can be damaged, resulting in the whole of the eye having reduced energy and function. If it is caught early enough (within 3 months of the illness), long-term damage to the retina can be avoided. To our knowledge, orthodox medicine has little to offer, and unfortunately there are few alternative practitioners who treat eye conditions, but it is well worth searching for a practitioner who is prepared to help. Therapies to consider are acupuncture, Chinese herbalism, and the Bates technique.

Deafness

The poison may invade the the inner ear, which leaves behind a severe injury. As with impaired vision, help should be sought immediately. The only therapies we know that can be of help are electroacupuncture and craniosacral osteopathy. If treatment is begun early, some hearing may be recovered.

ORTHODOX TREATMENT

As far as we know, the only treatment available in orthodox medicine is prophylactic antibiotics to prevent the occurrence of pneumonia and secondary bacterial otitis media.

■ MANAGEMENT

As soon as measles is confirmed, the child should be put to bed in a *darkened room.* He or she may show no signs of the eyes being affected, but this measure should be taken to prevent permanent damage to the eyes.

If you are a parent, spend as much time as you can with your child and provide comfort in times of distress. Careful nursing plays an important part in recovery from measles. Keep your child calm; read stories to your child rather than allowing him or her to watch TV or play computer games, which can strain the eyes and the brain.

Recovery

As the temperature starts to go down, the appetite will gradually return. Very simple food should be given at first, in very small quantities. Porridge or baby food is helpful as a first food (even for teenagers). As the appetite returns and the digestive system strengthens, a more varied diet can be given. In cases of great weakness, beef broth can be very helpful, as can vitamin and mineral supplements.

Recuperation

A child who has had measles is in a wonderland for a week or more after the fever has gone down. Commonly, the child will wander around with a dazed and wondrous look in the eyes. The child looks like someone who has emerged from a very deep sleep or someone who has been through a mystical experience. When you consider the changes that have taken place, this is not surprising. What is not always realized is how tender the child is during this important time. All defenses are down. If the child receives strong or violent impressions, they may have a lasting effect. For this reason, it can be helpful for a child to spend some time recovering in a quiet place in the country, if this is possible.

■ AVOIDING THE COMPLICATIONS OF MEASLES

All children are at risk for measles, even if they have been immunized. However, those who have not been immunized are at greater risk, and the parents should be informed about how to avoid any complications when their child gets measles.

General Advice

The main thrust of the advice is to keep the child healthy, and in particular to prevent the poisons from accumulating in the system. This has the following dietary repercussions:

- *Avoid artificial colorings and flavorings*, which should be kept out of children's foods as much as possible.
- *Avoid meat*, especially red meat, and completely eliminate *seafood*, such as *crabs and shellfish*. A child's digestive system is not as strong as an adult's, and it is difficult for children to digest meat completely without generating poison. In our opinion children should be mainly vegetarian up to the age of 7 years, except in special circumstances, such as recuperation after illness. This is not practical for most parents, but keeping meat to a minimum is worthwhile. According to the Chinese, seafood such as crabs, lobster, and shellfish all contain a certain amount of the poison that contributes to measles, so they should be avoided altogether.
- *Avoid oranges*, including orange juice and organic oranges. A child should not have more that one orange (or its equivalent in juice) a week. Oranges are said by the Chinese to contain poisons that irritate the brain in some children.

Avoiding Pneumonia

The obvious extra thing to look out for is mucus. Make sure that mucus has not built up and that the child does not get frequent coughs and colds. Dietary advice is the same as that for chronic cough and includes avoiding cow's milk products.

Avoiding Encephalitis

It has been ascertained that any attack of measles affects the brain and that the poisons released have a disrupting effect on brain activity. In the normal progress of the disease, this poison gives rise to a temporary dulling of consciousness, which passes as the poison levels subside. When the poison levels become too severe and the temperature of the brain too high, the resulting inflammation of the brain can lead to permanent damage; this will occur only if the brain is already too active and overstimulated. A child who already has a "hot head" is much more likely to suffer from encephalitis and its complications. Therefore the best way to reduce this risk is to ensure that the brain is as cool as possible. This means bringing up the child in as calm and peaceful a manner as possible. In particular, we advise avoiding brain stimulation by reducing the following:

- Exposure to TV
- Computer games
- Early learning methods (which overstimulate a child's brain)

On the positive side, encourage the child's imagination by reading to him or her and by encouraging painting, outside play, and simple daydreaming.

Avoiding Diarrhea

Again, the main advice is dietary. Ensure that the child eats regular meals. In younger children ensure that there is no buildup of the accumulation disorder.

■ OTHER TREATMENTS

Homeopathy

Homeopathy is of great benefit in children with measles. It is particularly helpful in bringing out the rash, thereby reducing the risk of encephalitis. Some information is given in Chapter 16. Besides remedies to help reduce the fever, both Aconite and Pulsatilla help relieve the rash.

Essential Oils

Use the following herbs to wash the skin:

German chamomile *Chamomilla matricaria*   5 drops
Lavender *Lavandula officinalis*   5 drops

Mix the oils in 1 pint of water and wash the body. This will soothe the rash and calm the child. If there is a risk of secondary infections, add the following to the water:

Tea tree *Melaleuca alternifolia*   5 drops

Vaporizer in the Room

You may also consider using a vaporizer in the child's room. Put the following oils in the vaporizer:

Eucalyptus *Eucalyptus globulus*   10 drops
or
Hyssop *Hyssopus officinalis*   10 drops

▪ POSSIBLE BENEFITS OF MEASLES

When measles goes well (i.e., the child does not experience any complications and is given time to recuperate), the child is changed afterward. The changes are most obvious on the emotional level and in the nature of the child. Many a mother and teacher have noticed how a child becomes more open, more generous, and more friendly. Provided the child is allowed to recuperate, benefits are seen on the physical level in terms of more stamina and better resistance to disease. In contrast, if a child does not get the measles until after the age of 10, the severity of disease is greater and there is an increased risk of complications.

Do You Have to Have Measles to Be Healthy?

Measles is the surest way of eliminating poisons from the body, but you do not have to have measles to be healthy. There are some children who are exposed to measles yet do not get it or get only very mild symptoms. These are the children whose systems have adapted to growing up without the need for a dramatic illness.

There is also another chance at puberty to eliminate the poisons that would normally be eliminated by measles. At this momentous transition, there is the chance of correcting imbalances that have been present since early childhood, and measles is one of these. The poison may come out between the ages of 12 and 14 years in the form of unexplained rashes, which have some similarity to the rash of measles in that they are red but they are not usually raised. This rash is often diagnosed as eczema but has a very different appearance and function from normal eczema.

21

Mumps

Of all the traditional children's diseases—mumps, measles, whooping cough, and polio—mumps is the least feared. As a disease it is hardly ever life threatening, and usually there is less discomfort than is experienced with other illnesses that occur annually in the spring. For a few children the pain and discomfort of the disease are severe. Mumps can also make some children feel tired and depressed for a long time (6 to 8 weeks while the illness lasts plus another 6 to 8 weeks after recovery). Treatment with herbs is very effective for restoring children's energy and cheering them up.

Causes

Once again a discrepancy exists between the orthodox view of mumps and the alternative view. In orthodox medicine mumps is thought to be caused by a virus. The alternative view is that the virus is the trigger for releasing poisons that are already there and that once these poisons are eliminated from the body, the child will be healthier (as in the case of measles). For mumps, toxins in the glandular system are being eliminated.

Beneficial Aspects

Just as measles eliminates a really nasty poison from the system, mumps eliminates a slightly less nasty poison. Its effect is to clear the poison out of the glandular system. If a child does not get mumps (either because of lack of exposure to the active disease or because of immunization), then he or she will be more prone to have glandular fever at a later age, or if mumps occurs at a later age,

it is likely to cause orchitis (swelling and inflammation of the testicles) or ovaritis (inflammation of the ovaries).

■ SYMPTOMS

The symptoms of mumps vary. They can be broadly divided into three categories: mild, medium, and strong.

Mild

When a child has mild mumps, at first you may not be sure that the disease is really mumps. The symptoms you might see include the following:

- The child is tired.
- The child may be somewhat grumpy.
- The forehead may feel hot.

On examination you will find that the parotid glands are slightly swollen. What will make you suspect mumps is the finding that the child was exposed to the disease about 2 weeks earlier.

Medium

This is the more classic manifestation of mumps. The incubation period is about 2 weeks. Then the child gets a mild fever, and one of the parotid glands starts to swell. In addition, the following are seen:

- The child has difficulty opening the mouth.
- The parotid gland is tender or even a bit painful.

- The child is lethargic, tired, and irritable.
- The child's appetite is reduced.

The swelling in one gland lasts for about 10 to 14 days, and then almost always the other gland swells for another 10 to 14 days. After the swelling subsides, it is normal for the child to feel tired for another 2 weeks.

Strong

This is a severe manifestation of mumps. The basic symptoms for strong mumps are the same as those for the medium type, but they are much more severe. You will see the following:

- The child has a high fever.
- The parotid gland is hot and painful all the time.
- The child cannot open his or her mouth and has to consume liquid foods.
- The child has to go to bed.
- The swelling may last for more than 14 days.

After these symptoms resolve, it is normal to be tired for another 3 to 4 weeks.

RELATIVE INCIDENCE
The mild type of mumps is now much more commonly seen.* The strong pattern appears to be seen rarely.

Complications

ORCHITIS OR OVARITIS
If mumps occurs after puberty, a small risk of complications—orchitis or ovaritis—exists. Orchitis is extremely uncomfortable and a cause of concern for men because they fear that they may become impotent or sterile. In fact, even a bad attack of orchitis rarely causes impotence or sterility.

EXHAUSTION
In most medical books the description of mumps stops at the active phase of the illness. What is omitted is the fact that effects of the illness may remain for a long time. The reason this information is missing may be that when the books were written, the course of illnesses was more straight-forward—children got ill and then got better again. This pattern is gradually shifting; thus now you see children with the following pattern: They are never really well; then when they get ill, they are not really very ill; and then they never quite get well again. This pattern may be seen with mumps too. Often, children are sent back to school long before they are well, and they never miss a day of school even throughout the course of the illness. In this situation the glands stay swollen for a much longer time, and when the swelling finally diminishes, the child may feel exhausted, in much the same way as after a bout of glandular fever (mononucleosis).

▪ TREATMENT*

The dosages we give are for children aged 3 years (Table 22-1) and are *suggestions only*. Each child may need something different.

Mild

For mild cases, no treatment is needed beyond keeping the child at home from school and allow-

Table 22-1

AGE	MULTIPLY 3-YEAR-OLD DOSE BY
6-12 months	× $\frac{1}{3}$
1-2 years	× $\frac{1}{2}$
2-4 years	× 1
4-7 years	× 1$\frac{1}{2}$
7-14 years	× 2
14+ years	× 3

---

*According to a nurse working in a Swedish hospital, the mild version now accounts for more than 30% of all cases of mumps.

*For more detailed information about dosages, see Chapter 8.

ing him or her to rest. The latter may be more difficult to enforce because the child probably does not feel very ill and wants to make the most use of the time off school.

Medium

| Yarrow *Achillea millefolium* | 20 drops tincture |
| Poke root *Phytolacca decandra* | 10 drops tincture |

If the child has completely stopped eating and drinking, add the following:

| Gentian *Gentiana lutea* | 5 drops tincture |

DOSAGE
Dosages are given for 3-year-olds. Use Table 22-1 to determine the correct dose for the age of child. Give the herbs in warm water three to four times a day.

Explanation. Yarrow is the all-purpose herb for fevers and is a tonic. If the fever is minimal, this herb may be omitted. Poke root is the specific herb for mumps. It helps clear the glandular system and reduces the swelling and pain of mumps. It is normal for the appetite to be reduced, so no special treatment is needed unless the child completely stops eating, in which case gentian will help stimulate the appetite.

RESULTS
If the child has a fever with chills, yarrow should help resolve these symptoms within 12 hours. After the fever is gone, yarrow may not be needed. However, poke root will be needed for at least a week and possibly longer. It will have the effect of reducing the swelling and pain. It may cause loose stools temporarily as the mucus comes out.

Strong

Elderflower *Sambucus nigra*	As an infusion
Peppermint *Mentha piperata*	As an infusion
Poke root *Phytolacca decandra*	As a tincture

DOSAGE
The best way to give elderflower and peppermint is as an infusion. Make a tea from 1 tsp of each herb in 1 cup of water and sweeten well. Give half the mixture while it is still warm every 2 hours (for 3-year-olds; for other ages, see Table 22-1), and then make some more.

Poke root is best given as 10 drops of tincture (for a 3-year-old; multiply for different ages) three or four times a day.

Explanation. The prescription is the same as the previous one, with yarrow replaced by elderflower and peppermint, because with strong mumps, the child usually has a high fever, which needs to be reduced.

RESULTS
The treatments will bring down the fever and reduce the severity of the illness, making the child much happier.

EXTERNAL APPLICATIONS
When the swelling is very painful and the child is miserable, there are herbs that may be used as an external application. These are as follows:

- Poke root *Phytolacca decandra:* Poke root may be given for all conditions. The best way to use it is to make a poultice from moistened powdered root. A good alternative is to soak a cloth in tincture and apply it to the swelling. Keep the cloth in place for as long as possible. The poultice should be taken off if the skin becomes discolored or if pustules appear.
- Ginger *Zingiber officinalis:* Chop or crush fresh ginger root and apply it as a poultice to the swelling. Remove the poultice before the skin becomes too red. Ginger root is effective when the swelling is not inflamed. One advantage of the use of ginger root is that it is readily available.
- St. John's wort *Hypericum perfoliatum:* Use oil or cream prepared from the herb and rub it into the swelling.

Complications

ORCHITIS
The herb of choice is the following:

Poke root *Phytolacca decandra*   The adult dose is 20 to 40 drops of tincture, together with herbs for fevers.

EXHAUSTION
If the child is still exhausted after the illness subsides, the toxins may not have been completely eliminated, so continue giving the herbs. At this stage you will probably also need to add herbs to improve the appetite (see Chapter14).

▪ ESSENTIAL OILS

Tea tree *Melaleuca alternifolia*   2 drops
Lavender *Lavandula officinalis*   2 drops
Lemon   *Citrus limonum*   2 drops

Put the drops in 30 ml (1 oz) of massage oil (e.g., olive oil, almond oil) and use for a compress on the swelling.

▪ IMMUNIZATION POLICY

Mumps is a comparatively mild disease; moreover, it is beneficial to the body. Therefore it seems to us quite unnecessary to immunize. This point of view is reinforced by recent observations suggesting that the protective effect of immunization can wear off after a few years. Thus by immunizing you may avoid mild disease in childhood but risk more severe disease in puberty or later and increase the risk of orchitis in adulthood.

22

Whooping Cough

Whooping cough as a disease is greatly feared. The reason is easy to understand: The sight of a child with the spasmodic cough of whooping cough is truly terrifying, even for an experienced practitioner. The way the veins stand out on the neck, the purple color of the child's face, and the gasping for breath give the impression that the child is about to die. In fact, this picture is misleading because these days children rarely die from whooping cough. Even in the past children did not usually die from the disease itself but from secondary infections, such as pneumonia, that occurred along with the whooping cough. Although these facts may be borne in mind, the sight is nonetheless frightening.

Who Is Most at Risk?

Babies and very young children are most at risk. Those who have a Weak energy pattern and those with weak lungs are especially at risk. After the age of about 3 years, the symptoms may cause much suffering, but they do not normally present any dangers.

> Those younger than 1 year of age with weak lungs or a Weak energy pattern are most at risk.

■ DESCRIPTION

Whooping cough traditionally has three stages.

First Stage (7-14 Days)

The first stage is just a cough. In some children the cough is harsh but not really severe. At this stage it may be unclear whether the child has whooping cough unless an epidemic is going round or a sibling has it too.

Second Stage (40-60 Days)

The second stage is when it becomes apparent that the child has whooping cough. The cough has the characteristic whoop, and all the other horrible symptoms are present. At this stage the sputum is so thick and sticky that it is almost impossible to cough up.

Third Stage (Recuperation Stage) (20-30 Days)

In the third stage it is clear that the child is going to recover. The child is getting stronger week by week. The appetite increases dramatically.

■ CAUSES

Many children are born with large amounts of mucus in the body. This tendency may have been acquired from their parents, or it may simply be something that they have brought with them when they were born. When a child gets whooping cough, the body goes through a process of eliminating this mucus. It is true that the illness is triggered by a bacterium, *Bordetella pertussis,* but the fundamental process that is occurring is elimination of mucus. In this way whooping cough is similar to the "transition" type of acute cough mentioned in Chapter 19. It is also similar to measles in that it can greatly benefit the child.

Despite the fact that whooping cough strikes suddenly and seems like an acute cough, it is really a transition process during which the body is eliminating large quantities of mucus.

As we saw in Chapter 2, digestion is often disturbed when a child has a cough. This is especially true for whooping cough, which is as much a disease of the digestive system as it is of the lungs. Moreover, when the disease runs without complications, the child becomes generally stronger, and the lungs and digestive system are both stronger. This can be seen in the appetite, which is usually much better after a child has had whooping cough.

▪ PATTERNS OF STAGE 2

Stage 2 is the long drawn-out period of whooping cough (the Chinese call it the *100-days cough*). This stage of the disease seems static because nothing seems to change for week after week. In many textbooks the cough is simply described as a "crowing cough," but in our experience, there are three ways that it can manifest. From the point of view of herbal medicine, it is worth making the distinction between these three ways, for each corresponds to a different pattern and will require slightly different herbs.

▪ SYMPTOMS

The three patterns are the following:

- Hard mucus
- Large amounts of mucus
- Exhaustion

Hard Mucus

This is the classic whooping cough.

- The child is strong.
- When the child is not coughing, he or she may look healthy, with rosy cheeks.
- The child has periods when there is no cough, punctuated by spasms of coughing, which can last for up to 5 minutes, during which the

child becomes increasingly distressed. The veins stand out on the neck, the child's face turns red or even purple, and it appears as though the child will suffocate.
- Even during the cough, little mucus is brought up, perhaps only some "ropy" or slimy sputum.
- The child often vomits during an attack of coughing. The vomit may be food and drink recently taken, or it may just be mucus.

Large Amounts of Mucus

This is a variation seen in children who have had a lot of mucus for most of their lives.

- The child does not look as healthy and strong.
- The child's face may be pale.
- There are obvious signs of mucus, and the child may even be coughing most of the time—little gurgly coughs, which are punctuated by spasmodic coughing fits. The whoop is still there, but it is less pronounced.
- Nasal discharge is often present.
- The child often has a history of lung problems.

Exhaustion

In the case of exhaustion, the child has used up most of his or her energy even before getting whooping cough. There are two presentations: straight weakness and weakness with nervous energy.

- The child looks pale, even white.
- The child is very thin.
- The child has a history of poor appetite.
- The child is lethargic.
- The child may have fits of coughing, but they are weaker than those in Strong children.
- After the spasmodic fit of coughing, the child may not crow or "whoop" at all.

VARIATION: EXHAUSTION WITH NERVOUS ENERGY
The symptoms are very similar; the main differences are the following:

- The child is always on the go.
- The child hates to rest.
- When the coughing fits occur, the child weeps in despair.

◼ TREATMENT

General Principles

The principles of treatment of whooping cough are similar to those of chronic cough. This may be surprising, for whooping cough strikes suddenly, is known to be caused by a bacterium, and would seem to be like an acute cough. The reason it is treated like a chronic cough is that the symptoms cannot be cured simply by overcoming the bacterium. They will disappear only when mucus has finally been cleared from the body.

The main principle of treatment is to relieve the severe symptoms. In particular, the aim of treatment is to reduce the severity of the cough and stop the vomiting so that the child is not weakened too much by the illness. The difference between whooping cough and chronic cough is that with whooping cough the digestive system is more severely affected and vomiting is common. Thus different herbs are needed for treating the digestive system. These herbs help eliminate mucus through the stools, so to a certain extent they shorten the course of the illness.

Dosages*

The dosages we give are for children aged 3 years (Table 22-1) and are *suggestions only.* Each child may need something different.

◼ Table 22-1	
AGE	MULTIPLY 3-YEAR-OLD DOSE BY
6-12 months	× $\frac{1}{3}$
1-2 years	× $\frac{1}{2}$
2-4 years	× 1
4-7 years	× 1$\frac{1}{2}$
7-14 years	× 2
14+ years	× 3

*For more detailed information about dosages, see Chapter 8.

HARD MUCUS

Sundew *Drosera rotundifolia*	4 drops tincture
Thyme *Thymus vulgaris*	4 drops tincture
Lobelia *Lobelia inflata*	2 drops tincture
Black root *Leptandra virginica*	2 drops tincture

A good alternative to sundew is the following:

Gum weed *Grindelia camporum*	4 drops tincture

For spasmodic vomiting, add the following:

Guelder rose *Viburnum opulus*	2 drops tincture

Explanation. The first three herbs are somewhat interchangeable, and if all three cannot be obtained, one may be omitted. Sundew is one of the most popular herbs for whooping cough, and it is specific. However, it can be hard to find because it is an endangered species, and therefore one has to have a license even to sell cultivated plants. For this reason, we have given a substitute. Thyme is an antispasmodic rather than a relaxant. It has the additional advantage of being a digestive tonic. Lobelia is an expectorant, with a relaxing effect on the entire body. Black root does not work on the lungs specifically but is essential to the prescription because it clears mucus from the digestive system. If it cannot be obtained, then some substitute must be found, such as Oregon grape *Berberis aquifolium.*

Gum weed is a relaxing expectorant with the special effect of relaxing a tight chest. Guelder rose helps relax the entire digestive system.

Results. In a child who starts out reasonably healthy, the results are very good. Within a few days there is a noticeable reduction in the frequency and severity of the whoops. After 7 to 10 days, the cough may be so mild that the parents think they can discontinue the medicine. However, they should not do so. The herbs must be taken for at least 1 month, because if they are stopped too soon, the cough will come back. The herbs need to be taken until all of the mucus has been eliminated.

In other children, particularly those who already have a history of lung infections, the results are not so pronounced. If they take the herbs, the strength and severity of the cough should be greatly reduced and the vomiting almost eliminated. The herbs may not eliminate the symptoms entirely but will change the child's condition from severely ill to mildly ill.

If changes of this kind are not seen, the next step is to increase the dose of herbs—by as much as four times.

LARGE AMOUNTS OF MUCUS

White horehound *Marrubium vulgare*	3 drops tincture
Mullein *Verbascum thapsus*	3 drops tincture
Elecampane *Inula helenium*	3 drops tincture
Aniseed *Pimpinella anisum*	2 drops tincture
Golden seal *Hydrastis canadensis*	2 drops tincture

If there is severe whooping and spasms, add the following:

Gum weed *Grindelia camporum*	2 drops tincture
or	
Lobelia *Lobelia inflata*	2 drops tincture
or	
Sundew *Drosera rotundifolia*	2 drops tincture

Explanation. This prescription focuses more on eliminating mucus from the lungs than on stopping the whoop and spasms. The first three are expectorant tonics. Elecampane is included because of its antiseptic and antispasmodic properties. Aniseed is a tonic to the digestive system, and golden seal removes mucus from the entire system. It is preferred here to black root *Leptandra virginica* because it is more stimulating, which is what these children usually need. If the spasms are significant, gum weed, lobelia, or sundew may be added as an antispasmodic.

Results. Progress is slower in this disease pattern because two things need to be done at the same time. The body needs to get rid of thick mucus while simultaneously clearing looser mucus from the lungs. Over the first 7 to 10 days, one can expect the lungs to clear considerably and thus the child will have more energy. The appetite should improve a bit over this time. After the mucus is eliminated from the lungs, the cough may change and become more like the traditional whooping cough. At this stage it may be necessary to change the prescription to the previous one.

WEAKNESS

Thyme *Thymus vulgaris*	3 drops tincture
Elecampane *Inula helenium*	3 drops tincture
Aniseed *Pimpinella anisum*	2 drops tincture
Angelica *Angelica archangelica*	2 drops tincture
Licorice *Glycyrrhiza glabra*	2 drops tincture

If the child has significant spasms or whoops, add the following:

Gum weed *Grindelia camporum*	2 drops tincture
or	
Sundew *Drosera rotundifolia*	2 drops tincture

If the child is cold and pale, add the following:

Ginger *Zingiber officinalis*	2 drops tincture

Explanation. There is more emphasis here on tonics. Thyme, elecampane, aniseed, and angelica are all digestive tonics. Thyme and elecampane also clear the lungs of mucus. Gum weed and sundew are antispasmodics for the chest, and ginger warms the digestive system and the entire body.

Results. There may be real difficulty in getting children to take the herbs. If they refuse to take by mouth, then use correspondingly larger quantities in a bath so that the herbs are absorbed through the skin. Alternatively, apply essential oils externally.

Provided that the herbs are taken, one should notice some change after a few days. Continue to give the herbs for 10 days. If there is still no change, try another therapy. This may sound like a short time for a trial, but 10 days seems like a very long time to the parents of a Weak child.

▪ OTHER TREATMENTS

Thyme Tea and Thyme Baths

Thyme is one of the main herbs for treating whooping cough, and moreover, it is widely available in the cookery section of a supermarket. If no other herbs are available, make a tea from 1 tsp of dried herb. Allow the tea to stand until lukewarm and then sweeten it. Get the child to drink as much and as often as possible, at least three times a day, and also in the night when the coughing spasms start.

The longer the herb is left to steep during in making the tea, the more bitter and rubbery it tastes. This taste makes it harder to get the child to drink it, but it is better for the digestive system. Parent will have to work to strike a balance between these two.

Thyme may also be used in the bath. A lot more of the herb is needed—about 1 to 2 Tbsp to 10 L (2 gallons) of water. This treatment is very effective for babies whose bath amounts are still small. Putting babies in this bath several times a day is just as effective as giving the herbs and is a lot easier.

Garlic on the Feet

An old remedy is to crush a whole garlic, put it inside a cotton bag or handkerchief, and tie it onto the soles of the feet overnight. The garlic helps to soften the mucus and reduce the severity of the cough. This treatment is necessary only if the herbs discussed earlier are not available.

--- A Word of Caution ---

Test the child's sensitivity to garlic. Some children break out in blisters if the garlic is left on for more than 2 hours.

■ ESSENTIAL OILS
For Massage

Lavender *Lavandula officinalis*	5 drops
Hyssop *Hyssopus officinalis*	5 drops
Thyme *Thymus vulgare*	5 drops
Cypress *Cupressus sempervirens*	5 drops

For the Weak pattern, add the following:

Fennel *Foeniculum vulgare*	5 drops

For the mucus type, add the following:

Eucalyptus *Eucalyptus globulus*	5 drops

Add to 30 ml (1 oz) of massage oil and rub into the chest. These oils may be used simply as an application, or a more active massage may be given as described in Chapter 18.

For a Diffuser

Thyme *Thymus vulgare*	10 drops
Hyssop *Hyssopus officinalis*	10 drops
Eucalyptus *Eucalyptus globulus*	10 drops

Put these oils into a diffuser or drop them into very hot water and allow the vapor to fill the room.

■ MANAGEMENT

The child should be kept warm. It is good for the child to go outside in the fresh air, but be sure that the child is clothed properly and is not exposed to wind. The child should have extra rest during the day to make up for sleep lost at night.

Treatment in Orthodox Medicine

There is no treatment for the whooping cough itself.* Many physicians advise giving prophylactic antibiotics, in small doses, to prevent opportunistic bacterial infection. Other physicians advise giving antibiotics only when an opportunistic infection occurs. This reduces the risk of developing of antibiotic-resistant bacteria.

When Is a Child Infectious?

The infecting agent for whooping cough is the bacterium *B. pertussis*, and it is present only in the first

---

*This is not strictly true. It has been found that erythromycin kills the bacterium *B. pertussis*. Unfortunately, this does not shorten the course of the illness. It is believed that killing the bacterium will reduce the spread of the illness to other members of the family.

stage of whooping cough—the stage when it is still a mild cough and the whoop has not developed. Once the cough is obviously whooping cough, the child is no longer infectious.

When Can the Child Go Back to School?

Children should be kept at home during the first stage of the disease, when they are infectious, and for the first part of the second stage, when the cough is very severe and they are losing a lot of sleep. Once their energy has recovered, they can go back to play school or day care—if the school will accept them back and if they do not get overtired.

■ ADVICE

One of the main dangers of whooping cough is that the child becomes exhausted and undernourished because of repeated vomiting. One way to overcome this problem is to give the main meal of the day before noon. The later in the day that the food is given, the more likely it is to be vomited back.

The Dr. Bach Rescue Remedy can be very helpful in allaying the fear and panic surrounding a coughing attack. We advise putting a glass of water with a few drops of Rescue Remedy beside the child's bed at night so that it is easy for the child to take a few sips in the night. If the mother is also overwhelmed by fear, it will be beneficial for her too.

■ DANGERS

The main dangers from whooping cough are exhaustion and opportunistic bacterial infection. There is another danger as well—that the child suffocates; however, this is an extremely rare occurrence.

Exhaustion

Those most at risk from the dangers of whooping cough are children who become exhausted. Infants (those younger than 1 year) are easily exhausted. Older children who are Weak to start with or those

for whom the long duration of the cough leads them to become thin and weak may become exhausted. When children are exhausted, they may easily succumb to another infection or even lose the will to live and stop breathing. Whooping cough should be monitored very carefully in these exhausted children. Children who show signs of turning blue, of very faint breathing, or of stopping breathing should be taken straight to the hospital.

Opportunistic Bacterial Infection

An opportunistic bacterial infection is unlikely to occur if the child starts taking herbal medicine early enough. It is likely to happen later on if the child has become exhausted. To start with, the symptoms may be similar to those of acute bronchitis. The difference is that the infection occurs in addition to whooping cough, and this combination makes progression to pneumonia likely.

SYMPTOMS
- Red face
- Fever
- Painful cough

When these symptoms appear, rapid treatment is necessary to prevent the development of pneumonia. In principle this condition can be cured with herbs, but we have no experience with it. The herbs of choice would be those given for the Hot pattern of acute cough. If these do not work or if you are unsure of what to do, it may be appropriate to give the child antibiotics.

Long-Term Problems

Whooping cough can go the "wrong way" when the complications are so great that they create long-term health problems. The most common is that the lungs are weakened. After a bad attack it may take years for the lungs to recover. We have even had adult patients who have become asthmatic after 50 years of age, whose asthma could be traced back to whooping cough when they were young. However, our experience is that with good care and the use of herbs, these problems can nearly always be averted.

Long-Term Benefits

When whooping cough is overcome without the child becoming exhausted or the lungs being damaged through so much coughing, the child's health can improve. In particular, the appetite is much improved. Even before the coughing is completely over, the child starts to eat more and a wider variety of foods. This improved appetite is reflected in other areas as well, as evidenced by the child becoming more enthusiastic and more robust.

◾ PREVENTION

As we have explained, whooping cough is a way the body gets rid of thick mucus from the digestive system. The long-term effects can be beneficial. Therefore we should ask ourselves whether we should really be trying to prevent the disease from happening at all. The answer is probably yes, or at least we should attempt to reduce its severity, but in our opinion it should not be through mass immunization. The immunization is only 80% to 90% effective, according to a conventional pediatrics textbook.* Others give a much lower figure.† Therefore the risk of development of the disease is still significant. The immunization is known to have many side effects, which can be detrimental to the health of the child and can even predispose a

child to development of asthma, a far more serious disease. In addition, it has been our experience that immunized children may get a cough with many symptoms similar to those of whooping cough, but which is much harder to cure.

A more effective method of management is to give treatments that will reduce the severity of the disease when it appears. Not generally recognized is the fact that in the past most people got whooping cough, but only a few exhibited the whooping symptoms. For most children, all that happened was that they got a bad cough; that is, the disease never progressed beyond the first stage. The children for whom this happened were those who did not have very much mucus in the body initially. There was no possibility of the disease progressing to the second stage because these children simply did not have any ropy mucus in the body.

This situation points the way to "prevention" of whooping cough. One does not try to prevent infection from the bacterium, but one tries to eliminate as much thick mucus out of the body as possible so that when infection occurs, the symptoms are only mild.

Mucus can eliminated with herbs. Some prescriptions are given in Chapter 23. These prescriptions can be given by anyone, although we recommend consulting an herbal practitioner. It is difficult to be objective about one's own child when trying to strengthen the constitution.

An alternative is the "homeopathic immunization." This is given by homeopathic practitioners.

---

*Quoted in Lissauer T, Clayden G: *Illustrated textbook of paediatrics,* London, 1997, Mosby.
†Coulter HL, Fisher BL: p New York, 1987, Avery Publishing Group.

23

Immunizations

In this chapter we describe some of the side effects, both acute and chronic, that are seen after an immunization. We give ways to strengthen a child before an immunization to reduce the severity of side effects and also provide treatments for when they do occur.

■ THE DEBATE ABOUT IMMUNIZATIONS

The debate over immunizations has been fierce since the first immunization was developed by Jenner for smallpox. Those who support immunization are rarely willing to admit that any side effects whatsoever occur, either short term or long term. Opponents of immunization are rarely willing to admit that there are any benefits. Arguments seem to start from the conclusion and to choose facts that support the conclusion. Both sides use scare tactics to recruit supporters.

This situation is unfortunate. Playing on people's fears in this way precludes rational debate. Thus we will not present a detailed discussion of the pros and cons of immunization. The subject is too complex to be covered in a book of this size without distorting our aim, which is to present the best treatment for children.

Our personal opinion is that the dangers of immunizations far outweigh the benefits for most children. This opinion on its own is not of much value, for it is up to the parents to decide the best course for their child. They are the ones who have to look after their child through illness—whether this comes from the immunization or the disease itself. Parents have very different opinions, based on their own fears and experiences and on their ability to handle acute illness.

We suggest that practitioners and parents inform themselves about the pros and cons of immunization (see Bibliography at the end of this book) and also learn how to treat the childhood diseases when they occur. We believe that it is unethical to advise parents not to have their child immunized if they do not have a way of treating the diseases when they occur. Moreover, we believe that it is essential for parents to have access to as much unbiased information as possible so that they can make an informed decision.

What Happens in Immunization

The principal of immunization is to give a child a mild version of the illness you wish to protect against. For example, for whooping cough, dead cells (or serum) of *Bordetella pertussis* are injected. The immune system recognizes the dead cells and develops antibodies against them, which are also effective against live cells. For polio, the virus is first attenuated by being given to monkeys. The virus that is adapted to monkeys is less harmful to humans.

Thus, when a baby is immunized, a disease is actually being given. The hope is that the disease given will be a mild version and that the baby will get over it quickly, but nevertheless a disease is being given. This fact explains the reactions, which are the same as those one would expect if a child suddenly got an infection. The symptoms appear immediately after immunization or during the next day or two. Longer-term effects are also seen.

Who Is Likely to Be Adversely Affected by Immunizations?

One of our colleagues summed up his interpretation of the literature on immunization as follows: "It is the weak children who are likely to be badly affected by the childhood diseases, but it is these same children who are at risk from the immunizations!" We believe this statement to be largely true, and our approach to the childhood diseases is to strengthen the child. Parents must ultimately choose whether to immunize the child.

Why Immunizations Lead to the Echo Pattern

Immunizations are now the most common cause of echo patterns. There are many possible reasons for this. One reason commonly put forward by alternative practitioners is that immunizations are given by an unusual route. When a child contracts measles or whooping cough, it is from infection taken in through the nose and mouth. They suggest that if the disease is injected directly into the bloodstream, it produces a different result. Our observation is that the inflammation and mucus in the system, two key signs of the echo pattern, increase.

Another reason is that immunizations are now given intensively to very young babies. A common age to start is 2 months old, with additional injections at 4, 6, and 12 months. In most of Europe and the United States, the standard practice is for a child to have received at least 16 immunizations, often with several given at one time, by the age of 12 months. An onslaught like this will overstrain all but the strongest constitutions.

The question of immunizations is complex. You should study all facets of the problem before making your decision. Find out what the real dangers of the childhood illnesses are in your area. Above all, we advise practitioners and parents alike to learn how to nurse and treat childhood illnesses when they occur.

Immunizations and the Herbalist

Although immunizations are introduced by an abnormal route, the imbalances they cause are not very different from those that can appear naturally after a severe illness in the form of an echo pattern. Understanding this opens the way for resolving any imbalances caused by immunizations. The immunizations leave a clearly recognizable pattern that can be treated.

For this reason, we devote this chapter to ways of preparing a child for immunizations so that any adverse effects will be minimized. We also give some information about how to identify longer-term side effects and what can be done about them.

▪ PREPARATION FOR IMMUNIZATION

Many children receive their immunizations with few immediate ill effects. A minority of children have terrible side effects, including brain damage.

In others there are short- and long-term effects. We have repeatedly stressed in this book the importance of the child's overall health in fighting disease. If a child is reasonably well in balance, an attack of a childhood disease will be milder and the disease course will be shorter than if the child is out of balance before the illness starts. The same principle holds for immunizations, so the preparation for immunization is to build up the child's strength and to correct the major imbalances.

There are many imbalances that a child may have, but there are three main patterns to look out for both before and after an immunization. Children with these symptoms and signs before immunization will be more likely to have a bad reaction to it. Likewise, after the immunization, these patterns will probably still be there. If a child has these symptoms and signs before immunization, the best advice is to urge parents to delay the immunization until the worst symptoms have been resolved. This may take approximately 1 month.

The three main patterns are the following:

- Mucus
- Heat
- Weakness

This discussion is a great oversimplification, but it is nevertheless a good place to start.

Why These Three?

We have chosen these three imbalances to look for because they are the ones that will probably cause the most trouble when a child is immunized. These three imbalances are likely to be aggravated by any infectious illness and thus also by any immunization.

This is certainly what we find in clinical practice. Some children get horrendous side effects from immunizations, but the vast majority do not. On the other hand, the vast majority *do* get a fever after immunizations; they *do* get a lot of mucus production, with a cough or cold, or at least a runny nose; and they *do* get exhausted and tired, often having a poor appetite for some time. Other changes also are seen, and each child reacts differently, but these three patterns are very common. If a child already has a significant imbalance in one of these patterns, the immunization will make it much worse and this may be the factor that turns a healthy child with a slight imbalance into a sick child. For example, if a lot of mucus is present and this amount is increased, the child can easily develop a bad cough, which may eventually turn into asthma. Likewise, if the child is already very Hot, the extra heat generated by the fever after the immunization may be enough to cause febrile convulsions.

■ SYMPTOMS AND SIGNS*

Typical symptoms and signs of these patterns have been given elsewhere, but we repeat them again here:

---

*Facial color reveals a lot about a child's energy. See p. 54 for a discussion of facial colors and variations among racial groups.

Mucus

- Repeated coughing
- Nasal discharge
- Swollen lymph nodes
- Gray face

Heat

- Has a red face and lips
- Is easily angered but is lovely when not angry
- Is uncomfortable in hot weather
- Is restless
- Sweats easily
- Hates wearing a lot of clothes
- Is a light sleeper
- Throws bedclothes off at night
- Sleeps on back with arms and legs stretched out

VARIATION: STAGNANT FOOD PATTERN

The child will also have the following:

- Swollen abdomen
- Red cheeks
- Irregular stools (constipation or diarrhea)
- Foul-smelling stools

VARIATION: ECHO PATTERN

The echo pattern may be locking in the heat, in which case the following will be seen:

- Swollen lymph nodes
- Dry or rough skin
- Discolored patch on cheek
- Recurrent illness such as tonsillitis or recurrent cough

Weakness

- Pale face; possibly slight yellow tinge to the face
- Rather droopy
- Often shy
- Not very forceful
- Poor appetite, very picky and choosy about food
- Often constipated; occasionally loose stools
- Easily cries

- Thin arms and legs or rather squashy arms and legs (without good tone)
- Easily tired
- May sleep during the day

VARIATION: OVERSTIMULATED
The symptoms as the same as for the previous pattern except for the following:

  - Has boundless energy
  - Does not want to go to bed
  - Seems to get his or her own way all the time

▪ TREATMENT*

In keeping with our standard practice in this book, the dosages we give are for children aged 3 years (Table 23-1), even though most immunizations are given to children much younger than this age. The prescriptions we give are only samples to provide a starting point and may be altered for the individual child. The dosages we suggest are *suggestions only*. Each child may need something different.

Mucus

Hyssop *Hyssopus officinalis*	3 drops tincture
Elecampane *Inula helenium*	3 drops tincture
Golden seal *Hydrastis canadensis*	2 drops tincture

Table 23-1	
AGE	**MULTIPLY 3-YEAR-OLD DOSE BY**
6-12 months	$\times \frac{1}{3}$
1-2 years	$\times \frac{1}{2}$
2-4 years	$\times 1$
4-7 years	$\times 1\frac{1}{2}$
7-14 years	$\times 2$
14+ years	$\times 3$

*For more detailed information about dosages, see Chapter 8.

Two other herbs may also be of use:

Elderflower *Sambucus nigra*	$\frac{1}{4}$ tsp herb or 3 drops tincture
Aniseed *Pimpinella anisum*	$\frac{1}{4}$ tsp herb or 3 drops tincture

Elderflower and aniseed may be given as a tea or as drops of tincture

Explanation. Hyssop is an all-purpose tonic for the lungs. Elecampane clears mucus from the lungs and stimulates the digestive system. Golden seal clears mucus from the entire system and is a mild stimulant. Elderflower clears chronic mucus from the lungs, and aniseed tones the digestive system. These two may be added to help remove mucus, or if supplies are difficult to obtain, these two may be used on their own.

Results. At first the child may have a slight increase in mucus discharge. The child may appear to have caught a cold as a result of taking the herbs. This symptom may persist for up to 1 week, and then it should gradually subside, leaving the child with less mucus. The time needed for the mucus to be cleared varies. It can take 1 or 2 months, so do not be in too much of a hurry. When the mucus has been cleared, the child may be given the immunization.

Heat

Pasque flower *Anemone pulsatilla*	1 drop tincture
Catnip *Nepeta cataria*	2 drops tincture

VARIATION: STAGNANT FOOD PATTERN
This should be treated with the addition of the following:

Black root *Leptandra virginica*	3 drops tincture

In addition, advice should be given about the diet. If the child has insomnia, consult Chapter 25 for suitable herbs.

VARIATION: ECHO PATTERN

Add the following:

Poke root *Phytolacca decandra*	2 drops tincture
Blue flag *Iris versicolor*	2 drops tincture

Explanation. Pasque flower is cooling and also helps bring heat to the surface. Catnip is also cooling. Black root is specific for the stagnant food pattern. Poke root and blue flag together are very good for the echo pattern and have the effect of softening thick mucus.

Results. The child should gradually calm down. If pasque flower is given, it sometimes increases restlessness for 1 or 2 days.

If the child has the stagnant food pattern, a significant discharge of stools will be seen. The dosage of black root should be adjusted accordingly. See Chapters 10 and 11 for a more detailed discussion of these short-term effects.

When poke root and blue flag are taken, one should look for an increase in mucus. Sometimes the only sign that the herbs are working is that the child has to clear the throat a few times upon arising in the morning. Then, as the herbs start to work over the next few weeks, rough skin should disappear and behavior should start to change. In some children the initial dosage of herbs is too high, and they may have a sudden evacuation of mucus, which makes you think they have diarrhea. If this happens, stop the herbs and start them again at a lower dosage when the stools have returned to normal. When a significant reduction in the heat signs occurs, the child is as prepared as possible for the immunization.

Weakness

Fennel *Foeniculum vulgare*	4 drops tincture
Sweet sedge *Acorus calamus*	2 drops tincture
Licorice *Glycyrrhiza glabra*	2 drops tincture

If the child will take it, add the following:

Gentian *Gentiana lutea*	2 drops tincture

If vomiting, constipation or diarrhea, or bad appetite is present, see the relevant chapter.

VARIATION: OVERSTIMULATED

The herbs are the same. However, you may have difficulty in persuading the child to take them, but do persevere. A child's long-term health is more important than temporary likes and dislikes. If the child absolutely refuses to take the herbs, then a massage with essential oils, as described in Chapter 14, may be a suitable alternative.

Explanation. Fennel is a general tonic for the digestive system. Sweet sedge is a bitter tonic and improves the appetite. Some children find its taste too bitter, but many have no problem taking it. Licorice is another sweet tonic, and it influences the whole body. Gentian is very bitter but is a marvelous tonic for the stomach and to build up the whole body.

Results. The child should have more energy and more enthusiasm for life. He or she should start to take much more interest in food and hopefully will have a better appetite. The key sign for deciding whether it is all right to proceed with immunization is an improvement in the child's energy and enthusiasm. It is not necessary to wait until the child's appetite is definitely improved. The other signs, such as mood, energy, and color of the face, determine whether the child is strong enough to take the next round of immunizations.

■ THE IMMUNIZATION

Common Reactions

When a child receives an immunization some sort of reaction is usually seen. The following are common reactions during the first few days:

- Swollen lump at site of injection
- Cough, cold, or nasal discharge
- Fever, restlessness, or crying

- Crying at night or excessive sleepiness
- Diarrhea (stools green or variable in color, often with bad smell or lumps of mucus)
- Poor appetite

Some of the less common but more serious reactions to immunizations are the following:

- Seizures: conv.ulsions, epilepsy, or infantile spasms
- Brain inflammation
- Loss of muscle control (paralysis), often one-sided
- Aching joints
- Thrombocytopenic purpura or hemolytic anemia
- Diabetes and hypoglycemia
- Cot death (sudden infant death syndrome)

Contraindications to Immunization (from the Orthodox Medical Point of View)

Do ensure that your physician has established that your child has no contraindications to immunization. Much depends on the individual case, but in general, immunizations are contraindicated if any of the following criteria are met:

- The child has had convulsions (fits).
- There is a family history of epilepsy.
- The child has already had the disease.
- The child is hyperactive.

If immunizations are given to these children, they may have a very violent reaction, possibly with convulsions, development of epilepsy, paralysis on one side of the body, or brain damage. In many places doctors are overworked and do not have the time to check to see if a child has any of these contraindications. Note also that if the child is allergic to eggs, a specially prepared vaccine may be necessary because many ordinary vaccines are made using egg protein.

Other Points to Watch for

- Does the child twitch? If so, this is an indication that he or she might get convulsions from an immunization.
- Is the child teething? If so, wait until this has passed.

▪ AFTER THE IMMUNIZATION

During the first week, the child may have many symptoms, such as a bad fever or an acute cough. These symptoms should be treated in the ways described in the relevant chapters.

After the first week, the main side effects of immunization should have worn off, but some children still may not be quite well. The three most common patterns seen at this stage are the same ones given earlier—mucus, heat, and weakness—and the treatment is exactly the same. Especially common is the variation of echo pattern. Besides these patterns or sometimes in addition to them are some specific symptoms for different immunizations. Symptoms we have observed are described in the following sections.

Measles

The onset of the effects is usually sudden. The child is often extremely hot. The skin is red, and it looks as though the child has a fever. It is common for the child to have a yellow nasal discharge and a productive cough. From time to time one sees a dry, scaly eczema. For the details of treatment of these symptoms, see the relevant chapters.

Polio

About 3 or 4 weeks after the immunization, the child develops a bad cough, often with white opaque nasal discharge. This effect may be seen in children who have never had a cough before, and it comes so long after the immunization (4 weeks is a long time when you have a growing baby or child) that the connection is easy to miss.

This effect should be treated like a chronic cough (see Chapter 17). Sometimes the herbs work initially, but they never seem to get rid of the mucus altogether. In our experience the next therapy to try is homeopathy, and the remedy that has been effective is the nosode Polio 30C. One or two doses of this remedy will often eliminate the last stages of mucus in a week or so.

A Word of Caution

Do not give the homeopathic remedy immediately after the immunization unless you are experienced in using homeopathy. This remedy should be given only in the last stages, after all the herbs have been given but a plateau in the treatment has been reached and the child's condition is still not improving. A better alternative is to consult a homeopathic practitioner before homeopathic remedies are used.

Whooping Cough

The reaction to the immunization for whooping cough is just as strange. Besides leaving a dry cough, which is an echo of the original disease, some children get a feverish illness regularly once a month after the immunization. A common reaction is for the child to get either a fever or otitis media about every 30 days. We do not know the reason, but we have found that this pattern of cyclical illness points to the whooping cough immunization. It also points to the treatment. Once again, we recommend starting with herbs for the symptoms of cough. When a plateau in the treatment is reached, it is time to go to a homeopathic nosode. In this case it is Pertussin 30C. The reaction to the homeopathic remedy can be severe, with a fever and aggravation of the cough during the first week so. Again, we advise consulting a homeopathic practitioner if you do not have experience in using these remedies.

■ OTHER THERAPIES

There are many other therapies that can be of benefit in preparing a child for immunizations. One that we would single out is craniosacral osteopathy. There are two situations in which this is of special use: (1) when a child has had a difficult birth or a severe blow to the head and (2) when there are spinal lesions.

When a child has had a difficult birth or a severe blow to the head, there may still be mild brusing in the brain and the cranial rhythms may still be disrupted. If a child is a given an immunizatoin in this condition, there is severe risk of brain damage. Craniosacral osteopathy can help restore the cranial rhythms and reduce this risk.

When a child has a spinal lesion (a displacement of one or more of the vertebrae from the proper position), this results in a blockage of energy in the spine. If a child then has a polio immunization or indeed the disease itself, there is a higher risk of paralysis developing, focused on the lesion. If any sort of osteopathy is given, it can reduce the risk of paralysis.

■ MAIN POINTS FROM THIS CHAPTER

- A healthy child is less likely to suffer side effects and more likely to receive beneficial effects from the immunization.
- Wait until your child is healthy. Do not be pressured to immunize when a child is still sick.

24

Ear Infections (Otitis Media)

Ear infections are common in babies and young children. Most children have an earache at one time or another, but some children have earaches repeatedly. In other children the pain is almost continuous, with added acute flare-ups. Ear infections are regarded with fear by most people. One reason is that pain in the ear is very distressing and can easily lead to panic in the child and the parents. Another reason is the fear of complications, although for most children this fear is unfounded: The great majority of earaches resolve by themselves and cause no damage. The occurrence of mastoiditis, the most common complication of the past, has almost disappeared. Hearing loss is very rarely caused by ear infections.*

What Is an Ear Infection?

Anatomically, the ear is divided into three parts, which are more or less separate and can develop problems independently (Figure 24-1). Generally, three types of ear infections are seen:

Otitis externa: inflammation of the ear canal
Otitis media: the most common type of ear infection in which the middle part of the ear becomes inflamed
Otitis interna: an extremely rare condition in which the innermost part of the ear becomes inflamed, usually with the mastoid

The external ear up to the eardrum can be seen with an otoscope (auriscope). Looking directly at the eardrum provides a great deal of information.

In this chapter we consider otitis media, which is the most common ear infection in children. We give remedies for treating pain during an acute episode and also for treating the underlying condition to prevent recurrent attacks.

■ CAUSES AND PATTERNS

Middle ear infections are thought to be caused by a virus or bacterium, which migrates from the upper respiratory tract along the eustachian tube. Various reasons are suggested for the particular susceptibility of children. Among these are the small size of the tubes relative to the ear, which allows them to be blocked easily; another is that babies who are fed in a supine position are at risk because this position encourages reflux of milk into the eustachian tube.

Ear infections are often seen in conjunction with throat or respiratory infections. The eustachian tube connects the throat and from there the respiratory tract to the ears; therefore it is easy for infections to pass from one location to the other.

These simple anatomic details alone cannot explain why some children are so susceptible to earaches. The reason, as noted throughout this book, is that the way a child reacts to a bacterium or virus depends on the underlying health of that particular child. Therefore to understand earaches we must look beyond the external causes to the internal imbalances in the body. When we do this

*Mendelsohn RS: *How to raise a healthy child*, New York, 1984, Ballantine.

265

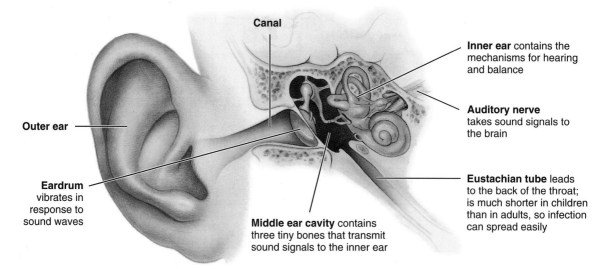

Canal

Inner ear contains the
mechanisms for hearing
and balance

Auditory nerve
takes sound signals to
the brain

Outer ear

Eustachian tube leads
to the back of the throat;
is much shorter in children
than in adults, so infection
can spread easily

Eardrum
vibrates in
response to
sound waves

Middle ear cavity contains
three tiny bones that transmit
sound signals to the inner ear

Figure 24-1   Anatomy of the ear. (Modified from Thibodeau GA, Patton KT: *Anatomy & physiology*, ed 4, St Louis, 1999, Mosby.)

we find very clear reasons and patterns of energy. By treating these patterns we can help resolve otitis media permanently.

Internal Factors

The internal factors that predispose children to ear infections include the following:

- Excessive buildup of mucus
- Internal heat
- Local or general Weakness of energy

EXPLANATION

If there is excessive mucus in the system, the eustachian tubes become full of mucus. The air no longer circulates there, and thus a breeding ground for bacteria and viruses is created.

Internal heat in the body particularly affects the head and ears. If a child is hot, it is common to find subacute inflammation in the ears. Only a small trigger is then needed to set off a full inflammatory response in the form of an acute earache.

When the energy is Weak, the immune system is also weakened, so the child cannot easily fight infection.

CAUSES

Diet. Diet has a direct effect on digestion, and if the digestive system is not working well, the entire system may become full of mucus or may become too hot or Weak. Common dietary causes are intolerance to cow's milk, greasy foods, and peanuts, all of which predispose to earaches. In children younger than 3 years, there are additional factors of overeating and irregular eating, which may contribute to the stagnant food pattern.

Immunizations and Echo Diseases. Immunizations can produce an acute attack as an immediate aftereffect but can also cause the echo pattern with thick mucus and heat, predisposing a child to ear infections. Pertussis immunization is a common cause of monthly recurring attacks of otitis media. Echo patterns also arise when a disease does not fully resolve. This situation is common when an acute earache is treated with antibiotics because the bacteria or virus never quite gets expelled from the ear. With each earache the ear becomes a little weaker and is more likely to succumb to another attack.

Weak Energy. The causes of Weak energy are outlined in Chapter 2.

Stress and Emotions. Stress and emotions are rarely mentioned in association with earaches, but we have found that holding in strong feelings can predispose children to earaches. The mechanism seems to be that the repressed feelings or stress causes Heat in the child. In today's society children are often told that expressing anger is unacceptable behavior, and they subsequently "boil up with rage." The Heat causes subacute inflammation in the body, with the ears being particularly affected. (Chinese medicine has long recognized this situation and for many centuries has listed suppressed emotion as a cause for ear infections.)

External Triggers

With these internal predispositions, any small external trigger can cause an acute attack. Some common triggers are the following:

- Exposure to cold wind
- Upper respiratory tract infection
- Water in the ears (from swimming or washing the hair)
- Teething
- Aftereffects of any immunization
- Pertussis immunization, which may cause monthly recurring attacks*

If a child has a tendency for earaches, recommend that you strengthen him or her before giving immunizations, especially pertussis. See Chapter 23.

■ SYMPTOMS OF ACUTE EAR INFECTION

Symptoms of acute otitis media vary considerably but may include the following:

- Pain, ranging from mild discomfort to excruciating
- Crying, rubbing, or tugging at the ear

---

*This is an observation we have made in our own clinic, for which we have no explanation.

- General misery, loss of appetite, irritability, and poor sleep
- Panic (with severe attacks)
- Raised temperature
- Partial deafness
- Discharge from the ear
- Swollen lymph nodes under the ear

Diagnosis

The specific orthodox diagnosis is often complex. The key questions for diagnosis and treatment with herbs are the following:

- Is the eardrum very red and bulging?
- Is there pain?
- Is there discharge from the ear? If so, is it clear or yellow?
- Is the middle ear permanently blocked?

■ TREATMENT DURING ACUTE PAINFUL ATTACKS

Treatment with herbs presents a welcome contrast to the glaring absence of any effective treatment in orthodox medicine other than pain-killing drugs and the use of antibiotics.

Calming Panic

Severe pain in a child is usually accompanied by panic—both in the child and in the parents. This panic causes the energy to rush up to the head, and while the child is in a state of panic, the pain is difficult to relieve. The panic is part of the illness. Often, merely calming the mother and child opens the way for the ear infection to resolve.

PRESCRIPTIONS
- Dr. Bach Rescue Remedy

Place 1 or 2 drops under the tongue or on the lips of the child every 5 minutes until the panic subsides. The panic should subside within 15 to 20 minutes. If it does not, then an alternative remedy is needed. If the mother is affected by the panic, she too may take the Rescue Remedy.

HOMEOPATHY
- Aconitum 6X or 6C, *or*
- Arnica 6X or 6C

Place a dose under the child's tongue every 5 minutes until the panic subsides. You should not usually have to do this more than three times. When the panic has subsided, the child may still be quite distressed because the pain will still be there. However, the whole demeanor of the child will be different.

Stopping the Pain

The most effective treatments involve warm eardrops, usually oil based. The drops are easily warmed to the right temperature by first placing a teaspoon in hot water and then pouring the oil into the warm spoon. Take care not to burn the ear with overheated oil or the hot spoon.

── A Word of Caution ──

Do not overheat eardrops! Do not put eardrops into a perforated ear because of the danger of introducing infection into the middle ear.

EARDROPS
The following are some suggestions for eardrops:
- Olive oil by itself
- Olive oil with garlic and mullein
- Olive oil with essential oils
- Tincture of ribwort

The simplest prescription is olive oil by itself. Warm some on a spoon and drop it into the ear. This may be improved upon by including the following:

- Garlic *Allium sativum*
- Mullein *Verbascum thapsus*

Garlic heals and contains an antibiotic.* Mullein is very soothing to the mucous membranes. In many places garlic and mullein oil is commercially available in convenient dropper bottles. Otherwise, it is easy to make. Details are given in Chapter 8.

HERBAL TINCTURES
Ribwort plantain *Plantago lanceolata*   As a tincture

A few drops of tincture, preferably diluted 1:10 and warmed, may be placed in the ear. Like garlic, ribwort contains an antibiotic; thus, in addition to being soothing for inflammatory conditions, it is appropriate for bacterial conditions as well.

ESSENTIAL OILS FOR EAR INFECTIONS
Lavender *Lavandula officinalis*   3 drops
Chamomile *Chamomilla matricaria*   3 drops
Ti-tree *Melaleuca alternifolia*   6 drops

Add all of these ingredients to a bottle containing 30 ml (1 oz) of a base oil. Place a few drops into the affected ear. These three oils effectively reduce the pain and infection. All are bactericidal, and ti-tree is also an antiviral.

EMERGENCY PRESCRIPTION
If none of these remedies is available, use any medicine that is prescribed for sore eyes. For example, Optrex, although designed for reducing inflammation in the conjunctiva, also reduces inflammation of the eardrum.

Besides using herbal remedies, simply warming the ear is often helpful. Use either a hot water bottle or a hot pack, made by filling a sock with rice and putting it in a microwave oven for 1 or 2 minutes. (Test it on yourself first to see whether it is too hot. Babies have very delicate skin that burns easily.)

---

*In the 1970s, the Chinese developed a procedure for treating ruptured eardrums. It involved putting a slice of garlic in the ear to provide a support for the new membrane. This procedure was so successful that it became the standard treatment in many hospitals.

RESULTS

The worst of the pain should pass within about 30 minutes. Pain may still linger after this and inflammation is likely, but the pain will be bearable. In a healthy child an ear infection usually resolves without the need for further treatment.

If the child has a fever, it should be treated accordingly. See Chapter 16.

VARIATIONS

If the child has a cough or cold, this should be treated as well. See Chapter 19.

EAR CANDLES

Hopi "ear candles" have a good reputation for soothing pain in the ears. They consist of a tube of cardboard about 20 cm (8 inches) long impregnated in beeswax. The tube is inserted in the ear canal, and the other end is ignited. As the candle slowly burns down, the warmth and slight suction have a beneficial effect.

A Word of Caution

There are obvious dangers in using fire so close to a child, so the method is suitable only for children who can be relied on to stay still. Take care also that the surroundings are not flammable (e.g., avoid using the candle in bed or on a flammable floor).

Complications and Dangers

HEARING LOSS

Hearing loss usually occurs as a result of repeated ear infections and buildup of mucus in the middle ear.

BURST EARDRUM

When the pressure increases in the middle ear, the eardrum may rupture. This condition is very painful initially. At first blood comes out, followed by the liquid—serum or pus—that caused the rupture in the first place. In acute otitis media this happens very quickly. In chronic otitis media, there may be more or less continuous discharge from the ear.

If the eardrum bursts once or twice, it is not normally a cause for alarm because it nearly always heals itself. Only repeated bursting of the eardrum is likely to impair hearing.

MASTOIDITIS

Uncommon but serious problems arise if the inflammation spreads to other areas, such as the mastoid process, because it may lead to meningitis. These problems are extremely rare but must be treated immediately in the hospital.

▪ RECURRENT EAR INFECTIONS AND "GLUE EAR"

If a child has an ear infection once or twice during the first 7 years of life, this is normal. If a child has repeated infections, this is abnormal. Something is out of balance and needs to be addressed. We have discussed the general internal factors that predispose a child to ear infections. These tend to manifest as one of the following underlying patterns. After these patterns are resolved, the ear infections no longer occur.

In "glue ear," a viscous gluelike fluid collects behind the ear. The child experiences a sensation of blocked ears and has difficulty hearing. In severe cases hearing loss may be significant, and the child may begin talking later than normal and may not be successful in school, simply because he or she cannot hear clearly. Following are underlying patterns that cause glue ear and allow otitis to recur:

- Excessive mucus
- Stagnant food pattern (children younger than 3 years)
- Weak energy
- Weak energy with overstimulation
- Echo pattern

Each of these patterns can give rise to one of the factors—mucus, Heat, or weakness—that predisposes children to infection.

■ SYMPTOMS AND SIGNS*

Excessive Mucus

- The child usually has mucus in the lungs and blocking the ears.
- If the eardrum is ruptured, there may be discharge from the ears.
- Often, some hearing loss occurs because the ears are full of fluid or mucus.
- Often, the child has a rattly cough or a runny nose.
- The sinuses are congested.
- The mucus may be clear or yellow or green.
- Often, the child is a mouth breather because the respiratory tract and nasal passages are blocked with phlegm.

In extreme cases children are not living up to their potential and possibly may be doing badly in school because they have difficulty hearing the teacher.

Stagnant Food Pattern (Children Younger Than 3 Years)

- The child is sturdy and has red cheeks.
- The child usually has a good appetite.
- The stools smell sour or foul, and bowel movements may be irregular.
- The abdomen is often distended.
- The child's behavior is usually boisterous, with a tendency for irritability and anger.
- The child is usually warm or hot.
- Ear inflammation may come with teething.

Weak Energy

- The child tends to be rather thin and pale.
- The child is rather picky about food and has a poor appetite.
- The child often gets one infection after another.

VARIATION: WEAK ENERGY WITH OVERSTIMULATION

The symptoms are the same as those for the Weak energy pattern with the addition of the following:

- The child's energy is better, which does not fit with the amount of food eaten.
- The child dislikes going to bed.
- The child may insist on getting his or her own way all the time, is demanding, and challenges all boundaries.

Echo Pattern

- The child may have a history of chronic cough or a history of repeated illness treated with antibiotics.
- A patch of slightly depigmented skin is seen on the cheek.
- Some parts of the body have rough skin.
- There is a slightly glazed look in the child's eyes.
- The glands are swollen.

■ TREATMENT*

The dosages we give are for children aged 3 years (Table 24-1). The dosages we suggest are *suggestions only.* Each child may need something different.

Excessive Mucus Type

The following three herbs are generally very effective:

Elecampane *Inula helenium*   4 drops tincture

■ Table 24-1

AGE	MULTIPLY 3-YEAR-OLD DOSE BY
6-12 months	$\times \frac{1}{3}$
1-2 years	$\times \frac{1}{2}$
2-4 years	$\times 1$
4-7 years	$\times 1\frac{1}{2}$
7-14 years	$\times 2$
14+ years	$\times 3$

*Facial color reveals a lot about a child's energy. See p. 54 for a discussion of facial colors and variations among racial groups.

*For more detailed information about dosages, see Chapter 8.

Golden seal *Hydrastis canadensis*	2 drops tincture
Hyssop *Hyssopus officinale*	2 drops tincture

Explanation. Elecampane moves mucus from the digestion and also from the mucous membranes of the respiratory system. Golden seal is a wonderful herb that stimulates the entire system and rids the body of mucus. Hyssop works on the mucous membranes of the lung system.

Alternatives to Hyssop include the following:

Mullein *Verbascum thapsus*	2 drops tincture
or	
Elderflower *Sambucus nigra*	2 drops tincture

These herbs may be used instead of or in addition to hyssop. Mullein benefits all of the upper mucous membranes and reduces inflammation in them. Elderflower helps remove mucus from the upper respiratory tract.

Results. When you first give this remedy, a lot of mucus discharge may be seen. It may come out of the nose, or the child may even start to get a cough. In the first few weeks the child should have a bit more energy; then after 2 or 3 weeks, this energy may develop into stubbornness. After a few weeks of this, the child will feel a lot better. During this process the child may get another ear infection. Avoid giving antibiotics at this time if possible because they will set back the treatment.

Stagnant Food Pattern (Children Younger Than 3 Years)

Regulating what the child eats is of utmost importance. This is discussed at length in Chapters 2 and 3.

For children with this pattern, the following prescription will be helpful:

Black root *Leptandra virginica*	3 drops tincture
Butternut *Juglans cinerea*	2 drops tincture
Hyssop *Hyssopus officinale*	2 drops tincture

Explanation. These herbs together will help restore the digestive function. Black root regulates the liver and has a gentle laxative effect. Butternut also has a laxative effect. (Both of these herbs may be used when mild diarrhea is present, provided they are used in small quantities. For a further discussion of their usage, see Chapter 9). Hyssop works on the mucous membranes. As was discussed for the previous pattern, hyssop may be replaced by mullein or elderflower.

Results. When the herbs are first given, there may be an enormous discharge of stools, so be careful. This is not a bad thing, but it needs to be kept under control. During this process the child is often very irritable. Once the mass of partly digested food has been evacuated, the child will be much better. This should take only 1 or 2 weeks. During this time the child may be more irritable, and there may be some sleep problems.

Weak Digestion

Children with weak digestion are the hardest to help, particularly if they are the sort of children who manage to get their way all the time. They often try to maintain control by refusing to take the herbs. Thus you may have to eliminate some of the best herbs and give only those that taste "nice."

PRESCRIPTION 1

Angelica *Angelica archangelica*	4 drops tincture
Gentian *Gentiana lutea*	2 drops tincture
Aniseed *Pimpinella anisum*	2 drops tincture
Licorice *Glycyrrhiza glabra*	2 drops tincture

Explanation. This combination is a rather bitter-tasting prescription, but it is a strong tonic. Angelica removes mucus from the upper respiratory tract, gentian is a tonic for the stomach and the digestive system, aniseed is a gentler tonic for the whole digestive system, and licorice is a sweeter-tasting herb that tones the whole body.

PRESCRIPTION 2

Elderflower *Sambucus nigra*	4 drops tincture
Mullein *Verbascum thapsus*	3 drops tincture
Fennel *Foeniculum vulgare*	2 drops tincture
Licorice *Glycyrrhiza glabra*	2 drops tincture

If the child is constipated (passes stools less frequently than once a day), add the following:

Butternut *Juglans cinerea*   2 drops tincture

Explanation. Elderflower removes mucus from the upper respiratory tract. Mullein removes mucus and also reduces inflammation in the upper respiratory tract. Fennel is more of a tonic than aniseed. Again, licorice tones the whole system. Butternut is a gentle tonic laxative.

VARIATION: OVERSTIMULATED

The herbs are the same, but some ingenuity may be needed to get the child to take them. The child may have strong preferences for one herb over another. When this happens, you may include some herbs and leave out others. The final prescription should contain at least one herb for the digestive system and at least one for the upper respiratory tract. An alternative is to give massage with essential oils, as described in Chapter 14.

Results. It takes time to build up a child's energy. During the first month or two, it is not uncommon for the child to get another infection. The parents often get discouraged when this happens and need encouragement to continue treatment. It can be helpful to point out to them how some symptoms (e.g., appetite, mood, sleep) have in fact been gradually improving.

Echo Pattern

Poke root *Phytolacca decandra*   2 drops tincture
Blue flag *Iris versicolor*   2 drops tincture
Elecampane *Inula helenium*   2 drops tincture
Golden seal *Hydrastis canadensis*   2 drops tincture

Explanation. Poke root and blue flag are the two main herbs for softening the thick mucus associated with the echo pattern. Elecampane is included to keep the lungs and the other mucous membranes of the upper respiratory system free from the mucus that is released by the poke root and blue flag. Golden seal

is a digestive stimulant and tonic, with the special effect of removing mucus from the system.

Results. The herbs normally need to be taken for a few months. When poke root and blue flag are taken, one should look for an increase in mucus. Sometimes the only sign that the herbs are working is that the child has to clear his or her throat a few times upon arising in the morning. Then, as the herbs continue to work over the next 1 to 3 months, rough skin should disappear and the child's behavior will begin to change. In some children the initial dosage of herbs is too high, and they may have a sudden evacuation of mucus, which makes you think they have diarrhea. If this happens, stop the herbs and start them again at a lower dosage when the stools have returned to normal.

Even though the child is becoming healthier, setbacks may occur, so do not get discouraged if the child gets another infection after a few weeks. This does not mean that the herbs are not working; it means that they have not had enough time to work. More details of what to look for over a period of time are given in Chapter 17.

If it is known that the initial cause for recurrent infections was an immunization, these treatments may be enough, but also read Chapter 23 on the aftereffects of immunizations.

▪ ORTHODOX TREATMENT AND DISCUSSION

The treatment you are likely to be offered varies considerably from place to place. Some practitioners recommend conservative treatment, using only decongestants, whereas others always give antibiotics.

Discussion

There is much debate about the efficacy of using antibiotics for ear infections. Some people believe that they do little to help because the cause of ear infections is often viral. In addition, antibiotics encourage the growth of yeast infections, contribute to the creation of antibiotic-resistant strains of bacteria, and predispose the child to further occurrences of earaches.

In contrast, natural medicines actually help the immune system of the child, and more important, they relieve the pain quickly. Therefore it makes sense to manage ear infections in the home using herbal medicine. Moreover, once a child has overcome one ear infection without the debilitating effects of antibiotics, he or she is a little stronger and more able to overcome the next infection. Gradually, the repeated earaches so feared by parents become less and less frequent and then disappear.

▪ ADVICE AND COMMENTS
Glue Ear and Partial Hearing Loss

Herbs can be of great benefit in treating glue ear and partial hearing loss from mucus accumulation. In this condition mucus is always present, and it might be thought that one should start with herbs that clear mucus. In practice, better results are obtained if treatment is given on the basis of which of the patterns discussed earlier dominates. If the child is Weak, you must first build up his or her strength before there is any chance of eliminating the mucus blocking the transmission of sound.

General Advice during Acute Attacks

If the child has a fever, he or she should be kept in bed and kept warm enough for the sweating to continue (see Chapter 16). In addition, the child should drink plenty of liquid to replenish what is being lost through sweating. The best drink is honey* and lemon, but any sweet drink is good. The drink should be given at room temperature or warmer and never ice cold.

If the ear is painful, make sure the child is not in a draught. Even if the child does not have a fever, he or she should nevertheless be kept at home and allowed to rest to help the infection to pass.

---

*The honey should be pasteurized for children younger than 1 year of age. See note on p. 67.

A Commonly Diagnosed Condition

Ear infection is probably the most common diagnosis for children. It has taken the place that tonsillitis had a generation or two ago. If a child is "under the weather" and just about ill enough to be taken to the doctor, it is likely that the ears will be examined. Often, the eardrum is found to be mildly inflamed, and the child will be diagnosed as having an "ear infection"—the source of all the child's misery. A generation or two ago, the same procedure was focused on the throat, with tonsillitis being considered the source of misery. Our observation is that children often get a mild fever with inflammation in the head. Wherever you look—throat, gums, ears, or nose—you find inflammation.

Consequently, if you are a parent, your child may have had a diagnosis of ear infection when really the child had a generalized mild inflammation in the head. Likewise, as a practitioner, you may find a disproportionate number of your patients with a diagnosis of ear infection.

Advice for Other Times
DIET

If there are any signs of mucus (as there usually are), mucus-producing foods should be avoided. This point cannot be overemphasized. Research done at Georgetown University Medical School showed a strong link between ear infections and food allergies. For some children a simple change in diet is enough to put an end to a history of repeated ear infections (see Chapter 15).

Foods to avoid include the following:

- Cow's milk products of all kinds
- Peanuts
- Oranges
- Bananas

In addition:

- Make sure the child gets enough sleep.
- Make sure the child avoids swimming and exposure to cold winds.

▪ ALTERNATIVE VIEWS

Ear inflammations are especially common in the first year of life if the child's birth was difficult. During a difficult birth, the head can be distorted quite severely and the cranium can be pushed badly out of shape. Inevitably, this causes some blockages to the flow of energy in the head. During the first year of life ear infections may arise while this birth trauma is healing. If recurrent ear infections do not respond to herbal treatment, the next therapy to try is craniosacral osteopathy, which has a good reputation for resolving birth trauma to the head.

25

Sleeping Problems

Insomnia by itself is not a disease, but it is nevertheless a major problem. Strangely enough, it is not a large problem for the child because very often the child manages to snatch a few more hours of sleep during the next day. However, it is a major problem for the rest of the family. For the parents in particular, night after night of broken sleep gradually undermines their strength. At the very least, it takes the enjoyment out of life for them and leaves them irritable all the time. In extreme cases it can lead to violence and injury to the children.

The main treatment of orthodox medicine is the use of hypnotics, such as diazepam (Valium) or in earlier times opium in the preparation known as *laudanum*. These drugs do have limited use in medical emergencies, but they are not suitable for children's long-term use. In this chapter we explain some of the underlying reasons why children do not sleep, and therefore point the way to the herbs that will cure them of this debilitating condition.

What Is Insomnia?

This is not a silly question. Many people do not know the age at which they can expect their child to sleep through the night. In England many parents take for granted that their children cry at night; thus it may be a surprise that there are remedies available to aid sleep throughout the night. Other parents expect their 2-year-olds to sleep through every night until 8 in the morning and are outraged when they are awakened at 6.

In Box 25-1 we give some guidelines on what are considered normal sleep patterns. However, each child will develop his or her own pattern. Healthy

children can possibly sleep through the night (8 PM to 6 AM) when they weigh more than 15 pounds.

What Age to Treat

In general, sleep disturbances should not be treated during the first 3 months after birth. It takes time for the baby to recover and settle into a routine after birth. If the child is obviously having problems with sleeping after about 3 months, then it is time to treat.

REASONS CHILDREN DO NOT SLEEP

Following are some common reasons why babies and children do not sleep:

- Heat
- Colic

275

- Emotional or physical shock
- Low energy
- Overactive brain
- Headache related to a difficult birth
- Habitual insomnia

Explanations for why these lead to insomnia follow.

Heat

When too much heat is present inside or outside the body, it is difficult to sleep. It is a common experience that it is difficult to sleep when the air temperature is very hot. When the heat is internal, one can experience the same difficulty. (For a discussion of what is meant by *internal heat*, refer to Chapter 1.) Another way of looking at this situation is that the heat in the brain and nervous system leads to a mild irritation and consequently increased mental activity.

Colic

The child wakes not because of mental activity caused by heat but because of pain. Colic that wakes a child during the day is obvious to both parents and practitioners. What is more difficult to determine and what is often overlooked is mild colic that only appears at night. It only occurs at night because that is when metabolism slows down, so any problem related to a sluggish digestion is likely to be worse then.

Emotional or Physical Shock

The child does not sleep well because he or she is suffering from the shock of some sudden and terrifying incident, such as a car accident. The baby or child wakes frequently at night during terrifying dreams. The shock that the mother experiences in the later stages of pregnancy can also be transmitted to the unborn baby.

Another way in which shock can become embedded is if the child experiences something sudden and unpleasant but does not cry at that time. An example of this is a patient who broke his leg at the age of 11 months. This was a very unpleasant experience, but what caused the shock to settle in the child's system was that he was unable to cry at all at the time of the accident.

Low Energy

In children with low energy the cause for insomnia is the metabolism slowing down at night. In these children it may slow down to the point that they wake up. The distinctive feature of this type of insomnia that a small drink—perhaps just a drink of hot water—is enough to get these children back to sleep again. This small drink gets the metabolism going enough to allow sleep. In elderly people in England one sees this same pattern; many older people find that when they wake in the middle of the night, the only thing that can help them get back to sleep is the stimulating effect of a cup of hot tea.

Overactive Brain

Some children simply cannot switch their minds off at night. Some children are born with this problem, whereas some acquire it from the high levels of mental stimulation that are now common. An adult can easily become hardened to the stimulating effects of modern life, but a baby or young child does not have these defenses. A simple car drive or trip to the supermarket can be an enormous stimulation for a child so open to impressions.

Headache Related to a Difficult Birth

The cause in these children is a bruised head from a difficult birth. When the womb contracts too strongly before the cervix has opened wide enough, the baby's head is pushed hard. This strong pressure on the cranium during birth may lead to a headache that may continue for years after birth if not treated. This problem is particularly common when birth is induced because the artificially stimulated contractions are sometimes very strong.

Habitual Insomnia

Once a pattern of insomnia has started, it may continue out of pure force of habit. Many parents come to the clinic complaining that they are awakened every night by their child coming into bed with them, and they ask whether there is an herbal remedy for it. Sometimes there is, but sometimes the child's insomnia is a habit that has developed.

■ SLEEP PATTERNS OF THE DIFFERENT TYPES

The sleep patterns of the different types are characteristic (Box 25-2). Very often, asking about the sleep pattern will give all the information needed to prepare a prescription.

Heat

There are three characteristics signs of the heat pattern. One or all may be present.

- Difficulty falling asleep
- Light sleep
- Fear of darkness

It is difficult for these children to fall asleep. They may be awake for 1 or 2 hours, tossing and turning as they try to fall asleep. Once they are asleep, they may sleep lightly and be awakened by the slightest noise.

When they wake during the night these children are usually cheerful. If they are sleeping in another room, they may simply call out for their parents, and it is only when their parents do not come that they start to cry in real earnest. When the parents do finally come, the child is delighted and may want to play for as long as 2 hours. The baby or child is quite happy to be up in the middle of the night, provided that there is someone to play with.

These children may be afraid of the dark. If they wake up in total darkness (rare in most city environments), they are terrified and disorientated, and it may take them a long time to be comforted. What distinguishes this pattern from the fright pat-

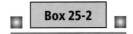

Box 25-2

Sleep Patterns of the Different Types

Hot
Has difficulty getting to sleep
Is a light sleeper, wakes during the night
Fears the dark

Colic
Writhes in pain and is restless even before waking
Wakes with a scream

Emotional or Physical Shock
Has bad dreams
Wakes up frightened

Low Energy
Wakes regularly during the night, possibly every hour
Goes back to sleep after a small drink

Overactive Brain
Has difficulty getting to sleep, but once asleep, stays asleep

Headache Related to a Difficult Birth
Has to be bounced up and down very vigorously to go to sleep
Bangs head against pillow or headboard to get to sleep

Habitual Insomnia
Gets into parents' bed while half asleep
Protests vigorously if made to stay in own bed

tern is that if there is a night-light, these children are not terrified when they wake.

This pattern used to be the most common. It responds well to hypnotics, such as hops *Humulus lupulus*, lettuce *Lactuca virosa*, and even orthodox insomnia pills.

Colic

Children with colic are awakened by abdominal pain. Even before they wake up, they may be writhing and restless and starting to whimper as the pain builds up. When they finally wake up, it may be with a dreadful shout. The insomnia may respond slightly to hypnotics, which may deaden the pain, but in some children these may actually make the insomnia worse.

Emotional or Physical Shock

The main characteristic of the sleep pattern is that the child has bad dreams. It seems that during the dreams the child relives again and again the moment when the shock occurred. As a practitioner you may not know whether the child has dreams, and the parent sometimes does not know. If there is doubt, ask the parent to observe the child during sleep. There are obvious signs of vivid dreams, such as restless movements and talking in the sleep. On waking, the child is often very frightened and "in another world" and is quite unaffected by the presence of a night-light. Sometimes the child resists going to sleep for fear of the dreams. This type of insomnia may respond slightly to orthodox medicines, but the effects soon wear off.

Low Energy

A distinguishing feature of the sleep pattern is that the child can easily go back to sleep if given something warm to eat or drink. The substance does not have to be nourishing food; often, warm water is enough. For nursing babies a small suckle at the breast is often enough to get them back to sleep.

If the child drinks only water or only a small amount of milk, this is not enough to provide nourishment for very long, nor is it enough to keep the metabolism going for very long. As soon as the effect wears off, the child wakes up again. In severe cases the child may wake up every hour during the night. As one parent described it: "every hour on the hour." This sleep pattern is devastating for most parents.

Overactive Brain

These children have difficulty in going to sleep because their brains are always working. After lying in bed for a few minutes, or sometimes as long as an hour, they get bored and get up. They may then go and find their parents, although sometimes they are content to stay in their bedroom and read books. Once they are asleep, they usually sleep soundly.

Headache Related to a Difficult Birth

These babies may have special difficulty going to sleep. The reason is that when babies go to sleep, the intracranial pressure increases for approximately 15 seconds at the moment of going to sleep. This rise in pressure causes the low-grade headache to become violent, causing the almost-asleep baby to wake up suddenly crying. The only way to get these babies to sleep is to bounce them up and down very vigorously to provide a distraction from the pain. Older children may bang their heads against the pillow or headboard.

Habitual Insomnia

Babies commonly wake for food, especially if they are being breast-fed. In half-sleep the baby senses the presence of the mother's milk and seeks it more with a thought of pleasure than from real need. If the baby sleeps with the father, this pattern may simply stop. When the child is old enough to get out of bed, he or she may hardly wake at all and, in half-sleep, walks into the parents' bedroom and snuggles into bed with them.

▪ OTHER SYMPTOMS AND SIGNS*

Heat

- The child has difficulty going to sleep.
- A night-light aids sleep.
- The child cries out for attention rather than from distress.
- The child sleeps lying face up.

---

*Facial color reveals a lot about a child's energy. See p. 54 for a discussion of facial colors and variations among racial groups.

- The bedclothes are often thrown off.
- The child sleeps lightly.
- Early awakenings are common.
- Upon waking, the child is wide awake at once, wanting to play.
- Often, the child's behavior is almost hyperactive.
- Some red color is seen in the features—face, lips, or tongue.

VARIATION: STAGNANT FOOD PATTERN

- The cheeks are red.
- Green nasal discharge is present.
- The abdomen is swollen.
- Stools are irregular and smell bad.
- The child is irritable.

VARIATION: HEAT FROM ECHO PATTERN

- The child has a history of immunization or high fever.
- The child has a history of recurrent infections.
- The lymph nodes in neck are enlarged.

CAUSES

The child may be born with this imbalance, especially if the late stage of pregnancy coincided with exceptionally hot weather. More commonly seen is heat from the stagnant food pattern or from the echo pattern.

When the heat comes from the digestive system, you will see the characteristic signs of the stagnant food pattern. Overeating, irregular feeding, or unsuitable food leads to fermentation in the abdomen, with corresponding generation of heat (see Chapter 2).

When the heat comes from the echo pattern, a history of febrile disease or a history of repeated lung infections or immunizations may be found, any one of which may leave heat in the system. Many parents report that the onset of insomnia occurred immediately after an immunization.

Colic

- The child wakes screaming because of pain.
- Crying and moaning often precede waking.

- The fists are clinched and the back arched.
- The face appears white, possibly blue above the lips.
- The child prefers to sleep face-down.
- The appetite may be poor.
- The child may look healthy and strong.

CAUSES

The most common cause for colic is giving the child Cold-energy food such as cucumbers and yogurt (see Chapter 3). Other foods that can cause colic are mentioned in Chapter 12, but we must mention here foods that contain a lot of fiber, such as brown bread and beans. This pattern also occurs when the baby starts taking new foods, for example, a new kind of milk or the first solid foods.

Other common causes of colic are anxiety in a nursing mother, the anesthetic used in childbirth, and excess consumption of Cold-energy food in pregnancy. Sometimes an immunization (particularly that for polio) can precipitate the colic pattern. Sometimes colic is the main symptom of a head injury from a difficult birth, and this pattern requires very different treatment (see later discussion).

Emotional or Physical Shock

- Upon awakening, the child is frightened and inconsolable.
- The child often has nightmares.
- The child fears going to sleep.
- The bridge of the nose or under the eyes is slightly colored blue.
- The face appears white or a pale blue-gray color.
- The child is clingy.
- The child is often jumpy and nervous.
- There is some history of fright or trauma.

CAUSES

As explained earlier, this pattern is related to seeing or experiencing something frightening. It is particularly likely to occur if the child does not cry at the time of the incident. The pattern can also be caused by the mother experiencing a sudden shock during pregnancy.

Low Energy

- The face is pale.
- The child often looks rather thin.
- The appetite is poor, or the child is picky about food.
- The child may be small for age.
- The pattern is often seen after some illness.
- The child may have a history of frequent infections.
- There may be a history of blood loss or anemia during pregnancy or birth.

CAUSES

The causes for this pattern are discussed at length in Chapter 2. Here we review the main headings: anemia or exhaustion during pregnancy, exhaustion of the nursing mother after childbirth, any long illness, immunizations, unstructured nursing, and frequent snacking.

Overactive Brain

- The face is pale.
- Dark rings are often seen round the eyes.
- The child is restless.
- The child has an inquiring mind.
- The child may have rather a large head.

CAUSES

In some children the main cause of insomnia is not found in any of the aforementioned patterns but is something innate in the child—an overactive brain. In the past this pattern was so uncommon that it was not mentioned at all. The pattern is seen now for several reasons. The main reason is that there is a tendency to stimulate children's brains in early learning programs. This tendency is also encouraged by the computer industry, which produces computer programs for 3-year-olds. Brain stimulation comes from many other causes, such as a trip around a supermarket with its myriad of stimulating advertisements. In many families, stimulation is provided by the TV being on all the time.

Headache Related to a Difficult Birth

- The head is very sensitive (the baby or toddler cries much more than expected if the head is accidentally hit).
- The child likes to be bounced up and down vigorously to help go to sleep.
- The child may bang the head against a pillow or headboard to help go to sleep.
- The child may have colic.

CAUSES

The cause is usually found in childbirth. Intense pressure on the cranium that occurs when the contractions are too strong causes the headache. This pressure is likely to occur if the contractions are stimulated too quickly before the cervix has opened fully.

Habitual Insomnia

There are no special symptoms and signs for this pattern, beyond the children wanting the comfort of their parents' bed. In fact, the very absence of signs points to this pattern.

CAUSES

Once a pattern of insomnia has started, it may continue out of pure force of habit.

▪ TREATMENT

Dosages*

Dosages are given for 3-year-olds (Table 25-1). The dosages we suggest are *suggestions only*. Each child may need something different.

The tinctures are given three times a day in about 25 to 50 ml of warm water. The medicine may be sweetened.

Heat

As we mentioned in the section on causes, two factors can lead to heat in the system: the stag-

---

*For more detailed information about dosages, see Chapter 8.

Table 25-1

AGE	MULTIPLY 3-YEAR-OLD DOSE BY
6-12 months	$\times \frac{1}{3}$
1-2 years	$\times \frac{1}{2}$
2-4 years	$\times 1$
4-7 years	$\times 1\frac{1}{2}$
7-14 years	$\times 2$
14+ years	$\times 3$

nant food pattern and the echo pattern. The herbs for treating the main symptoms of heat-type insomnia are the same, but to cure the condition the underlying cause must be addressed. This requires different herbs for the two different patterns.

First, herbs to treat the heat pattern of insomnia are the following:

Hops *Humulus lupulus*	3 drops tincture
Passion flower *Passiflora incarnata*	2 drops tincture
Chamomile *Chamomilla matricaria*	2 drops tincture

The herbs may be given as a tincture in sweetened warm water, or they may be given as a sweetened tea. The herbs should be given about 30 minutes before the child goes to bed. In some children it is helpful to give several additional doses throughout the afternoon. All of these herbs help a child go to sleep. When the child wakes in the night, he or she can be given this prescription again and again without risk of addiction.

Explanation. Hops is a general sedative. Passion flower is good for very imaginative children, who are overstimulated—they have a tendency to get overexcited, almost to the point of hyperactivity. Chamomile is for overexcitement, for example, after a party and for general heat. Thus these three herbs together cover most situations. Other herbs of benefit include the following:

Lime flowers *Tilea europea*	One or all of these herbs
Vervain *Verbena officinalis*	may be used. Make a
Lemon balm *Melissa officinalis*	tea by pouring a
	teacup of boiling
	water onto one
	heaped teaspoon of
	the dried herb, and
	sweeten.

Verbena is especially useful for those children who are unable to stop what they are doing.

Results. These herbs are often very effective in getting the child to sleep. The effects wear off if the underlying condition—stagnant food pattern or echo pattern—is not treated.

VARIATION: STAGNANT FOOD PATTERN
Give hops, passion flower, and chamomile, as listed earlier, with the following:

Black root *Leptandra virginica*	2 drops tincture
Aniseed *Pimpinella anisum*	2 drops tincture

The herbs are given three or four times a day in warm water.

Explanation. Black root is specific for the stagnant food pattern. Aniseed helps reduce any flatulence and pain that might occur when the stools start to move.

Results. If only the calming herbs are given, the child's sleep will improve slightly. Black root can then be introduced to start clearing out the stagnant food pattern. When this happens, the sleep may get worse. How much worse it gets will depend on the child's reaction to the black root. If the food clears out very quickly, total insomnia may occur for one night. If it clears out more slowly, the sleep will not be so badly affected but the small aggravation lasts longer. Typically, it takes between 1 and 3 weeks for this pattern to clear. It takes longer if the parents are unable to change the child's diet easily. (See Chapters 2 and 3 for dietary advice.)

VARIATION: HEAT FROM ECHO PATTERN

If there is heat in the lungs with cough, refer to Chapter 17 for treatment. When the heat has affected the lung system but there are no special signs of cough, in addition to the calming herbs mentioned previously, add the following:

Pasque flower *Anemone pulsatilla*	1 drop tincture
Poke root *Phytolacca decandra*	2 drops tincture
Blue flag *Iris versicolor*	2 drops tincture
Elecampane *Inula helenium*	2 drops tincture

The herbs are given three or four times a day in warm water.

Explanation. Pasque flower helps bring the heat to the surface. Once at the surface, it may be removed by the hops. Poke root and blue flag both soften thick mucus and thus help release heat that has been trapped. Elecampane eliminates any excess mucus through the digestive tract.

Results. Once again, if only the sedative herbs are given, the child's sleep will improve somewhat but the insomnia will return once the herbs are discontinued. Likewise, when blue flag and poke root are given, the sleep may worsen for a short while as the heat is cleared out.

In some children the heat remains stubbornly where it is for a long time. In these children one has to look for small changes to determine whether the herbs are working at all. It is common for the heat to be cleared in the form of a fever some months after treatment has commenced. If this fever is treated in the proper way, the child's sleep will take a turn for the better. In the echo pattern it is sometimes beneficial to combine herbs with homeopathy.

For general indications of what to look for during the process of expelling an echo pattern, see Chapter 17.

Advice and Comments

- Make sure that the child drinks enough water.
- Make sure that constipation, if present, is relieved.

Colic

Give herbs to warm and move digestion, such as the following:

Valerian *Valeriana officinalis*	4 drops tincture
Aniseed *Pimpinella anisum*	4 drops tincture
Ginger *Zingiber officinalis*	2 drops tincture
Prickly ash *Zanthoxylum americanum*	2 drops tincture

The herbs are given three or four times a day in warm water, either before or after feeding. They may also be given at night when the baby or child wakes.

Explanation. Valerian is a gentle relaxing antispasmodic that helps induce sleep when it is needed. Aniseed warms the digestive system and helps relieve flatulence. Ginger warms the digestive system as well, and prickly ash warms the entire system and improves general circulation.

In mild cases a tea from the following herbs and sweetened with honey* is very helpful:

Fennel *Foeniculum vulgare*	2 drops tincture
Ginger *Zingiber officinalis*	2 drops tincture
Dill *Anethum graveolens*	2 drops tincture
Lemon balm *Melissa officinalis*	2 drops tincture

A preparation similar to this (without the lemon balm) is sold in pharmacies in England under the name "Gripe water."[†]

Results. The results vary. Some babies and children have immediate relief, whereas in others an effect is noticed after several days. There should be a definite improvement within 10 days, though. If nothing has happened by this time, the prescription is not working. The problem sometimes returns when a new food is introduced or during a growth spurt.

---

*Note: The honey should be pasteurized for children younger than 1 year. See note on p. 67.

[†]Before prescribing gripe water, check the label to see that there are no unwanted ingredients.

Advice. Avoid giving the child bananas, yogurt, ice-cold food and drinks, and food with a lot of fiber. If a new food has recently been introduced to the diet (e.g., a new milk formula or the first solid foods), reduce the quantity of the new food. If the child is constipated, this should be treated (see Chapter 10). See also Chapter 12 for a more detailed discussion and advice about foods.

Emotional or Physical Shock

The treatment of choice is the following homeopathic remedy:

Arnica *Arnica montana*   See following text for dosage

We advise consulting a homeopathic practitioner. If this is not possible, give one pill of 30C potency every night for 3 nights and then no further remedy for at least a month. If the fright has been there for a very long time or was the result of a shock the mother experienced before the baby was born, a higher potency may be needed, or the Dr. Bach Flower Remedy may be tried.

Yet another alternative is the Rescue Remedy. Put 4 drops in a glass of water beside the baby or child's bed and give sips during the night. In addition, moisten the baby's or child's lips with the water at least four times during the day for up to 1 week.

Results. The results of treatment can be rather dramatic. Sometimes the child relives the shock in the daytime and is very clingy and frightened for a few days. Sometimes, when the shock has been there for many months, it has affected the whole body and caused heat to build up. When the shock is released, so is the heat and the child may get heat signs during the next week, such as the following:

- Fever
- Irritability
- Foul-smelling stools
- Sore anus or urethra

If the shock was severe, the child's entire energy may have become depleted by the lack of sleep and the debilitating effects of the shock. Thus the child may not have enough energy to have a fever or to expel the shock. For these children a combination of herbs may be needed to strengthen the body. Then after a few weeks, the child will have enough energy for the healing to take place. This may take the form of repeated low-grade fevers.

Low Energy

The main herbs for the treatment of low energy are the following:

Hawthorn *Crataegus oxyacantha*   4 drops tincture
Licorice *Glycyrrhiza glabra*   2 drops tincture
Fennel *Foeniculum vulgare*   2 drops tincture

Explanation. Hawthorn is a tonic for the circulation, and it improves the metabolism, whereas licorice benefits the energy generally. Fennel is a tonic for the digestive system. Another suitable herb, but which has a bitter taste, is the following:

Gentian *Gentiana lutea*   2 drops tincture

Gentian helps improve the appetite. Some children, especially those who are a bit jumpy and oversensitive, benefit from taking additional herbs that strengthen the nervous system, such as the following:

Vervain *Verbena officinalis*   3 drops tincture
Oats *Avena sativa*   3 drops tincture
Passion flower *Passiflora incarnata*   3 drops tincture

Whichever prescription is chosen, the herbs are given three or four times a day in warm water.

Results. As with all Weak conditions, some weeks or even months are needed for a complete cure, but some effects should be noticed during the first week.

Overactive Brain

This type of insomnia can be very difficult to cure because of the stimulating nature of most people's lives. Few are the houses without a TV and other electronic gadgets. A characteristic of this pattern is that the child likes to be involved in mental activity, at the expense of physical activity, and this points the way to a treatment. The child should be encouraged to be more in touch with his or her body. This may be done with activities such as horseback riding, swimming, and any physically agreeable pastime. There is also an anthroposophic remedy manufactured by Weleda, called *Fragador*, which helps this condition.

Headache Related to a Difficult Birth

The most appropriate treatment is craniosacral osteopathy. In some cases the following herb may help:

St. John's wort *Hypericum perfoliatum*   2 drops tincture
3 times a day

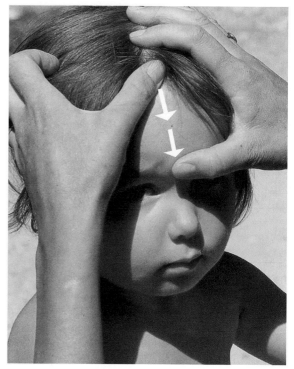

Figure 25-1   Massage down the forehead helps the child to go to sleep.

Habitual Insomnia

Changing a habitual sleep pattern is more of a parenting problem than a medical one. There are many books available that give guidance on how to solve the problem without too much trauma for the child or parents.

■ OTHER TREATMENTS

Massage: Down Forehead

Gently stroke the child's forehead from the hairline down to the point in between the eyebrows. The frequency should be one or two strokes per second. This is a traditional Persian massage for babies, and the skin is normally lubricated with sesame oil (Figure 25-1).

Correction of the Magnetic Field

Some children are very sensitive to magnetic fields. The direction that their head points determines whether sleep is peaceful or disturbed.

Lead Mattress

Some children benefit from placing a sheet of lead under their mattress. The mechanism by which it works is not understood, but some children are helped enormously.

Hop Pillows

Another way that hops *Humulus lupulus* can be administered is by filling a pillow with them and putting it in the child's bed. The vapor exuded by the hops helps the child sleep.

▣ ESSENTIAL OILS

Essential oils are very useful in the treatment of insomnia and can help calm a child before bedtime. They may be particularly helpful when used with a general massage.

The following prescriptions are helpful:

Chamomile *Chamomilla matricaria*	5 drops
Lavender *Lavandula officinalis*	5 drops

These are added to 30 ml (1 oz) of massage oil. Another prescription follows:

Lavender *Lavandula officinalis*	5 drops
Chamomile *Chamomilla matricaria*	5 drops
Clary sage *Salvia sclarea*	2 drops

These are added to 30 ml (1 oz) of massage oil.

The following oil may be added to the bath:

Chamomile *Chamomilla matricaria*	1 drop per year of age

Put the oil in the bath given before bedtime.

26

Eczema

Eczema is a highly irritating and distressing condition. The continual itch can cause the child to scratch until the skin bleeds. It can disturb sleep and interfere with relationships. Among children, eczema has become much more common than it used to be. Its increased incidence has paralleled the increase in the incidence of asthma. From the point of view of natural medicines this is not surprising, given the close link between the skin and the lungs (see Chapter 2).

An Internal Condition

The normal orthodox treatment for eczema is external application of creams. At present, few other treatments are available. This external treatment is misguided because it is another case of treating the symptom and not the cause. As with asthma, the cause of eczema is internal. There may be an external trigger such as soap, but the cause of the hypersensitivity comes from an internal energy imbalance.

Dangers

The main danger from eczema occurs when the skin is broken. Great care must be taken to ensure that broken skin remains clean, for it can provide an entry point for infection.

■ UNDERLYING FACTORS

The symptom of eczema is on the skin, but internal imbalances lead to this external appearance. Among these imbalances are the following:

- Skin and lung weakness
- Poor circulation of fluids
- Buildup of mucus
- Heat and mild inflammation

Skin and Lung Weakness: Hereditary or Acquired

A hereditary disposition for eczema is often found, with an entire family having skin problems. Eczema is often seen with asthma. The skin and lung weakness may not be hereditary but may be acquired through a series of bad infections.

Poor Circulation of Fluids

When something interferes with the normal circulation and elimination of fluids, the excess may accumulate under the skin, causing it to be puffy and moist. This condition is commonly seen when the digestive system is not working well.

Buildup of Mucus

A buildup of mucus obstructs the circulation of nutrients to the skin, which then becomes dry and flaky. This mucus buildup is often associated with fluid imbalance; thus the skin may be flaky, yet ooze fluid. Mucus is often seen in lymphatic congestion, which goes with the echo pattern. It is also the result of the consumption of too many mucus-forming foods or a food allergy.

Heat and Mild Inflammation

When heat is present in the system, the entire body, including the skin, becomes somewhat irritated.

The skin itches and becomes hypersensitive. These symptoms are seen in the echo pattern and can also be caused by a food intolerance or allergy.

■ CONTRIBUTING FACTORS

Eczema is rarely a straightforward condition, so it is not surprising that a long list of possible causes in life exists. Each of these causes initiates one of the patterns discussed later in the chapter. Treating these patterns is the starting point for treating eczema.

Broadly speaking, what we have observed in our clinic is that there are internal causes, which tend to initiate an imbalance in the body condition. In addition, there are external causes, which provide a trigger, in the same way as we have seen with asthma. In some patients the internal cause is enough to produce eczema without any trigger.

Internal Causes

A child may have one or many of the following causes:

- Digestive imbalance
- Irregular eating and overeating
- Food intolerance or allergy
- Consumption of poor-quality food
- Repeated infections treated with antibiotics
- Immunizations
- Buildup of toxins from the environment
- Stress in the family and hidden emotional causes

DIGESTIVE IMBALANCE
The digestive system is at the heart of a child's health. When digestion is out of balance, fluid or heat accumulation or may be present. When the digestive system is weak, it does not provide enough energy and the child may be prone to frequent infections. All of these imbalances contribute to eczema.

IRREGULAR EATING AND OVEREATING
Irregular eating and overeating can affect the digestive system, as discussed in Chapter 2. They may initiate the stagnant food pattern or the weak digestion pattern.

FOOD INTOLERANCE OR ALLERGY
Food intolerance or allergy is one of the most common factors leading to eczema. The intolerance or allergy leads to the buildup of heat or fluid or mucus. In many patients, simply changing the diet can cure eczema. Food allergies that are especially common are those to cow's milk, oranges, peanuts, peanut butter, and chicken. Food allergies are covered in more detail in Chapter 15.

CONSUMPTION OF POOR-QUALITY FOOD
Much of the food on sale now contains a variety of poisons, from industrial pollutants to herbicides and insecticides. Some children cannot tolerate such toxins in the body, and heat and irritation build up. In addition, factory-farmed food is lacking in components such as microminerals, which are essential for the health of the skin.

REPEATED INFECTIONS TREATED WITH ANTIBIOTICS
Antibiotics are given freely to children, without any thought about the possibility of side effects. Alternative practitioners have found that antibiotics can be a contributory cause of eczema. One possible reason was given in Chapter 2, in which we saw how broad-spectrum antibiotics have the unwanted effect of killing beneficial bacteria in the gut. The loss of these beneficial bacteria upsets the digestive system and can also aggravate leaky gut syndrome. It can also aggravate food intolerance or allergies.

IMMUNIZATIONS
As discussed in Chapter 5, immunizations often have the effect of causing an echo pattern and thus congesting lymphatic circulation. In some children they also introduce heat into the system, with corresponding irritation.

BUILDUP OF TOXINS FROM THE ENVIRONMENT
Unnatural chemicals can find their way into the system by a variety of routes. Many building mate-

rials and furnishings, soaps, and bubble baths contain strange chemicals. Exhaust fumes hang like a pall over many cities. These toxins may cause a variety of imbalances, including fluid imbalances, buildup of mucus, and heat.

STRESS IN THE FAMILY AND HIDDEN EMOTIONAL CAUSES

It is one of the basic principles of holistic medicine that every energy imbalance has an emotion associated with it, and this is particularly true for eczema. Stress and hidden emotions are often important factors in eczema but are rarely the sole cause. More commonly, they are aggravating factors. They are very significant in treatment, though, because they can completely stop herbs from working and are the main reason why eczema is so difficult to treat after it has taken hold.

The emotional cause may be obvious but is sometimes hidden. For example, the stress of parents may be felt subconsciously by the child. Likewise, any deep shock or trauma to either the child or the parents can be a contributing factor. Emotional stress during pregnancy (e.g., abandonment by the father) may lead to the early appearance of eczema, possibly even at birth. This early appearance is especially seen with the echo pattern, where negative feelings get buried and do not find suitable expression. The following case history gives an example.

▪ Case History

One of my first child patients was a beautiful little girl of 18 months. Not only was she beautiful, but she also had a lovely nature and never complained, even though she had a nasty rash on the backs of her knees and her elbows. The mother had done some work herself, eliminating one food after another, and had come to the conclusion that her baby was allergic to chicken.

The child had the echo pattern and with treatment recovered completely. In addition, her allergy to chicken went away.

To my surprise, the mother was not altogether pleased. As far as she was concerned, treatment had some undesirable side effects. Her sweet, docile child with lovely brown curls had turned into a very forceful child. She knew exactly what she wanted and screamed if she did not get it.

The poor mother even asked me one day, "Can you bring the eczema back? I know she is much healthier and that really she has a forceful character, but she was such a *sweet* girl before!"

Some Triggers That May Lead to Eczema

As we have mentioned, these triggers are usually of secondary importance. However, it makes sense to keep children away from these triggers until they are able to cope with them. In our experience, when the underlying imbalance has been corrected, most children can tolerate the substance that caused them so much misery before. Some triggers include the following:

- Animal hair
- Pollen
- Soaps and detergents
- Food allergy

▪ PATTERNS

For treatment, the starting point is to find the pattern that best fits the child. Some common patterns are the following:

- Fluid imbalance with mucus
- Heat
- Weak energy
- Echo pattern
- Stagnant food pattern (children younger than 3 years)

▪ SYMPTOMS AND SIGNS*

Fluid Imbalance with Mucus

The dominating cause is fluid gathering beneath the skin. When the child scratches a lot, the skin

---

*Facial color reveals a lot about a child's energy. See p. 54 for a discussion of facial colors and variations among racial groups.

may become hot, but at other times, Cold signs may predominate.

- The skin rash is often moist and in severe eczema is oozing pus.
- The skin is puffy with retained fluid in the area around the rash.
- Copious nasal discharge is present.
- The child has a productive cough.
- Wheezing and a rattly chest are sometimes seen.
- The face has a yellow, sallow hue.

Heat

The dominating cause is the high level of irritation in the body. Even when the child does not have a rash, many signs of a heat pattern may be seen.

- The face appears red.
- The skin rash is often angry and red.
- The child is hot to touch or feels hot all the time.
- The child likes to take his or her clothes off in the daytime and kicks the bedclothes off at night.
- The child is restless at night.
- The child is thirsty.
- The child has a good appetite.

Weak Energy

When the energy is Weak, many different functions can become out of balance, such as the digestive system, the immune system, and fluid elimination. Rather than address each of these individually, it is often better to address the overall energy level.

- The rash tends to be less severe and less red.
- The child tires easily.
- Sleep is disturbed, with the child waking many times during the night.
- The child's limbs are rather thin.
- The face appears pale or white.
- The child is often cold.
- Often, the child has shadows under the eyes.

- The child's appetite is poor.
- The stools can be loose or normal.
- The child may have a history of frequent infections.
- Any nasal discharge is clear and white.

Echo Pattern

In the echo pattern the skin is not properly nourished because the thick mucus prevents proper circulation to the skin. In contrast to the previous patterns, there are no significant signs of mucus in the child or significant weakness.

- The lymph nodes in the neck are swollen and often hard.
- The skin is dry and the rash rarely oozes, but the skin may be flaking.
- The child is reasonably strong and has good energy.
- The energy level occasionally drops for no apparent reason.
- The child's appetite is adequate and sometimes very good.
- The limbs are strong and well built.
- The face appears yellow, sometimes with a white forehead.
- The stools are loose or normal and possibly glistening.
- Any nasal discharge is green or yellow, thick, and hard to expel.
- The child's eyes may have a slightly glazed look.

Stagnant Food Pattern (Children Younger Than 3 Years)

Children younger than 3 years who have an echo pattern often have the stagnant food pattern as well. In these children digestion must be regulated before treating more complex issues such as an echo pattern. In theory, the stagnant food pattern can be the sole cause of the eczema, and once it is resolved, the eczema will resolve too. The reason for this is found in the consequences of the stagnant food pattern—mucus and heat in the body. However, in nearly every patient we have seen, an echo pattern underlies the stagnant food pattern.

- The rash is often red and oozing.
- The child is strong.
- The cheeks are red, and a green color is seen around the mouth.
- A green nasal discharge is present.
- The child has a swollen abdomen.
- The stools are irregular and foul smelling or smell of apples.

Eczema is a complicated disease, and this fact is reflected in the many patterns described. In this chapter we cover merely the most common ones. When it comes to a child you are treating or your own child, you may find that the symptoms point to more than one of the patterns we have given or to yet another pattern that bears no relation to the ones we describe. If you find the latter, treat the pattern that you see; do not try and fit the symptoms of the child into the patterns that we have given.

The complexity and variety of components causing eczema explain why the results of treatment are unpredictable. Some children get better much more quickly than expected, whereas others respond little, if at all, to treatment.

■ TREATMENT

Treatment involves various steps. However, before herb treatment is initiated, the following should be attended to.

Steps to Treat Eczema
- Eat organic food.
- Find out whether a food allergy is present.
- Take food supplements if necessary.
- Identify the main pattern.
- Take herbs.

Diet

There is little hope for successful treatment if the child is eating the wrong foods or eating poisons. This leads to the following strong recommendations.

EAT ORGANIC FOOD

We have seen many children in whom a rash develops if they eat "factory-farmed" food. All of this food, whether meat, vegetable, or fruit, contains pesticides. Children with a strong digestion can cope with the poisons introduced in this way, but if digestion is not strong, they may cause eczema. We strongly recommend that children eat organic food that comes from healthy animals and that contains the right proportions of nutrients essential for health. (See the discussion on essential fatty acids in Chapter 3.)

FIND OUT WHETHER A FOOD ALLERGY IS PRESENT

Common food allergies that cause eczema are allergies to milk, peanuts, oranges, and chicken. Throughout treatment, these foods should be kept out of the diet, even if there is little change when they are excluded at first. There are many other foods that some children are allergic to. An allergy test may be appropriate. For further details see Chapter 15.

Foods That Often Contribute to Eczema
- Cow's milk
- Peanuts
- Oranges
- Chicken

TAKE FOOD SUPPLEMENTS

If the child has been eating nonorganic food, he or she is likely to have a deficiency of trace elements and some other components essential for health, such as omega fatty acids (see later discussion). Even if the child is eating organic food, supplements are often beneficial. In particular we recommend the following:

- Flax seed oil or other oils such as evening primrose, almond, or borage, which are rich in omega-3 fatty acids
- Organic mineral and vitamin supplements
- Adequate zinc and selenium*

■ WORKING OUT A PRESCRIPTION

The presentation of eczema has so many possible variations that it is impossible to provide enough prescriptions to cover the majority of situations. Therefore we have chosen to give some principles on how to put together a prescription, followed by sample prescriptions for each pattern, and then further herbs that may be of use. The principles we use when treating eczema are the following:

- Treat the energy pattern.
- Treat the symptoms.
- Include alteratives.
- Do not use more than seven herbs in a prescription.
- Try to think of one "king" herb.

Treat the Energy Pattern

The energy pattern that accompanies eczema varies from child to child. Impurities in the blood may make one child feel weak and tired, may generate a lot of mucus in another, and may manifest as great heat and hyperactivity in yet another. In keeping with the principles that we expounded in Chapter 2, we select herbs according to the main energy pattern of the child.

Treat the Symptoms

In orthodox medicine the first thing to be addressed is the symptom. Here we consider it second,

for in many cases the particular way the eczema appears is of less importance than the underlying causes. If the causes are removed, often the symptom disappears. This is not to say that the symptoms are not important. They are, after all, what the child is complaining of. In addition to treating the particular way the eczema manifests, we include herbs for any other secondary symptoms.

Include Alteratives

What are alteratives? The term *alterative* is a classification of herbs that was in widespread use in the nineteenth and early twentieth centuries. It is based on the idea that the blood could become "impure" or "dirty." When this happens, external signs of the body trying to throw out the dirt, such as spots, boils, pus formation, and eczema, are seen. The patient themselves would be inclined to have mood swings, with perhaps depression or outbursts of rage. An alterative is an herb that "cleanses the blood."

This idea of "cleansing the blood" has been part of the herbalist's tradition for the last 200 years, but after the discovery of antibiotics, attention was focused more on the immune system than on the condition of the blood. The idea is becoming more popular again with the development of leaky gut syndrome, in which impurities are thought to leak into the blood through faulty functioning of the intestines (see Chapter 2). The idea is especially useful when it comes to treating eczema. Not only does broken skin look as though the body is trying to expel something, but also all the herbs that are alteratives have a good effect on the skin.

Always include some alteratives in the prescription. This is not difficult because by the time the pattern and the main symptom have been treated, an alterative has usually already been included.

Do Not Use More Than Seven Herbs in a Prescription

This is not an absolute rule. We have occasionally used more. The reason for this guideline is that the exercise of limiting the number of herbs used helps sharpen the mind and helps the practitioner focus

---

*Although these elements can be taken individually, they are best taken in multimineral combinations.

on the really important things that are going on in the child. Through the imposition of this restriction, the medicine is more specific for each child.

Try to Think of One "King" Herb

The exercise of choosing one most important herb (or pair of herbs that are often used together) focuses the mind even more. What is the most important change needed in the child? Once you have answered this question, the most important herb will become clear. Put proportionally more of this herb in the prescription. This principle is discussed more fully in Chapter 8.

■ USEFUL HERBS

Dosages*

Doses are given for 3-year-olds (Table 26-1). The dosages we suggest are *suggestions only*. Each child may need something different.

The tinctures are given three times a day in about 25 to 50 ml of warm water. The medicine may be sweetened.

Prescriptions for Different Energy Patterns

These prescriptions are intended as suggestions. All of them address the main pattern and contain an alterative.

Table 26-1	
AGE	**MULTIPLY 3-YEAR-OLD DOSE BY**
6-12 months	× 1/3
1-2 years	× 1/2
2-4 years	× 1
4-7 years	× 1 1/2
7-14 years	× 2
14+ years	× 3

*For more detailed information about dosages, see Chapter 8.

FLUID IMBALANCE WITH MUCUS

Nettles *Urtica dioica*	4 drops tincture
Cleavers *Galium aparine*	4 drops tincture
Agrimony *Agrimonia eupatoria*	2 drops tincture
Oregon grape *Berberis aquifolium*	4 drops tincture
Red clover *Trifolium pratensis*	3 drops tincture
Burdock *Arctium lappa*	2 drops tincture

Explanation. Nettles, cleavers, and agrimony all work on the fluid circulation. These are duretics and are drying. Oregon grape, red clover, and burdock clear mucus. Red clovers, burdock, and cleavers are alteratives and have the additional effect on the skin and the lymphatic system. If the skin is very wet and weepy, take the first three herbs and one herb out of the second three. If the skin is only slightly weepy but there are no signs of mucus, take the last three herbs and one herb out of the first three.

Results. There may be an increase in the amount of urine as the fluids start to circulate, and the child may also start to ask for more to drink. If the child has a cough or nasal discharge, this should gradually resolve. Some changes of this sort will be seen during the first week, but it can take 2 weeks or more before any significant change is noticed in the skin. Sometimes the first change seen is that the skin condition worsens.

HEAT

Violet *Viola odorata*	4 drops tincture
Marshmallow *Althea officinalis*	4 drops tincture
Pasque flower *Anemone pulsatilla*	1 drops tincture
Licorice *Glycyrrhiza glabra*	3 drops tincture

Explanation. Violet is the main herb in the prescription, being an alterative that is both cooling and of benefit to the skin. Marshmallow is a general cooling herb. Pasque flower helps mobilize the heat. Licorice is cooling and harmonizes the prescription.

Results. The burning heat should start to come out of the child during the first week. The treatment should continue for at least 1 month and possibly longer. If there is no change during the first 2 weeks, another approach should be tried.

WEAK ENERGY

Burdock *Arctium lappa*	3 drops tincture
Cleavers *Galium aparine*	3 drops tincture
Nettle *Urtica dioica*	3 drops tincture
Fennel *Foeniculum vulgare*	3 drops tincture
Licorice *Glycyrrhiza glabra*	3 drops tincture

Explanation. Burdock, nettles, fennel, and licorice are all tonics. Burdock and cleavers are alteratives with a special action on the lymphatic system and skin. Nettles is drying and is useful in treating skin complaints. Licorice is included to harmonize the prescription.

Results. Building up energy takes time, so no change may be noticed during the first 2 or 3 weeks. The first sign to look for is a change in the child's mood and also the interest shown in food. Sometimes, as the digestive system starts to work, the skin condition becomes a little worse at first. After a few weeks or months, as the appetite and elimination improves, there should be some improvement in the skin symptoms.

ECHO PATTERN

Poke root *Phytolacca decandra*	4 drops tincture
Blue flag *Iris versicolor*	4 drops tincture
Elecampane *Inula helenium*	2 drops tincture
Hyssop *Hyssopus officinalis*	2 drops tincture

Explanation. Poke root and blue flag are specific for softening thick mucus characteristic of the echo pattern. They are also alteratives and have a beneficial action on the skin. Elecampane helps resolve the mucus that is loosened by the first two herbs, and hyssop, a tonic for the lungs, is included to prevent a cough from developing when the mucus is loosened.

Results. The herbs for the echo pattern all have the effect of loosening thick mucus. Thus one of the first signs will be slightly loose stools or possibly some other signs of mucus, such as a need to clear the throat first thing in the morning. After 2 or 3 weeks the child may have a change in mood. It may take 1 month before changes start to be seen in the skin. The skin should become more supple and less dry. In some children the rough flaky skin may become more moist, which may make the eczema look like it is getting worse at first.

STAGNANT FOOD PATTERN (CHILDREN YOUNGER THAN 3 YEARS)

Black root *Leptandra virginica*	4 drops tincture
Burdock *Arctium lappa*	2 drops tincture
Yellow dock *Rumex crispus*	2 drops tincture

Explanation. Black root is the main herb for clearing the stagnant food pattern. Burdock and yellow dock also have a gentle effect in moving the digestive system. They are both alteratives and have a strong effect on the skin and the lymphatic system.

Results. The results are sometimes rather dramatic, with release of the buildup of stagnant food pattern. That is, many and very smelly stools are seen for the first few days. The dosage of herbs must be adjusted so that this occurrence is not too violent. It is common for the skin condition to get significantly worse as the poorly digested food is eliminated. Then after 1 or 2 weeks, the skin condition should start to improve.

Variation: Insomnia. If insomnia is present with any of the previous patterns, add the following to the prescription:

Passion flower *Passiflora incarnata*	3 drops tincture

Variation: Signs of Cold. If the child shows signs of Cold, such as a white face or a tendency for colic, in any of the aforementioned patterns, add the following:

Ginger *Zingiber officinalis*	3 drops tincture
Cayenne *Capsicum minimum*	3 drops tincture

Treating the Skin Symptoms

HOT SKIN

Give herbs internally to clear the heat. Externally, the application of calendula ointment may help.

WATER OOZING FROM SKIN
Give herbs internally to regulate the fluid imbalance.

DRY OR ROUGH SKIN
Give herbs internally for the echo pattern.

DRY SKIN WITH A WHITE TRANSLUCENT-LOOKING FACE
This may point to mild anemia.

FLAKING SKIN
Give herbs internally for a mucus imbalance.

ITCHING
Include herbs from the following list:

- Marigold *Calendula officinalis*
- Marshmallow *Althea officinalis*
- Chickweed *Stellaria media*
- St. John's wort *Hypericum perfoliatum*

These herbs may be taken internally, used externally as a wash, or added to the bath water. Alternatively, add chamomile tea to the bath water (15 g for a shallow bath).

BROKEN SKIN
- Marigold *Calendula officinalis*

Marigold is bacteriostatic. It reduces itching, and the tea may be safely applied to broken skin.

PUS OR INFECTION
Echinacea *Echinacea angustifolia*	4 drops tincture
Garlic *Allium sativum*	$\frac{1}{2}$ to 1 capsule per day

These herbs are taken internally.

ECZEMA IN EMOTIONALLY STRESSED CHILDREN
Eczema is worse in emotionally stressed children. The following additions to one of the previous prescriptions may be helpful:

Valerian *Valeriana officinalis*	3 drops tincture
Skullcap *Scutellaria lateriflora*	3 drops tincture
Passion flower *Passiflora incarnata*	3 drops tincture

These herbs, when taken internally, may help the symptoms, but the underlying emotional problems have to be addressed for a cure.

Treating Secondary Symptoms

Here we suggest just one extra herb to add to the prescription. If the secondary symptom is severe, we recommend reading the relevant chapter.

Diarrhea	Agrimony *Agrimonia eupatorium*
Constipation	Butternut *Juglans cinerea*
Cough	Elecampane *Inula helenium*
Insomnia	Passion flower *Passiflora incarnata*

Alteratives: Herbs That Are Good for All Skin Conditions

Herb	Additional Action
Blue flag *Iris versicolor*	Softens thick mucus
Burdock *Arctium lappa*	Hepatic; improves digestion
Cleavers *Galium aparine*	Diuretic
Figwort *Scrophularia nodosa*	Reduces urogenital irritation, heart tonic
Violet *Viola odorata*	Soothes cough, cooling, laxative
Poke root *Phytolacca decandra*	Softens thick mucus
Golden seal *Hydrastis canadensis*	Clears mucus from the whole body, is a stimulant
Oregon grape *Berberis aquifolium*	Clears mucus from the whole body, is a laxative
Red clover *Trifolium pratense*	Clears cough
Yellow dock *Rumex crispus*	Is a laxative

What to Do if the Cause Is Mainly Emotional

If the emotional aspect of the eczema is obvious, it is easy to address. However, when the emotional problem is deeply buried, this situation is more difficult because there is no obvious cause to address. It is hard to treat something that nobody admits is there. In these circumstances we have found that the following steps are sometimes helpful.

1. Diagnose and treat the physical symptoms as outlined in this chapter. Often, by merely correcting the main energy imbalance, the way is opened for a more positive approach to life. As we have seen with the cure of the echo pattern (see Chapter 5), the child often goes through emotional changes without the need for anything else other than the herbs. Once the energy flow has been reestablished, the child can withstand life's emotional blows.

2. An obvious emotional aspect should be addressed, perhaps with herbs, perhaps with the Bach Flower Remedies, or perhaps with some interactive therapy such as counseling.

External Treatments: Creams and Washes

Finally we give some substitutes for the ubiquitous corticosteroid creams.

- Calendula cream: Available at many pharmacies and health food stores.
- Graphites cream: Available at many pharmacies and health food stores.
- Chickweed *Stellaria* cream: Available at many pharmacies and health food stores.
- Chamomile wash: Make a tea from chamomile and put it in the bath.
- Calendula (marigold) wash: Make a tea from calendula and put it in the bath.
- Moisturizing cream: Make sure that the cream has an aqueous base and has no added perfume.

▪ ESSENTIAL OILS

A Word of Caution

In some children the use of oils can aggravate the skin condition.

The following oils are good for improving the skin quality:

- German chamomile *Chamomilla matricaria*
- Melissa *Melissa officinalis*
- Geranium *Pelargonium* spp.

These oils may be used separately or together. The amount to use is up to 6 drops if each oil is used separately or 3 drops each if all three are used together in 30 ml of oil. Use as a massage oil or put some oil in the bath.

For Itching

German chamomile *Chamomilla matricaria*	4 drops
Lavender *Lavandula officinalis*	4 drops
Melissa *Melissa officinalis*	2 drops

Add to 30 ml of base oil and apply to the skin.

Omega Fatty Acids

Omega fatty acids are found in many foods. Omega-3 and omega-6 are the two main omega fatty acids. They are similar in nature, but omega-6 is somewhat irritating to the system, whereas omega-3 is a counterirritant. Both are needed for good health. In addition, both are needed in the correct ratio.

The perfect ratio of omega acids is about 1 part omega-3 to 3 parts omega-6. This pattern is found in many foods. For example, this ratio is found in eggs, milk, and butter produced by traditional organic methods with animals fed on polyculture pastures.* In factory-farmed eggs, this ratio is about 1 to 30, and in factory-farmed milk it is more than 1 to 100. Margarine, which at one time was considered much healthier for individuals than butter, has virtually no omega-3. Thus a normal diet of food bought at a supermarket with margarine substituted for butter would contain virtually none of the counterirritant omega-3,[†] whereas a diet of organic food is likely to contain a satisfactory ratio. We strongly recommend

---

*Pasture land that has been used for hundreds of years is likely to contain 30 different species of plant in about 1.2 square yards (1 square meter), most of which would be gathered in one mouthful of a grazing cow. Pastures that are plowed and resown with a single grass variety (monoculture) produce higher yields of milk and meat but of inferior quality.

†This information was provided by a researcher in the field. When she tried to publish her work some 20 years ago, she found that publication was blocked by the then-powerful margarine industry.

all children with eczema to increase their consumption of omega-3 fatty acids.

Corticosteroid Creams

One of the orthodox treatments is the application of corticosteroid creams. In many children these are astonishingly effective in relieving the symptoms. Having said this, one must be aware that these are suppressing the symptoms, not curing the condition. In fact, if the creams are used for some months, they actually weaken the skin and irritate it. This means that when the use of creams is stopped, the eczema flares up worse than it was before the creams were used. Thus the cream becomes an addictive drug.

In some situations we recommend the use of creams. If a child has lost sleep for several nights because of persistent itching, the use of these creams for a few nights to enable the child to catch up on sleep is justified.

Other Treatments

As we have mentioned earlier, sometimes more than one kind of therapy is required to effect a cure. If herbs have been tried for at least 6 months without even a slight change, another therapy should be considered. Different therapies work on different levels, and a complicated condition such as eczema, may require treatment on many different levels for a cure. In particular, we recommend the following:

- Homeopathy
- Acupuncture
- Craniosacral osteopathy
- Relaxation techniques or meditation for older children

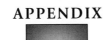

Calcium in Food

100-mg (3-oz) PORTION	CALCIUM (mg)
Kelp	1099
Sesame seeds	1100
Hard cheese	682
Dried wheat or barley grass	514
Sardines	443
Almonds	233
Amaranth	222
Parsley	203
Kale (cooked)	187
Sunflower seeds	174
Watercress	151
Chickpeas	150
Quinoa	141
Black beans	135
Kale	134
Pistachio nuts	131
Figs (dried)	126
Yogurt	121
Milk	119
Tofu	100
Salmon	79
Cottage cheese	60
Eggs	56
Broccoli	48
Ground beef	10

Note: These figures are approximate, and will vary from sample to sample, but they show that calcium can be found in many sources other than milk.

Further Reading List (Annotated)

Cook WH: *Physio-medical dispensatory*, Sandy, Ore, 1998, Eclectic Medical Publications (reprint of 1869 edition).

This and Felter and LLoyd (1898) are two excellent books on Materia Medica. They are written by men who had many years of experience as primary care practitioners using herbs. This book includes only herbs that are non-poisonous, but it makes up for that by the wealth of clinical experience and the excellent first part outlining the use of herbs.

Culpeper N: *Culpeper's complete herbal*, London, 1995, Foulsham.

A revolutionary book in its time (1649), it was written for common people to understand. It is still as relevant today as when it was written. The only real shortcoming is the limited range of herbs and the use of herbs that used to grow in the English countryside but no longer do.

Felter HW, Lloyd JU: *King's American dispensatory*, Sandy, Ore, 1983, Eclectic Medical Publications (reprint of 1898 edition).

See Cook, with which this book may be compared. It is written by an eclectic and thus includes not only poisonous plants but also highly toxic chemicals. The authors seem to delight in describing how much is needed to kill a farm animal or a human being and the nature in which they die. However, there is also a lot of information on the use of herbs and particularly on the use of essential oils and plasters.

Gerard J: *The herball*, rev ed, New York, 1975, Dover (London, reprint of 1636, Facsimile Edition).

This book is a sheer joy to read. The first Materia Medica in English, it gives the "temperature" of each plant and the "vertues." It relies heavily on the classics, but there is also a lot of personal experience here.

Grieve M: *A modern herbal*, London, 1931, Jonathan Cape.

Although written many years ago, this is still a standard reference book. If there were just one Materia Medica on your bookshelf, it should be this.

Weiss RF: *Herbal medicine*, Gothenburg, Sweden, 1988, Arcanum (and Beaconsfield Publishers, Beaconsfield). (English translation of *Lehrbuch der Phytotherapie*, 1985.)

This book is a joy to read. It is written by a very experienced doctor, who has used herbs for his whole life. It is one of the best modern books on herbal medicine in print.

Bibliography

HERBS FOR CHILDREN

Bove M: *Encyclopaedia of natural healing for children and infants*, New Canaan, Conn, 1996, Keats.

Gladstar R: *Herbal remedies for children's health*, North Adams, Mass, 1999, Storey.

McIntyre A: *The herbal for mother and child*, Shaftesbury, 1992, Element.

Scott J: *Natural medicine for children*, London, 1990, Unwin.

Tenney L: *Today's herbal health for children*, Pleasant Grove, Utah, 1996, Woodland Publishing.

HERBS

Bardeau F: *La pharmacie du bon dieu*, Paris, 1973, Marabout, Editions Stock.

Bartram T: *Bartram's encyclopedia of herbal medicine*, London, 1995, Robinson.

Beckett S: *Herbs for clearing the skin*, Wellingborough, 1973, Thorsons.

Bremness L: *The complete book of herbs*, London, 1988, Dorling Kindersley.

Bremness L: *Pocket encyclopedia of herbs*, London, 1990, Dorling Kindersley.

Carse M: *Herbs of the earth*, Hinesburg, Vt, 1989, Upper Access Publishing.

Ceres: *Herbs for acidity and gastric ulcers*, Wellingborough, 1976, Thorsons.

Chevallier A: *Encyclopedia of medicinal plants*, London, 1996, Dorling Kindersley.

Chieh R: *The MacDonald encyclopedia of medicinal plants*, London, 1984, MacDonald.

Fernie WT: *Herbal simples*, ed 3, Bristol, 1914, John Wright.

Flück H: *Medicinal plants*, English ed, Slough, 1976, Foulsham.

Girre L: *Les vieux remèdes naturels*, Paris, 2000, Ouest-France.

Gladstar R: *Herbal healing for women*, New York, 1993, Fireside.

Gosling N: *Herbs for colds and flu*, Wellingborough, 1976, Thorsons.

Griggs B: *Green pharmacy*, London, 1982, Robert Hale.

Griggs B: *The home herbal*, London, 1982, Jill Norman and Hobhouse.

Harper-Shove F: *Medicinal herbs*, ed 2, Saffron Walden, UK, 1952, CW Daniel.

Hemphill R: *Herbs for all seasons*, Harmondsworth, 1972, Penguin.

Hewlett-Parsons J: *Herbs, health and healing*, ed 2, Wellingborough, 1975, Thorsons.

Hobbs C: *Foundations of health*, Loveland, Colo, 1992, Interweave Press.

Hoffmann D: *The herbal handbook*, Rochester, Vt, 1987, Healing Arts.

Hoffmann D: *The new holistic herbal*, ed 3, Shaftesbury, 1992, Element.

Holmes P: *The energetics of western herb*, Boulder, Colo, 1989, Artemis.

Huxley A: *Natural beauty with herbs*, London, 1977, Darton Longman and Todd.

Jenney L: *Today's herbal health*, ed 4, Pleasant Grove, Utah, 1997, Woodland Publishing.

Jiangsu New Herbal Research Institute: *Zhongyao Da Cidian (Greater Encyclopaedia of Chinese Herbs)*, Shangai, Hong Kong, 1978, Shanghai Technical Press.

Levy, J de B: *Common herbs for natural health*, New York, 1972, Schoken.

Lust J: *The herb book*, Toronto, 1974, Bantam.

McIntyre A: *Alternative health herbal*, London, 1987, Optima.

McIntyre A: *The complete woman's herbal*, London, 1994, Gaia.

McIntyre A: *Flower power*, New York, 1996, Henry Holt.

Mességué D: *Les plantes de mon père*, Paris, 1973, Opera Mundi.

Mességué M: *Mon herbier de santé*, Paris, 1975, Opera Mundi,

Mességué M: *Mon herbier de beauté*, Paris, 1979, Opera Mundi.

Mills S: *The essential book of herbal medicine*, London, 1991, Arkana.

Mills S: *The complete guide to modern herbalism*, London, 1994, Thorsons.

Mills S, Bone K: *Principles and practice of phytotherapy*, Edinburgh, 2000, Churchill Livingstone.

Moore M: *The medicinal plants of the Pacific West*, Santa Fe, NM, 1995, Red Crane Books.

Mowrey DB: *Herbal tonic therapies*, New Canaan, Conn, 1992, Keats.

Mulot M-A: *Sécrets d'une herboriste*, Paris, 1984, Dauphin.

Nordal A, Rognlien B, Svaar T: *Urter til mat og medisin*, Oslo, 1988, Norsk Rikskringkasting.

Ody P: *The herb society's complete medicinal herbal*, London, 1993, Dorling Kindersley.

Ody P: *Complete medicinal herbal*, London, 1999, Dorling Kindersley.

Palaiseul J: *Grandmother's secrets*, London, 1976, Penguin.

Paris RR, Moyse H: *Matière médicale*, ed 2, Paris, 1976, Masson.

Powell EFW: *The natural home physician*, Holsworthy Devon, 1975, Health Science Press.

Rau HAD: *Healing with herbs*, New York, 1980, Arco.

Ritchason J: *The little herb encyclopedia*, Pleasant Grove, Utah, 1995, Woodland Publishing.

Roberts F: *Modern herbalism for digestive disorders*, Wellingborough, 1978, Thorsons.

Santillo H: *Natural healing with herbs*, Prescott, Ariz, 1992, Hohm Press.

Thomson WAR: *Healing plants*, London, 1980, Macmillan.

Tierra L: *Herbs of life*, Freedom, CA, 1992, The Crossing Press.

Tierra M: *The way of herbs*, New York, 1990, Pocket Books, Simon and Schuster.

Tierra M: *Planetary herbology*, Twinlakes, Wisc, 1988, Lotus Press.

Treben M: *Health through God's pharmacy*, Steyr, Austria, 1988, Ennsthaler.

Valnet J: *Phytothérapie*, Paris, 1972, Maloine.

■ ANTHOPOSOPHICAL MEDICINE

Bott V: *Anthroposophical medicine*, London, 1978, Rudolf Steiner Press.

Evans M, Rodger I: *Anthroposophical medicine*, London, 1992, Thorsons.

Grohmann G: *The plant*, Kimberton, Pa, 1989, Biodynamic Farming and Gardening Association.

Holtzapfel W: *Children's illnesses*, Spring Valley, NY, 1989, Mercury Press.

Steiner R: *Health and illness*, New York, 1981, The Anthroposophic Press.

Steiner R: *Pastoral medicine*, New York, 1987, The Anthroposophic Press.

Wolff O: *The anthroposophical approach to medicine* (in 3 volumes), New York, 1982, The Anthroposophic Press.

■ AROMATHERAPY

Davis P: *Aromatherapy: an A-Z*, Saffron Walden, UK, 1988, CW Daniel.

Ryman D: *Aromatherapy*, London, 1991, Piatkus.

Tisserand R: *The art of aromatherapy*, Saffron Walden, UK, 1979, CW Daniel.

Valnet J: *The practice of aromatherapy*, Saffron Walden, UK, 1982, CW Daniel.

Worwood VA: *The fragrant pharmacy*, London, 1990, Macmillan.

■ HOMEOPATHY

Borland DM: *Children's types*, London, British Homoeopathic Association.

Castro M: *Homeopathy for pregnancy, birth and baby's first year*, New York, 1993, St Martin's.

Clarke JH: *The prescriber*, Saffron Walden, UK, 1972, CW Daniel.

Curtis S: *A handbook of homoeopathic alternatives to immunisation*, London, 1994, Winter Press.

Hammond C: *How to use homoeopathy*, Shaftesbury, 1991, Element.

Hayfield R: *Homeopathy for common ailments*, London, 1993, Gaia.

Hayfield R: *Homeopathy, a practical guide to everyday health care*, London, 1995, Virgin.

Lockie A: *The family guide to homeopathy*, London, 1989, Penguin.

Puddephat N: *Puddephatt's primers*, Saffron Walden, UK, 1976, CW Daniel.

Smith T: *Homoeopathic medicine: a doctor's guide*, London, 1982, Thorsons.

Speight P: *Homoeopathic remedies for children*, Saffron Walden, UK, 1983, CW Daniel.

Speight P: *Homoeopathy for emergencies*, Saffron Walden, UK, 1984, CW Daniel.

Speight P: *Homoeopathic remedies for women's ailments*, Saffron Walden, UK, 1988, CW Daniel.

Ullman DU: *Homoeopathy, medicine for the 21st century*, Wellingborough, 1989, Thorsons.

■ BACH FLOWER REMEDIES

Chancellor PM: *Bach flower remedies*, Saffron Walden, UK, 1971, CW Daniel.

Harvey CG, Cochrane A: *Encyclopaedia of flower remedies*, London, 1995, Thorsons.

Hyne-Jones TW: *A dictionary of the Bach flower remedies*, ed 2, Saffron Walden, UK, 1977, CW Daniel.

Scheffer M: *Bach flower therapy*, Wellingborough, 1990, Thorsons.

Vlamis G: *Flowers to the rescue*, Wellingborough, 1986, Thorsons.

Weeks N: *The medical discoveries of Edward Bach*, Saffron Walden, UK, 1940, CW Daniel.

■ IMMUNIZATIONS

Chaitow L: *Vaccinations and immunisations: dangers, delusions and alternatives*, Saffron Walden, UK, 1987, CW Daniel.

Coulter HL: *Vaccination, social violence and criminality*, Berkeley, Calif, 1990, North Atlantic Books.

Coulter HL, Fisher BL: *D.P.T.—a shot in the dark*, New York, 1987, Avery Publishing Group.

Cournoyer C: *What about immunizations?* Santa Cruz, Calif, 1995, Nelson's Books.

Hume ED: *Pasteur exposed*, Bookreal, Australia, 1989, Beekman.

Miller NZ: *Immunization theory vs. reality*, Santa Fe, 1995, New Atlantean Press.

Miller NZ: *Vaccines: are they really safe and effective?* Santa Fe, 2002, New Atlantean Press.

Moskowitz R: *The case against immunisations*, England, The Society of Homoeopaths.

Murphy J: *What every parent should know about childhood immunization*, Boston, 1993, Earth Healing Products.

Neustaedter R: *The immunization decision: a guide for parents*, Berkeley, Calif, 1990, North Atlantic Books.

O'Mara P (ed): *Vaccination: the issue of our times*, Santa Fe, 1997, Mothering Magazine.

Scheibner V: *Vaccination*, Blackheath, Australia, 1993, V. Scheiber.

UK Department of Health: *Immunisation against infectious disease*, London, 1990, HMSO Publications.

Walene J: *Immunisation: the reality behind the myth*, Westport, Conn, 1988, Bergin and Garvey.

■ ORTHODOX MEDICINE

Gascoigne S: *The manual of conventional medicine for alternative practitioners*, Dorking, UK, 1993, Jigme Press.

Lissauer T, Clayden G: *Illustrated textbook of paediatrics*, London, 1997, Mosby.

Mendelsohn R: *How to raise a healthy child in spite of your doctor*, New York, 1984, Ballantine.

Index

Page numbers followed by f indicate figures; t, tables; b, boxes.